Haematology & Immunology

5th Edition
CRASH COURSE

SERIES EDITORS

Philip Xiu
MA, MB BChir, MRCP
GP Registrar
Yorkshire Deanery
Leeds, UK

Shreelata Datta
MD, MRCOG, LLM, BSc (Hons), MBBS
Honorary Senior Lecturer
Imperial College London,
Consultant Obstetrician and Gynaecologist
King's College Hospital
London, UK

FACULTY ADVISOR

Matthew Helbert
MBChB, FRCP, FRCPath, PhD
Clinical Immunologist

Vikramajit Singh
MBBS, MRCP, FRCPath (Haematology)
Consultant Haematologist
Aintree University Hospital NHS Foundation Trust
Liverpool
UK

Haematology & Immunology

Gus Redhouse White
BSc (Hons)
Medical Student
University of Leicester
Leicester, UK

Olivia Vanbergen
MA Oxon, MSc, MBBS (distinction)
Clinical fellow in anaesthesia at Hampshire hospitals

For additional online content visit StudentConsult.com

ELSEVIER

ELSEVIER

Content Strategist: Jeremy Bowes
Content Development Specialist: Alexandra Mortimer
Project Manager: Andrew Riley
Design: Christian Bilbow
Illustration Manager: Karen Giacomucci
Illustrator: MPS North America LLC
Marketing Manager: Deborah Watkins

First edition 1998
Second edition 2003
Third edition 2007
Reprinted, 2008, 2010 (twice)
Fourth edition 2012
Updated Fourth edition 2015
Fifth edition 2019

Notices

Practitioners and researchers must always rely on their own experience and knowledge in evaluating and using any information, methods, compounds or experiments described herein. Because of rapid advances in the medical sciences, in particular, independent verification of diagnoses and drug dosages should be made. To the fullest extent of the law, no responsibility is assumed by Elsevier, authors, editors or contributors for any injury and/or damage to persons or property as a matter of products liability, negligence or otherwise, or from any use or operation of any methods, products, instructions, or ideas contained in the material herein.

ISBN: 978-0-7020-7363-2
eISBN: 978-0-7020-7364-9

your source for books,
journals and multimedia
in the health sciences
www.elsevierhealth.com

Working together
to grow libraries in
developing countries

www.elsevier.com • www.bookaid.org

The
publisher's
policy is to use
paper manufactured
from sustainable forests

Series Editors' foreword

The *Crash Course* series was conceived by Dr Dan Horton-Szar who as series editor presided over it for more than 15 years – from publication of the first edition in 1997, until publication of the fourth edition in 2011. His inspiration, knowledge and wisdom lives on in the pages of this book. As the new series editors, we are delighted to be able to continue developing each book for the twenty-first century undergraduate curriculum.

The flame of medicine never stands still, and keeping this all-new fifth series relevant for today's students is an ongoing process. Each title within this new fifth edition has been re-written to integrate basic medical science and clinical practice, after extensive deliberation and debate. We aim to build on the success of the previous titles by keeping the series up-to-date with current guidelines for best practice, and recent developments in medical research and pharmacology.

We always listen to feedback from our readers, through focus groups and student reviews of the Crash Course titles. For the fifth editions we have reviewed and re-written our self-assessment material to reflect today's 'single-best answer' and 'extended matching question' formats. The artwork and layout of the titles has also been largely re-worked and are now in colour, to make it easier on the eye during long sessions of revision. The new on-line materials supplement the learning process.

Despite fully revising the books with each edition, we hold fast to the principles on which we first developed the series. Crash Course will always bring you all the information you need to revise in compact, manageable volumes that still maintain the balance between clarity and conciseness, and provide sufficient depth for those aiming at distinction. The authors are junior doctors who have recent experience of the exams you are now facing, and the accuracy of the material is checked by a team of faculty editors from across the UK.

We wish you all the best for your future careers!

Philip Xiu and Shreelata Datta

Authors

I have really enjoyed re-writing this book. Disentangling some of the thornier concepts of what can be a complex pair of medical specialties has been a welcome learning experience for me and I hope that medical students will equally benefit from the opportunity to assimilate the distilled essences of the basic concepts in both haematology and immunology. I'm grateful to Barbara Simmons and Alex Mortimer for their tireless support and expertise. Likewise Dr Vikram Singh and Dr Matthew Helbert for their expertise and guidance during the development of this book. Most of all, my partner and my son for always giving me their love, motivation and support.

Olivia Van Bergen

Many students have a hypersensitivity reaction to immunology. This is understandable - its broad molecular and cellular biology is tricky to teach as a single unit in many systems based medical school courses. Equally, immunology is relevant to all body systems and most disease processes that doctors encounter! Our edition has revised and restructured a lot of previous content, as well adding novel and relevant topics such as sepsis, allergy desensitisation and immunotherapy for cancer. What we hope we have produced is a text that makes immunology accessible and understandable, rather than lists to be recited.

Gus Redhouse White

Faculty Advisors

Clinical immunology develops very quickly. Since the last edition, new immunotherapy has improved the life expectancy for many cancer patients. New auto-immune mechanisms are being discovered for some types of schizophrenia, particularly those that do not respond well to conventional forms of treatment. The discovery that auto-immunity causes some of these cases may now lead to successful treatments.

On the other hand, there are areas where immunological solutions have still not been found. There is currently no effective vaccine for HIV, although Pre Expsoure Prophylaxis with anti retroviral drugs does appear to work. Who knows what the next few years will show?

Matthew Helbert

The world of Clinical Haematology has seen exciting changes in the past few years. While in the field of Haemato-Oncology, "targeted drugs" have revolutionised treatment for many haematological malignancies by replacing standard chemotherapy, in Haemostasis, the newer anticoagulants drugs are very rapidly replacing the traditional anticoagulants. The development of gene therapy for haemophilia B is also expected to alter the course of this disease.

While clinical haematology and management of haematological disorders and malignancies remains one of the very niche sub-speciality of medicine, many other aspects of haematology are relevant to most doctors. "Full Blood Count" is one of the most common and valuable blood test and its interpretation remains a basic medical skill. Similarly, coagulation tests are increasing being requested and most junior doctors will be expected to interpret these, just as they would be expected to prescribe anticoagulant drugs and manage patient taking them. Knowledge of blood transfusion is mandatory for most hospital doctors and along with it the management of transfusion reactions.

Vikramajit Singh

Acknowledgements

Authors

I have enjoyed co-authoring this book with Gus, and have been very well supported and guided by our faculty advisors Dr Helbert and Dr Singh. We've also benefited from fantastic support from Alex Mortimer and Barbara Simmons. I hope this book gives readers a route to navigate through what can be extremely complex areas of medicine.

My contribution is dedicated to my Mother, Hazel.

Olivia Vanbergen

Thanks to Dr Vanbergen for all your help and contribution throughout the creation of this book & to Dr Helbert for the opportunity and for meticulously improving my chapters.

Thanks also to family, friends and Katie for all the personal support!

Gus Redhouse White

Faculty Advisors

Thanks to Gus for being such a great author to work with.

Matthew Helbert

As a faculty advisor it has been a pleasure to work with Olivia. She has overhauled this edition of the book but has kept to the core principles of the series.

Vikramajit Singh

Series Editors' acknowledgements

We would like to thank the support of our colleagues who have helped in the preparation of this edition, namely the junior doctor contributors who helped write the manuscript as well as the faculty editors who check the veracity of the information.

We are extremely grateful for the support of our publisher, Elsevier, whose staffs' insight and persistence has maintained the quality that Dr Horton-Szar has set-out since the first edition. Jeremy Bowes, our commissioning editor, has been a constant support. Alex Mortimer and Barbara Simmons our development editors has managed the day-to-day work on this edition with extreme patience and unflaggable determination to meet the ever looming deadlines, and we are ever grateful for Kim Benson's contribution to the online editions and additional online supplementary materials.

Philip Xiu and Shreelata Datta

Contents

Contents

Principles of haematology

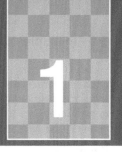

PRINCIPLES

Haematology is the medical specialty concerned with the study, diagnosis, treatment and prevention of diseases related to blood and is the subject of the first part of this book. This chapter discusses blood cells, their production (haematopoiesis), bone marrow and the spleen.

BLOOD

Blood is the fluid contained within the heart, arteries, capillaries and veins of the circulatory system. It delivers oxygen and nutrients to organs and tissues and carries carbon dioxide and metabolic 'waste' products to excretory organs such as the kidneys, liver and lungs.

Blood consists of several components:

- Plasma
- Cells (red cells, white cells, platelets)
- Electrolytes (e.g., Na^+, K^+, Ca^{++})
- Proteins (including hormones and immunoglobulins)
- Lipids
- Glucose

The cellular components of blood are synthesized in the bone marrow in a process called 'haematopoiesis'.

BLOOD CELLS

This section discusses mature blood cells found in the bloodstream.

Red blood cells

Red blood cells ('erythrocytes') are derived from the erythroid blast-forming unit (BFU-E) progenitor cell. Red cells lack a nucleus and have a biconcave discoid shape.

Their primary role is the transportation of oxygen (from lung to tissue) and carbon dioxide (from tissue to lung). They contain haemoglobin, a specialized molecule that avidly binds these gases under conditions of high partial pressure and releases them under conditions of low partial pressure, thus allowing bulk transport of O_2 and CO_2 to proceed in the appropriate direction. Red blood cells are discussed in further detail in Chapter 2.

Platelets

Like red cells, platelets lack nuclei. Platelets (thrombocytes) are derived from megakaryocytes, which derive from the colony-forming unit megakaryocyte (CFU-Meg) progenitor cell. They play a pivotal role in haemostasis (Chapter 6).

White blood cells

White blood cells (leucocytes) are large unpigmented cells with primarily immune roles. They are also found in the bloodstream, along with red blood cells and platelets. Leucocytes are further classified into granulocytes, monocytes/macrophages and lymphocytes. Each group fulfils different immunological roles, participating in immune defences against infection.

Granulocytes

'Granulocytes' is the collective term for white blood cells with granules in their cytoplasm. The term encompasses neutrophils, eosinophils and basophils. The specific chemical content of the granules (and thus the cell's function role) varies according to subtype. Note that some clinicians misleadingly use the term 'granulocytes' for neutrophils, which can cause confusion.

Neutrophils

Neutrophils (aka 'polymorphs') have multilobed nuclei. Neutrophils (diameter 12–14 μm) comprise ≈60% of the bloodstream white cell population. They leave the bone marrow, where they are synthesized, and circulate in the bloodstream for ≤10 hours before entering tissues.

Neutrophils are an essential component of the innate immune system, due to their ability to phagocytose (engulf) microorganisms and kill them by releasing cytotoxic molecules from their granules. Once they arrive at the site of an infection or inflammation, they also recruit further immune cells with chemotactic mediators (see Chapter 9: Neutrophils). Neutrophils therefore represent a key component of the first-line defence against bacterial infections.

Eosinophils

Eosinophils (diameter 12–17 μm) have bilobed nuclei. They stain strongly with acidic dyes and comprise ≈1%–6% of the bloodstream white cell population. Like other granulocytes, eosinophils release specific cytotoxic and messenger molecules. These are released directly into the extracellular space by degranulation. Note how eosinophils differ in this respect from neutrophils, which phagocytose pathogens *before* releasing cytotoxic molecules. Eosinophils migrate into areas of inflammation or infection, particularly infection with multicellular parasites, e.g., helminths (worms). They are also important in both innate (see Chapter 9: Eosinophils) and adaptive immunity and allergic responses.

Basophils

Basophils (diameter 14–16 µm) have bilobed nuclei and granular cytoplasm, like eosinophils, but stain strongly with basic dyes. Basophils represent ≤1% of the bloodstream's white cell population. In concert with eosinophils and mast cells, they contribute strongly to innate and adaptive immunity. Physiological histamine is derived in part from basophilic granules.

Monocytes/macrophages

Monocytes and macrophages are larger than granulocytes (diameter ≤25 µm). They have a large eccentrically placed reniform (kidney-shaped) nucleus. In the bloodstream, they are called monocytes and account for ~2%–10% of the white cell population. They circulate for 1–3 days, then leave the circulation and enter the tissues, where they differentiate further, developing into macrophages.

Macrophages comprise the reticuloendothelial system and are found in tissues throughout the body. They phagocytose cellular debris and pathogens and produce various cytokines. They also process and present antigens to lymphocytes as part of the adaptive immune response (see Chapter 10: MHC processing).

Lymphocytes

These white blood cells are small and have a relatively large, round nucleus relative to their nongranular, basophilic cytoplasm volume. They all originate from the lymphoid lineage.

B lymphocytes

These cells are small lymphocytes (diameter 6–9 µm) expressing the B cell receptor. They secrete immunoglobulins (antibodies). A large proportion of B lymphocytes reside in lymph node germinal centres, where they are known as memory B cells. Some B lymphocytes also mature further into plasma cells.

Plasma cells are larger than B lymphocytes and have a strongly basophilic cytoplasm and an eccentric round nucleus. They are mainly seen in the bone marrow, but a few may be seen circulating in the peripheral blood.

T lymphocytes

These cells are small lymphocytes (diameter 6–9 µm) expressing the T cell receptor. T cells are subclassified by type of surface glycoproteins they express, indicated by the CD prefix. Cytotoxic T cells (CD8 +ve) mediate destruction of cells infected by intracellular organisms, while T helper cells (CD4 +ve) release cytokines to regulate and assist in the adaptive immune response (Chapter 10).

Natural killer cells

These large granular lymphocytes are also cytotoxic lymphocytes, like T cells, but natural killer (NK) cells are larger. Their behaviour differs from that of T cells in that they do not require major histocompatibility complex (MHC) or antibody-bound antigen complexes to recognize and destroy foreign or infected cells. They are thus prominent in the innate immune response (Chapter 9).

HAEMATOPOIESIS

Haematopoiesis is the formation and development of blood cells. The haematopoietic system is composed of the bone marrow, spleen, liver, lymph nodes and thymus.

Pluripotent haemopoietic stem cells

All blood cells originally derive from a population of pluripotent, CD34 +ve haemopoietic stem cells, residing in haematopoietic tissues. These stem cells may either:

- Remain as pluripotent stem cells, dividing to form identical daughter cells, maintaining the haemopoietic population
- Differentiate into specific progenitor cells, which ultimately develop into specific cellular components of blood

After initially differentiating into either a myeloid or lymphoid progenitor cell, further developmental changes follow. As cells progress down their respective development pathways, they sequentially acquire characteristic receptors and functions, ultimately forming a mature blood cell (Fig. 1.1) with characteristics specific to the cell type.

Progenitor cells

The pluripotent stem cells can differentiate into one of the two multipotent progenitors:

- Myeloid lineage progenitor cell
- Lymphoid lineage progenitor cell

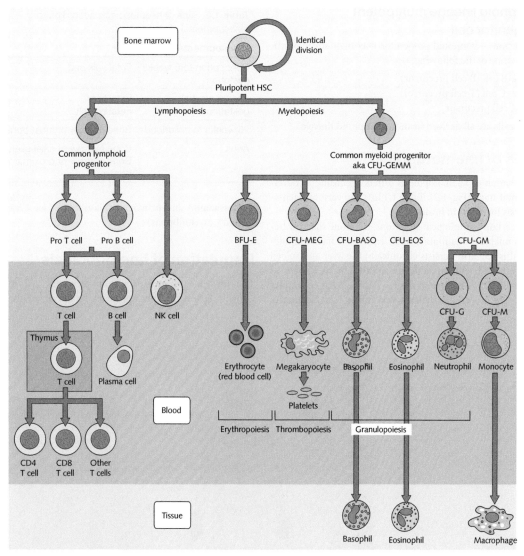

Fig. 1.1 Overview of haemopoiesis. Note the four relevant zones: bone marrow, blood, tissues and thymus. For information on growth factors important for various specific maturations, please see Table 1.2.
HSC, haematopoietic stem cell

Myeloid lineage multipotent progenitor cell

The CFU generating myeloid cells (CFU-GEMM) multipotent stem cell subsequently further differentiates into either:

- Red cell progenitor (BFU-E)
- Platelet progenitor (CFU-Meg)
- Eosinophil progenitor (CFU-Eos)
- Basophil progenitor (CFU-Baso)
- Neutrophil/monocyte progenitor (CFU-GM)

These cells are all derived from the myeloid lineage.

HINTS AND TIPS

COLONY-FORMING UNITS (CFU)

CFU describes a progenitor cell committed to the development of a particular blood cell. For example, CFU-Baso is a progenitor cell that ultimately develops into a basophil.

Lymphoid lineage multipotent progenitor cell

The common lymphoid progenitor may further differentiate into one of the following:

- Pre-B cell (B cell precursor)
- Pre-T cell (T cell precursor)
- NK cell precursor

These cells are all derived from the lymphoid lineage.

Sites of haematopoiesis

The location of haematopoiesis differs according to developmental stage (Fig. 1.2). Table 1.1 lists the various haematopoiesis locations in health.

In certain pathological situations, the bone marrow becomes unable to maintain a sufficient rate of haematopoiesis. If this scenario persists chronically, the liver and spleen may resume haematopoietic capability. This is known as extramedullary haematopoiesis. Two classic examples where this is seen are thalassaemia major (see Chapter 3: Thalassaemia) and primary myelofibrosis (see Chapter 5: Primary myelofibrosis).

Table 1.1 Sites of haemopoiesis according to developmental stage

Developmental stage	Site
Conception to 6 weeks' gestation	Fetal yolk sac
6 to 26 weeks' gestation	Fetal liver Fetal spleen
26 weeks to childhood	Bone marrow of most bones
Adult	Bone marrow of axial skeleton Bone marrow of proximal long bones

Regulation of haemopoiesis

The presence of growth factors promotes cell division. Growth factors are glycoproteins produced in the bone

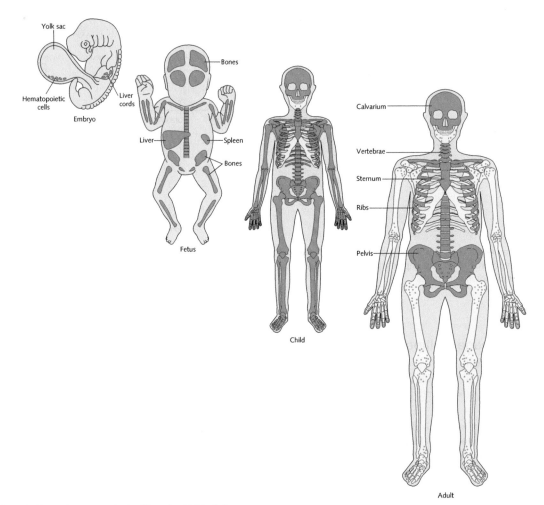

Fig. 1.2 Sites of haemopoiesis. (See also Table 1.1).

marrow, liver and kidneys. They bind to surface receptors on haemopoietic cells and can trigger replication, differentiation or functional activation, depending on the particular growth factor and the physiological context. In the absence of protective growth factor stimulation, cells undergo apoptosis (regulated cell death of old or dysfunctional cells). Specific growth factors and their respective responsive cells are indicated in Table 1.2. Note that some growth factors are used clinically.

CLINICAL NOTES

CLINICAL USE OF GROWTH FACTORS

Recombinant growth factors may be used clinically to increase the synthesis of a specific blood cell and compensate for a cytopenia. As an example, erythropoietin is used to increase red cell synthesis in the context of insufficient endogenous erythropoietin (such as in chronic end-stage renal disease). G-CSF stimulates the CFU-GM progenitors to differentiate into mature neutrophils. It is used when neutrophil count is dangerously low, for example following chemotherapy. Eltrombopag and romiplostim stimulate platelet synthesis via stimulation of the thrombopoietin receptor on megakaryocytes. They are used to increase platelet counts in immune thrombocytopenic purpura (ITP).

BONE MARROW

Bone marrow is the major haematopoietic organ in adults, producing ~500 billion cells daily and accounting for ~5% of body weight. It is divided into red marrow and yellow marrow. Red marrow is red due to haematopoiesis and yellow marrow is yellow due to fat. In situations where the existing red marrow is unable to perform haematopoiesis at a rate sufficient for normal physiological function, yellow marrow retains the ability to resume haematopoiesis, in which case it becomes red marrow.

Structure

Bone marrow tissue lies within central cavities of bones, supported by a matrix of bony trabeculae. Red marrow provides an optimal microenvironment for haematopoietic stem cell growth and development. It has two main components: haematopoietic parenchyma (developing blood cells) and supporting stromal tissue.

Stroma

In red marrow, stroma consists of vascular sinusoids and specialized fibroblasts. Vascular sinusoids consist of blood-filled spaces, fed by arterioles and interconnected by multiple fenestrated capillaries. Sinusoids ultimately drain (radially) into a large central vein from whence they enter the venous circulation. The fenestrations allow passage

---

Table 1.2 Growth factors

Growth factor	Source	Cellular target	Action
Erythropoietin	Kidneys	BFU-E and CFU-E	Stimulates the BFU-E and CFU-E to progress down the differentiation pathway of red cell precursors, ultimately forming mature red cells
Thrombopoietin	Liver	CFU-Meg, megakaryocytes	Enhancement of basal production rate of megakaryocytes (from CFU-Meg) and platelets (from megakaryocytes)
G-CSF	Endothelial cell, macrophages, lymphocytes	CFU-G	Differentiation into mature neutrophils
GM-CSF	Macrophages, T cells and mast cells	CFU-GM	Granulocyte and monocyte precursor growth and differentiation
Interleukin 2	Activated T cells, NK cells, macrophage	Pre-T cell	T cell growth and differentiation
Interleukin 3	T cells, thymic epithelium	CFU-GEMM	Haematopoiesis
Interleukin 5	T cells, mast cells, eosinophil	CFU-Eos	Eosinophil growth and differentiation
Interleukin 6	T cells, macrophages, some B cells	Activated B cells, plasma cells, T cells, macrophages	Inflammatory cytokine that induces acute-phase response

BFU-E, Erythroid burst-forming unit; CFU, colony-forming unit; CFU-Eos, CFU eosinophil progenitor; CFU-G, CFU neutrophil precursor; CFU-GEMM, CFU generating myeloid cells; CFU-GM, CFU granulocyte-myeloid precursor (the neutrophil/monocyte precursor); G-CSF, granulocyte-colony stimulating factor; GM-CSF, granulocyte-macrophage colony stimulating factor; NK, natural killer.

of matured blood cells out of the marrow and into the bloodstream by this route. Specialized fibroblasts (adventitial reticular cells) secrete reticulin (a subtype of collagen) fibres, which form a supportive mechanical framework for the haematopoietic tissue.

Haemopoietic tissue

Also known as 'haematopoietic islands' or 'haematopoietic cords', the synthetic tissue of red marrow contains stem cells, progenitors, precursors and mature bloods cells. This haematopoietic tissue fills the area between the vascular sinusoids. Anatomical compartmentalization occurs according to the type of blood cell being synthesized, e.g., red cell synthesis occurring in erythroblastic islands, megakaryopoiesis occurring in zones adjacent to the sinusoids, etc.

Haematopoietic cord macrophages

Macrophages, full of iron-rich stores of ferritin and haemosiderin, are centrally located within each cluster of haematopoietic synthesis. They have three main functions:

1. Provision of an iron supply for developing erythroblasts (for haemoglobin synthesis)
2. Phagocytosis of the cellular debris associated with haematopoiesis
3. Contributing to the cellular regulation of haematopoiesis

Lymphocyte differentiation

Bone marrow synthesizes lymphocytes and is thus termed a 'primary' lymphoid organ.

B cell differentiation

B cell development is dependent on bone marrow stroma. As B cell precursors develop, they migrate towards the central axis of the marrow cavity and become less reliant on stromal support. Any developing B cells that demonstrate binding to self-antigens are destroyed at this stage. The surviving B cells enter the circulation, travelling to the spleen/lymph nodes for final maturation.

T cell differentiation

T lymphocyte precursors leave the bone marrow earlier in their development. They enter the circulation and travel to the thymus for maturation.

Natural killer cell differentiation

NK cells undergo initial development in the bone marrow, but ultimately deploy to secondary lymphoid tissue (tonsils, lymph nodes and spleen) for further maturation.

THE SPLEEN

The spleen is the largest secondary lymphoid organ. In some ways, it may be thought of as a very large and sophisticated lymph node. The spleen is responsible for the following physiological roles:

- Removal of particulate matter from the bloodstream (e.g., opsonized bacteria, antibody-coated cells)
- Destruction of elderly and poorly deformable erythrocytes
- Initiation of the immune response to blood-borne antigens
- A storage zone for platelets (~1/3 of the platelet population is found in the spleen)
- Fetal haematopoiesis

Embryology

The spleen originates as a mesodermal proliferation from the primitive gut during the fifth week of fetal development.

Anatomy

The spleen is an intraperitoneal organ, measuring between 6 cm and 13 cm when healthy. It is wrapped in a dense fibro-elastic capsule that protrudes conspicuously into the organ, subdividing it. Blood supply to the spleen is via the splenic artery, which enters at the hilus. Venous drainage via the splenic vein also leaves via the hilus, ultimately entering the portal vein via the superior mesenteric vein. It is connected to the body wall by the lienorenal ligament and to the stomach by the gastrolienal ligament.

It is anatomically related to:

- Stomach, tail of pancreas, left colic flexure (anteriorly)
- Left kidney (medially)
- Diaphragm, ribs 9–11 (posteriorly)

There are two types of functional tissue: red pulp and white pulp. These are separated by the marginal zone.

Red pulp

Red pulp is a 3D meshwork of splenic cords (connective tissue) and numerous blood-filled sinusoids. Blood cells are extravasated into splenic cord filtration beds where lattice-like networks of connective tissue and macrophages perform the mechanical filtration function of the spleen, removing antigens, microorganisms, senescent blood cells and blood-borne particulate matter. Once through the filtration bed, cells return to the circulation via the sinusoids, which drain into the venous system.

White pulp

White pulp consists of B cell follicles and peri-arteriolar lymphoid sheaths (PALS), which protrude into the red pulp. PALS are dense areas of lymphatic tissue, mainly consisting of T cells, wrapped around splenic arterioles. The B cell follicles are continuous with the PALS.

Marginal zone

This region (histologically considered white pulp) delineates red pulp and white pulp. Some resident macrophages and marginal zone B cells are permanent features. Other B cells and T cells are only present temporarily, in transit between the circulation and their splenic domains (follicles or PALS respectively). This makes the marginal zone an optimal site for antigen processing and presentation and lymphocyte/dendritic cell interaction.

Disorders of the spleen

Splenomegaly

Enlargement of the spleen (splenomegaly) may arise in many different disorders, as illustrated in Table 1.3. Clinically palpable splenomegaly must be accurately assessed with appropriate imaging.

Table 1.3 Causes of splenomegaly

System/mechanism	Specific causes
Infection: bacterial	Tuberculosis Salmonella Brucella Syphilis Infective endocarditis
Infection: viral	Epstein-Barr virus[a] Hepatitis Cytomegalovirus HIV
Infection: parasitic	Malaria Toxoplasmosis Schistosomiasis Visceral leishmaniasis Trypanosomiasis
Inflammation/immune	Sarcoidosis Rheumatoid arthritis Systemic lupus erythematosus
Haematological malignancy (Chapter 5)	Lymphomas Leukaemias Myeloproliferative disorders (especially primary myelofibrosis)
Nonmalignant haematological causes	Haemoglobinopathies Haemolytic anaemia
Congestive (portal hypertension)	Liver cirrhosis[a] Right ventricular failure[a] Thrombosis of portal, hepatic or splenic veins
Trauma	Splenic intracapsular haematoma
Infiltrative	Lipid deposition disorders (e.g., Gaucher disease) Niemann-Pick disease Amyloidosis Glycogen storage disorders

[a] Most common causes for splenomegaly in the UK

CLINICAL NOTES

SPLENOMEGALY

The spleen must increase significantly in size in order for it to be palpated below the costal margins; so a palpable splenic edge always indicates splenomegaly.

Hypersplenism

Irrespective of the underlying cause of a splenomegaly, the enlarged spleen filters out more cells, resulting in excessive clearance of cells from the bloodstream. This reduces circulating numbers and results in cytopenias, resulting in the release of immature blood cells into the bloodstream from functionally normal bone marrow. This phenomenon is called hypersplenism and should be identified, because the effective treatment of the underlying cause of the splenomegaly can improve blood cell counts without resorting to a splenectomy.

Splenic infarction

Splenic infarction is the ischaemic death of splenic tissue due to occlusion of the arterial supply. It may affect part (partial infarction) or all (complete infarction) of the spleen. Emboli (secondary to atrial fibrillation) are the most common cause, but locally formed thrombi within the splenic artery or its major branches (associated with sickle-cell disease and myeloproliferative disorders) can also be responsible.

Following complete infarction (autosplenectomy), patients are rendered functionally asplenic and require asplenic management.

Rupture of the spleen

The spleen may rupture secondary to abdominal trauma, certain infections (e.g., Epstein-Barr virus; see Clinical notes) or disorders of haematopoiesis, e.g., primary myelofibrosis.

CLINICAL NOTES

EPSTEIN-BARR VIRUS

EBV infection (aka glandular fever or infectious mononucleosis) can cause splenomegaly for ≤8 weeks postinfection. Although it commonly causes mild/moderate splenomegaly, it is rarely serious. To prevent splenic rupture, patients with acute EBV infection are advised to avoid contact sports for at least 8 weeks.

Splenectomy

Indications for splenectomy (surgical removal of the spleen) include:

- Severe splenic trauma causing uncontrollable bleeding
- Splenic lymphoma
- Immune cytopenias (autoimmune haemolytic anaemia, immune thrombocytopenia)
- Nonimmune haemolysis when secondary to splenic RBC destruction (Thalassaemia major, hereditary spherocytosis)
- Splenic cysts (only rarely)

Autosplenectomy refers to the hyposplenism that develops when the spleen is rendered nonfunctional by disease. Splenic artery thrombosis is an illustrative example. Sickle cell disease is the one of the most common causes in infancy, due to cumulative localized small-vessel thrombosis. Coeliac disease is another well-known cause of autosplenectomy, although the exact mechanism is unclear.

Congenital abnormalities

Congenital asplenia (absent spleen) is rare and usually associated with other congenital abnormalities. Conversely, ~10% of people have accessory spleens (additional small areas of splenic tissue).

Management of the hyposplenic patient

Regardless of the cause of their hyposplenism, asplenic and hyposplenic patients are at an increased risk of infection, particularly infection by encapsulated bacteria (e.g., *Neisseria meningitides, Streptococcus pneumoniae, Haemophilus influenzae*). This is primarily because the spleen, being the largest lymphoid organ, is the major site for immunoglobulin synthesis, including IgM. IgM is necessary for opsonization of encapsulated organisms. Macrophages lining the meshwork of the red pulp also ingest and remove unopsonized bacteria. In the absence of a spleen, both these functions are lost. The clinical consequence is a patient with lifelong susceptibility to overwhelming postsplenectomy infections (OPSI).

To reduce the chance of OPSI, several interventions are required in asplenic/hyposplenic patients:

1. Vaccinations (courses to be completed >2 weeks prior to splenectomy or initiated >2 weeks post splenectomy). The first three vaccines must be protein conjugate vaccines, which are more effective than plain polysaccharide vaccines:
   - Pneumococcal vaccine (with boosters every 5–10 years afterwards)
   - Haemophilus influenzae vaccination course
   - Meningococcal vaccines
   - Influenza vaccination (repeated annually lifelong)
2. Lifelong prophylactic daily oral antibiotics: Penicillin V (clarithromycin if penicillin-allergic). Many patients unfortunately stop taking their daily antibiotics after a few years, only to die of overwhelming sepsis.
3. Clear advice regarding the need for urgent medical review if patients develop symptoms of infection, e.g., sore throat/fever/productive cough/lethargy/diarrhoea/vomiting, etc.

It is of paramount importance is that patients repeat the above vaccinations as required for the rest of their lives, as well as continuing to take their daily prophylactic antibiotics.

LYMPHADENOPATHY

Enlarged lymph nodes (lymphadenopathy) are normal when occurring in response to infection or inflammation. However, in the absence of these factors, lymphadenopathy may be an important indicator of neoplastic disease. An illustration showing the main groups of lymph nodes is given in Fig. 1.3. Acute, localized tender/painful lymphadenopathy is generally a helpful indicator of infection in the area drained by the enlarged nodes. Insidious, painless, nontender generalized (involving >1 anatomical region) node enlargement is more likely to be due to malignancy (see Chapter 5: Lymphadenopathy red flags) but may be due to a nonmalignant pathology. Examples are detailed in Table 1.4.

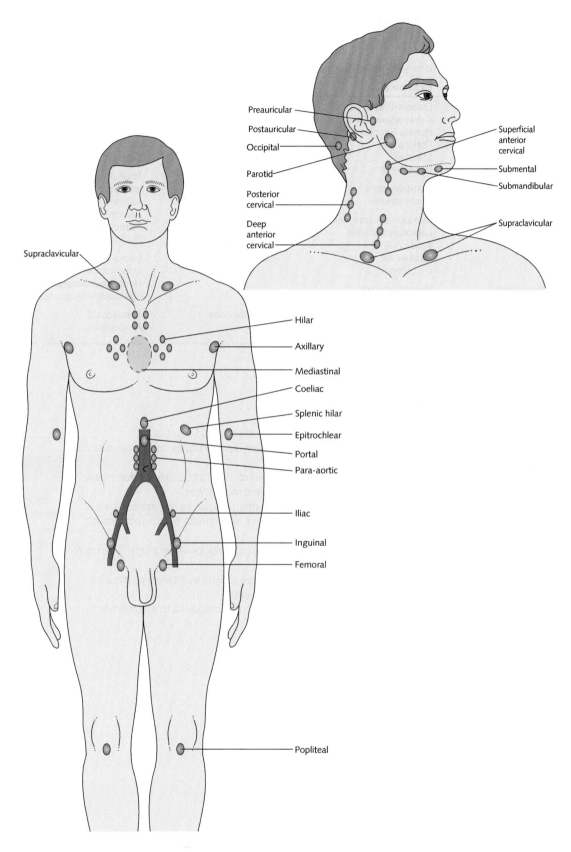

Fig. 1.3 Lymph node locations. Solid circles represent palpable lymph node(s), unfilled circles represent impalpable or internal lymph nodes. Note that the popliteal lymph nodes are palpable in the popliteal fossa on the posterior surface of the leg.

9

Table 1.4 Causes of generalized lymphadenopathy

Mechanism	Examples	Mechanism	Examples
Infection: viral	Epstein-Barr virus Cytomegalovirus Herpes Simplex 1 and 2 Rubella Measles Hepatitis B	Connective tissue disease	Rheumatoid arthritis Systemic lupus erythematosus Churg-Strauss syndrome Dermatomyositis
Infection: protozoal	Toxoplasmosis Leishmaniasis	Drugs	Phenytoin Isoniazid Aspirin
Infection: bacterial	Borreliosis (Lyme disease) Leptospirosis (Weil syndrome) Tularaemia Brucellosis		Penicillins Tetracyclines Sulphonamides
		Neoplasia	Leukaemias Lymphomas Nonhaematological metastatic malignancy
Infection: fungal	Histoplasmosis Cryptococcosis Coccidioidomycosis	Miscellaneous	Sarcoidosis Amyloidosis

● Chapter Summary

- Blood consists primarily of different cell types suspended in fluid plasma.
- Blood delivers oxygen and nutrients to cells of the body and removes carbon dioxide and waste products.
- There are several types of blood cells, each with characteristic structure and functions: erythrocytes, platelets, lymphocytes, granulocytes and monocytes.
- Blood cells are synthesized via a process of development known as haematopoiesis.
- Different development pathways for different cell types all originate from haemopoietic stem cells.
- Haematopoiesis occurs in different tissues according to developmental stage. This takes place in the bone marrow in adults.
- The spleen plays several important immunological roles as well as filtering particulate matter and removing aged red cells from the bloodstream.
- Lymph node enlargement (lymphadenopathy) may occur in response to infection or malignancy.

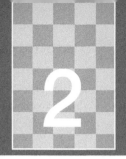
ERYTHROCYTES

Erythrocytes are mature red cells. Their average lifespan is 120 days. The normal concentration of erythrocytes in the blood is $3.9–6.5 \times 10^{12}$/L.

Structure

A typical red cell has an average diameter of 7.2 μm. Their three-dimensional shape is a biconcave discoid (Fig. 2.1), offering a high surface area:volume shape, which is optimal for gas exchange (the primary function of the red cell). It also facilitates rapid, reversible cellular deformation, necessary for squeezing through microvasculature where vessel diameter may be as small as 3 μm.

Contents

Erythrocytes have no nuclei or organelles. Instead, they are packed with haemoglobin, the oxygen-carrying, haem-containing metalloprotein, which gives blood its familiar red colour.

Function

The primary function of erythrocytes is gas exchange. In mammals, oxygen is transported from the lungs to peripheral tissues and carbon dioxide from the tissues to the lungs.

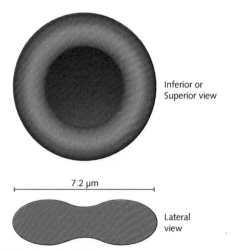

Inferior or Superior view

7.2 μm

Lateral view

Fig. 2.1 Erythrocyte 3D shape.

Oxygen transport

The vast bulk of O_2 transported from the lungs to the tissues travels bound to red cell haemoglobin; only a minute fraction is dissolved in solution in blood. Oxygen carriage by haemoglobin varies according to several variables:

- Haemoglobin concentration
- Haemoglobin affinity for oxygen (varies according to environmental factors such as pO_2, pCO_2)
- Haemoglobin saturation (determined by the arterial partial pressure of oxygen (pO_2))

Expressed as an equation where Hb = haemoglobin; pCO_2 = partial pressure of carbon dioxide and SpO_2 = blood oxygen saturation:

$$O_2 \text{ carried by Hb} = [Hb] \times SpO_2 (\%) \times 0.01 \times 1.34$$

Note that 1.34 represents Huffner's constant and describes the maximum amount of oxygen carried per gram of haemoglobin (i.e., mL/g). The 0.01 is a correction factor to account for using percentage.

The contribution of dissolved oxygen in solution is very small and is also a function of arterial pO_2:

$$O_2 \text{ carried in solution} = 0.0225 \times pO_2 (\text{in kPa})$$

The 0.0225 represents the amount in mL of oxygen per kPa of partial pressure. Combining the two components:

$$\text{Total oxygen carriage} = (O_2 \text{ carried by Hb}) + (O_2 \text{ in solution})$$

Using an example, let us assume that arterial pO_2 = 13.3 kPa, [Hb] = 15g/100 mL and SpO_2 is 100%:

$$(1.34 \times 15 \times 100 \times 0.01) + (0.0225 \times 13.3) = 20.4 \text{ mL oxygen per } 100 \text{ mL blood, or } \sim 200 \text{ mL oxygen per litre.}$$

Multiplied by an average resting cardiac output of 5 L/min, we can conclude that ~1000 mL/min of O_2 is delivered to the tissues. This well exceeds the minimum resting physiological O_2 requirement (~250 mL/min).

Carbon dioxide transport

CO_2 is a product of respiration (aerobic and anaerobic). Blood pCO_2 is tightly regulated by changes in ventilation. CO_2 is carried in the blood in three forms:

- Bicarbonate ions (~90%). Functioning as a biochemical CO_2 reservoir, these play a significant role in blood pH buffering.

- Direct solution (~5%)
- Carb-amino compounds (~5%): CO_2 combines with protein amino groups, primarily those of haemoglobin.

Secondary functions

Haemoglobin is also a key blood pH buffer, due to its ability to bind H^+ ions. The H^+ ions associated with haemoglobin are derived from bicarbonate generation and carb-amino compound formation (Fig. 2.2).

Another important (but secondary) erythrocyte role is vasodilation. This is mediated by release of biomediators including adenosine triphosphate (ATP), S-nitrosothiols, nitric oxide (NO) and hydrogen sulphide. This is triggered by red cell shear stress from collision with vessel walls, which occurs more in vasoconstricted vessels.

ERYTHROPOIESIS

Erythropoiesis (Fig. 2.3) is red blood synthesis, starting with the CFU-GEMM myeloid lineage progenitor (see Chapter 1, Fig. 1.1). Erythropoiesis occurs in erythroblastic islands within bone marrow. Macrophages situated here supply iron (needed for haemoglobin synthesis) to the surrounding developing cells. It takes ~1 week for a stem cell to differentiate fully into a mature erythrocyte.

Sequence of erythropoiesis

Maturation is characterized by the following key stages:

- Erythroid burst-forming units (BFU-E): colony-forming unit generating myeloid cells (CFU-GEMM) differentiation to a BFU-E commits to the erythrocyte development pathway.
- Pronormoblast: haemoglobin is absent, organelles are still present, and the nucleus is large relative to cytoplasm volume.
- Early, intermediate and late normoblasts. Overall cell size and nuclear size (relative to cytoplasm) decrease. Haemoglobin accumulates and the nucleus is ejected from the late normoblast to form a reticulocyte.
- Reticulocyte. These are released from bone marrow into the bloodstream. Some ribonucleic acid (RNA) is still present and the shape remains rounded.
- Erythrocyte. The biconcave discoid shape defines the mature erythrocyte. Intracellular organelles have been lost.

In a healthy person, bone marrow erythrocyte production rate is approximately matched by splenic erythrocyte removal rate. The total erythrocyte population therefore remains approximately constant.

An imbalance developing due to excessive destruction of red cells (e.g., acute haemolysis) can be compensated by

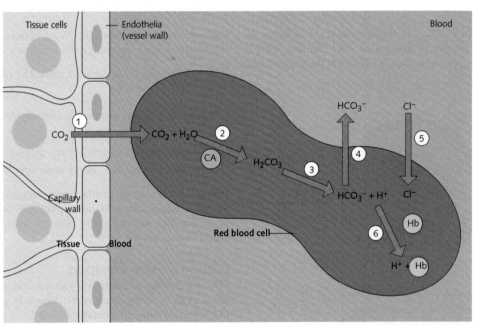

Fig. 2.2 Carbon dioxide transport in blood. (1) CO_2 travels down the partial pressure gradient (respiring cells → blood). (2) Red cell carbonic anhydrase enzyme catalyzes the formation of carbonic acid (H_2CO_3) from H_2O and CO_2. (3) H_2CO_3 dissociates into protons (H^+) and bicarbonate ions (HCO_3^-). (4) Bicarbonate ions diffuse down their concentration gradient into the plasma. (5) Chloride ions (Cl^-) enter the cell to maintain electroneutrality (the chloride shift). (6) H^+ (produced as a result by dissociation of H_2CO_3) bind to imidazole groups on the amino acids comprising haemoglobin. *CA,* Carbonic anhydrase.

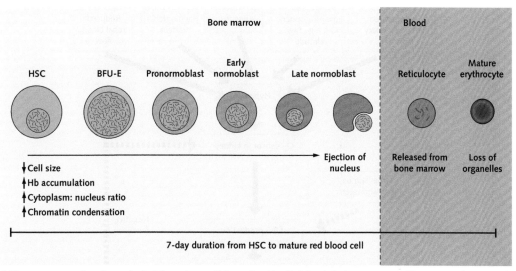

Fig. 2.3 The sequence of erythropoiesis takes place within erythroblastic islands in bone marrow. These contain macrophages, which supply iron to the surrounding erythroid progenitor cells. For intervening stages between the haematopoietic stem cell and BFU-E, please see Fig. 1.1. *HSC*, haematopoietic stem cell; *BFU-E*, Burst-forming unit-Erythroid.

an increase in erythropoiesis, so the red cell count remains constant. Enhanced erythropoiesis is suggested by the (abnormal) presence of nucleated precursors in peripheral blood (i.e., on a blood film) or an increased reticulocyte count.

Ineffective erythropoiesis

Each pronormoblast can potentially give rise to 16 erythrocytes, but some normoblasts fail to develop and are phagocytosed by bone marrow macrophages. In a healthy individual, the proportion of ineffective erythropoiesis is small. However, in certain pathological states, developmental abnormalities increase the proportion of ineffective erythropoiesis.

Regulation of erythropoiesis

The principal factor promoting erythropoiesis is a hormone called erythropoietin.

Erythropoietin

Erythropoietin (EPO) is a heavily glycosylated polypeptide, 165 amino acids in length with molecular weight $\approx 30,400\,kDa$. It is secreted by:

- Peritubular capillary endothelial cells (renal cortex; 90%)
- Kupffer cells and hepatocytes (liver; 10%)

Control of erythropoietin secretion

Hypoxia (low intracellular pO_2) is the main stimulus for EPO synthesis and secretion. Hypoxia is defined by insufficient oxygen delivery to meet cellular requirements. Hypoxia may arise due to a multitude of causes (Fig. 2.4).

Most causes can ultimately be categorized within one of the following underlying mechanisms:

- Reduction in the oxygen-carrying capacity of blood
- Impaired oxygenation at the pulmonary alveolar-arteriole interface
- Compromised tissue perfusion (i.e., oxygen delivery; which may be local or global)

A loss of functional renal tissue, e.g., nephrectomy or renal disease, will also result in decreased EPO production with the physiological consequence of anaemia. Conversely, renal cell carcinomas can produce excessive levels of EPO, resulting in a pathological increase in red cell production. Chronically raised EPO levels can also lead to extramedullary haematopoiesis (see Chapter 1).

Clinical indications for erythropoietin

Recombinant EPO (produced in animal cells) is used to increase the red cell count in specific anaemia scenarios, i.e., where the underlying pathology is due to a failure of serum (EPO) to increase appropriately in response to anaemia, e.g.,

- Anaemia secondary to chronic renal failure
- Some specific cases of anaemia of chronic disease, e.g., congestive heart failure
- Postchemotherapy
- Certain subtypes of myelodysplastic syndromes, where EPO may be combined with granulocyte-colony stimulating factor (G-CSF)
- To boost the red cell count prior to autologous blood transfusions

Altitude training

Athletes training at high altitude exploit the lower environmental pO_2 (due to reduced atmospheric pressure at elevation) to stimulate endogenous EPO production. This increases their

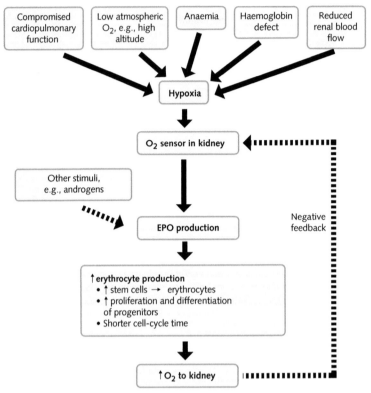

Fig. 2.4 Regulation of EPO synthesis. *EPO,* Erythropoietin.

red cell counts and thus the oxygen-carrying capacity of their blood, theoretically improving athletic performance. Synthetic EPO may be illegally administered with the same intention.

HAEMOGLOBIN

Structure

A haemoglobin molecule consists of four globin chains united by noncovalent interactions (Fig. 2.5). Each globin features a haem pocket, a hydrophobic crevice containing the haem moiety. Each haem group can bind one molecule of oxygen. Since there are four haem pockets (one per globin chain) a maximum of four oxygen molecules can be transported per haemoglobin molecule. Normal adult haemoglobin (HbA) is tetrameric, consisting of two α and two β globins. Each α first dimerizes with a β. Two identical αβ dimers then unite, forming a tetramer.

Haem (Heme)

Haem belongs to a family of compounds known as the porphyrins, which are characterized by the presence of a tetrapyrrole ring. The haem group consists of an Fe^{2+} (ferrous) ion at the centre of the tetrapyrrole ring protoporphyrin

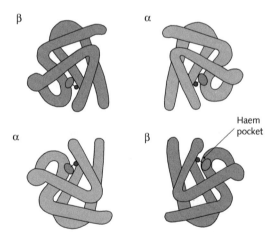

Fig. 2.5 Structure of adult haemoglobin. α polypeptides (globins) are 141 amino acids, whilst β polypeptides (globins) are 146 amino acids in length. Note the haem pocket featuring in each globin.

IX. This consists of four pyrrole rings, linked by methene bridges. Each ferrous ion is bonded to four N atoms, one from each pyrrole ring. The ferrous ion acts as an oxygen-binding site (described as the sixth coordination site). Importantly, the iron ion remains in the ferrous 2+ oxidation state, regardless of whether oxygen is bound or not.

Physiological properties of haemoglobin

Each Hb molecule is capable of binding four molecules of oxygen, one at each haem site.

Haemoglobin: deoxyHb and oxyHb

Haemoglobin with ≥1 haem-bound oxygen is termed oxy-haemoglobin (oxyHb). Haemoglobin without any haem-bound oxygen is termed deoxyhaemoglobin (deoxyHb).

Haemoglobin: tense versus relaxed

The haemoglobin molecule may exist in two structural configurations: relaxed (R-Hb) and taut (T-Hb). In the R-Hb state, there is increased mobility between globin chains compared with the T-Hb state. Oxygen molecules can more easily access the haem pockets and therefore the R-Hb state has a greater affinity for oxygen.

Factors consistent with the tissue environment [low pH, high pCO_2 and high 2,3-diphosphoglycerate (2,3-DPG)] favour the T-Hb conformation, which exhibits reduced oxygen affinity. In the presence of these environmental factors, bound oxygen is more likely to dissociate from T-Hb. This is ideal, since in the environment of respiring cells, oxygen offloads readily in environments where it is most needed. The mechanism underlying the variable affinity is that H^+ ions, CO_2 and 2,3-DPG covalently bind to haemoglobin, imposing conformational changes that are less favourable for the oxygen–haemoglobin association.

The converse scenario (high pH, low pCO_2 and low 2,3-DPG) favours the relaxed conformation R-Hb, which has increased oxygen affinity and thus binds oxygen more avidly. These factors are consistent with the gas exchange surface, i.e., the alveolar-arterial surface in the lungs, where it is physiologically advantageous for haemoglobin to bind oxygen avidly.

Cooperation

The binding of an O_2 molecule increases the haemoglobin molecule's binding affinity for any subsequent oxygen molecules. Thus the fourth oxygen molecule binds much more readily than the first. Conversely, unloading of O_2 from one haem group facilitates oxygen offloading from the other haem groups. This property accounts for the characteristic sigmoidal (S-shaped) shape of the oxygen dissociation curve (Fig. 2.6).

The oxygen dissociation curve

The oxygen dissociation curve is a plot of pO_2 (x axis) against haemoglobin oxygen saturation (y axis). Elevated pCO_2, 2,3-DPG, H^+ and temperature shift the curve to the right, i.e., reducing the affinity for oxygen and promoting oxygen offloading. These conditions are consistent with respiring tissues. For a given pO_2 value, the right-shifted curve exhibits a lower haemoglobin saturation.

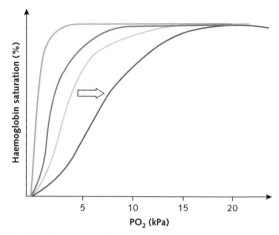

Fig. 2.6 The oxygen dissociation curve. Adult haemoglobin (dark blue curve), fetal haemoglobin (blue curve) and myoglobin (green curve) are illustrated. The arrow demonstrates the rightward shift seen in low pH (high [H^+]), high pCO_2, high 2,3-DPG and high temperature conditions (red curve).

Due to the sigmoidal nature of the curve, as the pO_2 falls, there is initially little change in the oxygen affinity and therefore haemoglobin saturation. However, below a certain pO_2 there is a sharp drop in oxygen affinity and therefore Hb saturation, resulting in greater release of oxygen as pO_2 lowers.

Fetal haemoglobin

Fetal Hb (HbF) is distinguished from adult Hb (HbA) by the substitution of two γ globins for the two β globins. HbF has greater affinity for oxygen than HbA. This ensures that even at very low pO_2 (such as the gas exchange surfaces of the placenta), where HbA would offload its oxygen cargo, HbF still binds oxygen avidly. At the placental gas exchange surfaces, oxygen is released from maternal HbA and is immediately bound to HbF, which still has a high affinity for oxygen, despite the low pO_2 environment. This effectively allows fetal Hb preferential access to maternal oxygen. The oxygen dissociation curve for HbF is shifted to the left (Fig 2.6). HbF is the predominant haemoglobin in fetuses and newborns. Different types of haemoglobin molecule predominate at different developmental stages (Table 2.1).

Haemoglobin variants

Different variants of haemoglobin exhibit variable oxygen affinities and thus have their own characteristic oxygen dissociation curves. Sickle haemoglobin (HbS) is a pathological form of haemoglobin, where a point mutation distinguishes it structurally and functionally from normal HbA.

Under normal pO_2 conditions, HbS and HbA have similar oxygen affinities. At low pO_2, HbS does exhibit a lower oxygen affinity than normal HbA. Importantly, however, the rightward shift in the dissociation curve that characterizes HbS is not solely due to this affinity variance at low pO_2. It is also due to abnormal HbS polymerization at low PO_2, causing structural

Table 2.1 Haemoglobin types present at different developmental stages

Developmental stage	Haemoglobin type	Globin components	Specific
Embryonic	Hb Gower I Hb Gower II Hb Portland	$\zeta_2\epsilon_2$ $\alpha_2\epsilon_2$ $\zeta_2\gamma_2$	From conception to 2nd trimester of fetal life
Fetal	Hb F	$\alpha_2\gamma_2$	From 2nd trimester of pregnancy to 12 weeks age
Adult	Hb A Hb A2	$\alpha_2\beta_2$ $\alpha_2\delta_2$	The primary type of Hb Typically represents $\leq 2\%$ of Hb

Hb, Haemoglobin

distortion and vaso-occlusion. Occluded, ischaemic cells increase their anaerobic activity, elevating the 2,3-DPG, which shifts the oxygen dissociation curve rightwards for HbS.

Haemoglobin genetics

The genes encoding the ϵ, γ, δ and β globins are found on chromosome 11. The ζ- and two copies of the α-chain genes are found on chromosome 16. Each globin gene consists of three exons each separated by an intron. Different globins are separately synthesized before uniting in various combinations to form a functional Hb tetramer.

MYOGLOBIN

The other major haem-containing protein in humans is myoglobin, which consists of a single globin with a single haem group. Myoglobin is found principally in muscle, where it only releases bound oxygen at extremely low pO_2, effectively functioning as an oxygen reservoir when oxygen demand exceeds delivery.

IRON AND HAEM METABOLISM

Total body iron is ~4 g, distributed as shown in Table 2.2. Dietary iron occurs as haem iron or nonhaem iron.

Iron metabolism

Absorption of haem iron

Dietary haem iron is almost exclusively derived from animal tissue such as meat or offal. In haem iron, the iron ion in the +2 (ferrous) oxidation state is incorporated in the haem group. This form of dietary iron is more completely and easily absorbed, since a receptor-mediated endocytosis absorbs the iron intact within the haem structure. The iron is intracellularly dismantled from the haem group within the enterocyte. Extrusion into the portal circulation from the enterocyte basal surface is via a common iron exporter.

Table 2.2 Physiological distribution of iron. Total body iron = 5 g

Total body iron (%)	Location
70	Component of haem moiety of haemoglobin
25	Reticuloendothelial macrophages, usually incorporated into iron storage proteins such as ferritin and haemosiderin
4.9	Component of iron-containing enzymes and proteins
0.1	In plasma, typically bound to transferrin

Absorption of nonhaem iron

Dietary nonhaem iron is obtained from dark leafy green vegetables. In nonhaem iron, the iron ion is in the +3 (ferric) oxidation state and is usually protein-associated. Nonhaem iron is less easily absorbed, since it must be divorced from its associated protein and then be reduced to the ferrous state prior to absorption across the enterocyte. This pre-absorption processing confers sensitivity to the chemical properties of coingested foods. Acid and reducing agents, e.g., ascorbic acid (vitamin C), increase absorption of ferric (nonhaem) iron by promoting the $Fe^{3+} \rightarrow Fe^{2+}$ reduction. The ferrous (Fe^{2+}) iron ions then enter enterocytes via the H^+/Fe^{2+} symport. Export into the portal circulation from the basal surface of enterocytes is via a common iron exporter.

Transport in the circulation

Once in the serum, ferrous ions (Fe^{2+}) oxidize, becoming ferric (Fe^{3+}) ions. In this form, they bind to transferrin, a transport protein. This delivers the iron to cells possessing transferrin receptors, including:

- Erythroblasts (within bone marrow) for incorporation into haemoglobin during erythropoiesis
- The liver and reticuloendothelial macrophages, where it is incorporated into ferritin or haemosiderin for storage
- Muscle, where it is incorporated into myoglobin

Ferritin and haemosiderin

Both ferritin and haemosiderin function as iron storage proteins, storing iron in the (Fe^{3+}) ferric form. Ferritin is a water-soluble compound of protein and iron. Haemosiderin is insoluble and consists of aggregates of ferritin that have partially lost their protein component.

Regulation of iron absorption

As there is no specific physiological iron excretion mechanism, iron levels in the body can only be regulated by variation of dietary iron absorption. This is mediated by hepcidin, a protein synthesized by the liver. Hepcidin binds to and internalizes (removes) the iron exporter from the basolateral enterocyte surface, limiting the iron's access to the circulation.

Excretion

Importantly, since a specific mechanism for excess iron excretion is absent, iron loss from the body can only take place via:

- desquamation of keratinocytes
- sloughed mucosal cells
- blood loss

Iron overload

Excess iron is deposited in the tissues, where it results in organ damage. The heart, liver and endocrine organs are particularly susceptible. Due to the lack of an iron excretion mechanism, iron overload is a significant hazard of iron administration or abnormally increased gastrointestinal iron absorption.

Increased absorption

Increased absorption may result from the following:

- Primary haemochromatosis (see below): normal amount of iron available for absorption, but excessive proportion absorbed
- Iron-containing supplement overdose: normal proportion of iron absorbed, but increased iron available
- High levels of ineffective erythropoiesis (e.g., as seen in thalassaemia)

Iatrogenic causes of excess iron intake

- Multiple blood transfusions (1 unit of blood contains ≈ 200–250 mg iron)
- Inappropriate or excessive oral or parenteral iron therapy

Treatment of iron overload

It is important to start therapy as soon as possible to prevent irreversible organ damage. Options include:

- Dietary advice (decrease iron intake, increase intake of natural chelators, e.g., tea)
- Venesection (1 mL blood represents 0.5 mg iron)
- Chelation therapy: desferrioxamine is an iron-chelating agent that is administered subcutaneously or intravenously. Deferipone and deferasirox are oral iron-chelating alternatives.

Haemochromatosis

This autosomal recessive disorder of iron metabolism arises from the failure of hepcidin synthesis due to human haemochromatosis (HFE) gene (chromosome 6) mutations. This results in a dramatic and pathological increase of enterocyte-absorbed dietary iron into the circulation (hepcidin usually *reduces* iron export from enterocytes to the circulation). Although a normal amount of iron may be ingested, a much higher proportion accesses the circulation.

Epidemiology

Around 0.5% of the population are homozygous for various HFE mutations. However, clinical penetrance shows considerable heterogeneity: only ~5% of homozygotes present symptomatically. Men present more commonly than women. Alcohol may enhance disease presentation.

Clinical features

Clinical features arise from inappropriate iron deposition in the relevant organs and include:

- Bronze skin pigmentation (skin)
- Hepatomegaly and/or cirrhosis (liver)
- Diabetes mellitus (pancreas)
- Cardiomyopathy, cardiac arrhythmias (heart)
- Arthritis (iron deposition in joints)

Management includes venesection, chelation with desferrioxamine and ultimately transplantation if cirrhotic failure is acute. Genetic testing of first-degree relatives is also advisable.

HAEMOGLOBIN METABOLISM

Haemoglobin consists of globin chains and haem groups that consist of ferrous iron complexed to a protoporphyrin ring.

Haemoglobin biosynthesis

Protoporphyrin biosynthesis occurs in the mitochondria of developing erythroblasts in the bone marrow (Fig. 2.7). The iron ion (derived from transferrin or ferritin) is integrated into the protoporphyrin in the cytoplasm, forming haem.

Globins are translated in the cytoplasm in the typical manner of protein synthesis. Each haem moiety is integrated into a globin and tetramerization results in a functional haemoglobin molecule.

Haemoglobin breakdown

Degradation of senescent erythrocytes occurs in the macrophages of the spleen, liver and reticuloendothelial system. The haemoglobin is dismantled to component haem and globins (Fig. 2.8).

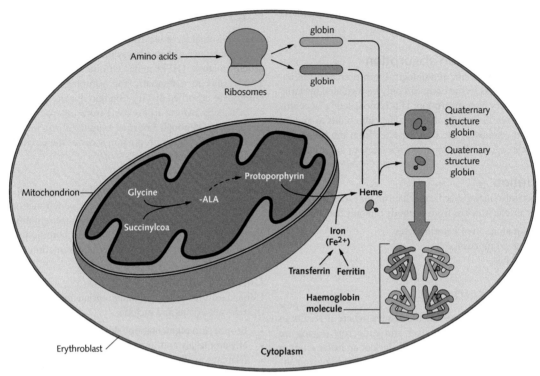

Fig. 2.7 Haemoglobin synthesis in erythroblasts. Within the mitochondria, glycine and succinyl CoA combine to form δ-aminolaevulinic acid (δ-ALA). This step is catalyzed by δ-ALA synthase/coenzyme vitamin B_6. δ-ALA is converted to protoporphyrin (dashed line) via multiple intermediates; not shown for simplicity. Protoporphyrin then exits the mitochondria and incorporates a ferrous iron to form haem. The iron may be derived from either ferritin or transferrin. Each haem molecule then combines with a globin chain (α or β) and tetramerization occurs to form the haemoglobin molecule. Please note the mitochondrion is not to scale relative to the cell.

Haem breakdown

Haem is further degraded to protoporphyrin and iron components. The iron is recycled and may be transported to bone marrow for erythropoiesis. Protoporphyrin is converted to bilirubin, which travels in the bloodstream to the liver bound to albumin (unconjugated bilirubin or indirect bilirubin on lab reports). Here it is conjugated to glucuronide (conjugated bilirubin), rendering it water-soluble, before being secreted into the gastrointestinal (GI) lumen.

If bilirubin is generated at a rate exceeding the liver's conjugation capacity, serum [bilirubin] increases. This is hyperbilirubinaemia, which may be clinically apparent as jaundice of the sclera, mucosal membranes and skin. This scenario occurs where red cell breakdown is excessive, i.e., haemolysis of any cause.

Unconjugated hyperbilirubinaemia may also occur where the liver's conjugation capacity is impaired, so even where bilirubin production rate is normal, unconjugated hyperbilirubinaemia occurs. Such conditions include Crigler-Najjar syndrome, Gilbert syndrome and physiological neonatal jaundice.

Conjugated bilirubin in the gastrointestinal tract is de-glucuronidated in the terminal ileum by commensal bacterial enzymes, forming urobilinogen. Urobilinogen may be reabsorbed into the bloodstream and ultimately excreted into urine by the kidneys or, alternatively, it may remain in the GI lumen where it is further reduced to stercobilin and stercobilinogen, which are excreted in faeces.

RED CELL CYTOSKELETON

Structure

The erythrocyte plasma membrane is supported internally by a dense, fibrillar, protein shell—the cytoskeleton. The cytoskeleton:

- Maintains resting cell 3-dimensional shape
- Confers the erythrocyte membrane with structural flexibility, allowing rapid and reversible deformity during passage through the microvasculature

The proteins of the plasma membrane are important constituents of the cytoskeleton (Fig. 2.9) and are categorized as integral or peripheral. Band numbers refer to the protein's electrophoretic mobility.

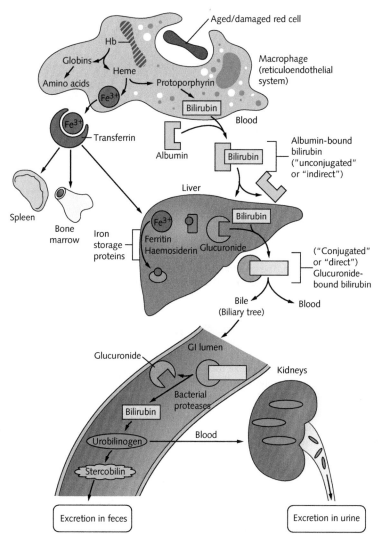

Fig. 2.8 Haemoglobin catabolism. Haemoglobin is separated into haem and globin components. Haem is broken down into iron and protoporphyrin. Iron is transported by transferrin to the bone marrow for erythropoiesis or to the liver for storage. Protoporphyrin is degraded to bilirubin, which is insoluble and bound to albumin in the blood (described as unconjugated bilirubin). On reaching the liver, bilirubin is conjugated to glucuronide before being excreted in bile into the GI lumen. Bilirubin is oxidized to urobilinogen in the GI lumen, which may be reabsorbed and excreted in the urine or further oxidized to stercobilin and excreted in the faeces.
GI, Gastrointestinal.

Integral proteins

Integral proteins span the cell membrane bilayer and are closely associated with it. These include band 3 protein and glycophorins.

Peripheral proteins

Peripheral proteins are loosely attached to the lipid bilayer and include spectrin, ankyrin, band 4.1 protein and actin. Dysfunction within the peripheral proteins is the basis of some inherited diseases that result in anaemia. The two most common are hereditary spherocytosis and hereditary elliptocytosis.

Surface proteins

There are numerous proteins projecting from the surface of the red cell. Many are anchored by the glucosyl phosphatidylinositol (GPI) molecular anchor. Somatic mutations in the gene for phosphatidylinositol glycan protein A (PIG-A) result in the condition paroxysmal nocturnal haemoglobinuria (see Chapter 3: Paroxysmal nocturnal haemoglobinuria).

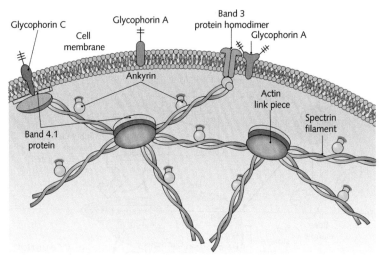

Fig. 2.9 Components of the cytoskeleton. The spectrin lattice is anchored to glycophorin C or band 3 protein dimers studding the red cell membrane by band 4.1 protein and ankyrin respectively. Spectrin is the primary structural component of the cytoskeleton.

RED CELL METABOLISM

As red cells lack mitochondria, they cannot oxidize metabolic substrates aerobically. Anaerobic glycolysis is the primary ATP-generating pathway in red cells, while the pentose phosphate pathway is the main generator of the NADPH+H⁺ needed for glutathione regeneration. Glucose is therefore the principal metabolic substrate for red cells. It is taken up by facilitated diffusion in an insulin-independent fashion.

Glycolysis

Glycolysis occurs in all living cells (Fig. 2.10). The fate of pyruvate, the end-product of the pathway, is ultimately determined by whether both oxygen and mitochondria are present. In aerobic conditions (where oxygen is available), pyruvate is converted to acetyl CoA and enters the TCA cycle within the mitochondrial matrix. Reducing equivalents generated by the TCA cycle then participate in oxidative phosphorylation, generating large amounts of ATP. However, in anaerobic conditions or cells lacking mitochondria (such as the red cell) pyruvate is metabolized to lactate with a net yield of two ATP molecules.

$$\text{glucose} + 2P_i + 2ADP \rightarrow 2\,\text{lactate} + 2ATP + 2H_2O$$

Defects of the glycolytic enzymes are rare. Approximately 95% are associated with pyruvate kinase and their consequences largely restricted to red blood cells. Within erythrocytes, one of the earliest casualties of restricted intracellular ATP is the structural integrity of the cytoskeleton. The outcome of this is an overly fragile red cell with a shortened life span. The most overt clinical manifestation relates to anaemia secondary to haemolysis (see Chapter 3: Enzyme defects).

Pentose phosphate pathway

In red cells, the supply of NAPH+H⁺ is generated by the pentose phosphate pathway (PPP), also called the hexose monophosphate shunt. NADPH+H⁺ (reduced NADP⁺) is vital in erythrocytes because it regenerates oxidized glutathione (GSSG) by acting as redox partner for the necessary reduction reaction. An available pool of intracellular reduced glutathione (GSH) is vital to protect the red cell membrane and intracellular proteins (including Hb) from oxidative damage. Defects in PPP enzymes (see Chapter 3: Glucose-6-phosphate dehydrogenase deficiency) may also manifest with shortened red cell lifespan.

METHAEMOGLOBINAEMIA

When the iron ion (within the haem component of haemoglobin) is oxidized ($Fe^{2+} \rightarrow Fe^{3+}$), Hb becomes methaemoglobin (metHb). Typically, ≤1% of a person's Hb is in this oxidized form. A higher proportion (≥1%) is known as methaemoglobinaemia. Levels >10% lead to a progressive blue-ish discolouration of mucosal membranes and skin. Levels >20% cause symptoms related to hypoxia. Treatment is oxygen supplementation and methylene blue. Pulse oximetry is unreliable in the context of methaemoglobinaemia.

Methaemoglobinaemia is dangerous, because MetHb is useless in terms of oxygen delivery, but more seriously the presence of MetHb shifts the normal Hb's dissociation curve to the left, i.e., rendering intact Hb less likely to appropriately offload its oxygen cargo at a given pO₂. This impairs oxygen delivery to the tissue on two levels. An NADH+H⁺-dependent enzyme (methaemoglobin reductase) is usually responsible for returning the ferric (3+) ion to the ferrous (2+) state.

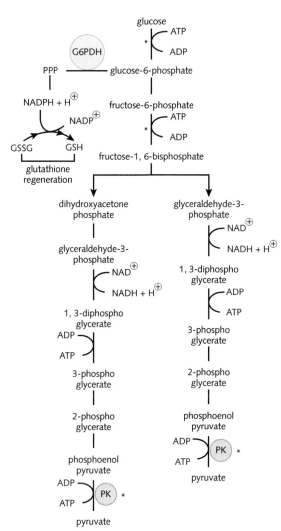

Fig. 2.10 Glycolysis. Starred arrows represent the rate-limiting steps.
ADP, Adenosine diphosphate; *ATP,* adenosine triphosphate, *G6PDH,* glucose-6-phosphate dehydrogenase; *NAD⁺/NADH+H⁺,* nicotinamide adenine dinucleotide/reduced nicotinamide adenine dinucleotide; *NADPH+H⁺/NADP⁺,* nicotinamide adenine dinucleotide phosphate/reduced nicotinamide adenine dinucleotide phosphate; *PK,* pyruvate kinase.

Causes

Elevated methaemoglobin may arise due to:

- Exposure to certain substances (see Box 2.1 later)
- Structurally abnormal haemoglobins rendering the ferric ion resistant to normal enzymatic reduction (e.g., HbM)
- Nicotinamide adenine dinucleotide (NADH) methaemoglobin reductase deficiency
- Glucose-6-phosphate dehydrogenase deficiency (see Chapter 3: Glucose-6-phosphate dehydrogenase deficiency)

CLINICAL NOTES

DRUGS KNOWN TO CAUSE METHAEMOGLOBINAEMIA

This category includes prilocaine, benzocaine, primaquine, chloroquine, nitroprussin, nitroglycerin, glyceryl trinitrate, amyl nitrite, dapsone and sulphonamides.

FULL BLOOD COUNT AND RETICULOCYTE COUNT

Blood samples are collected in EDTA-lined sample tubes (see Chapter 6: Calcium chelation for samples). The samples are tested by an automated analyzer, which provides the following parameters:

- Hb concentration, haematocrit, red-cell count, mean cell volume (MCV), mean cell haemoglobin (MCH) and mean cell haemoglobin concentration (MCHC)
- Red cell distribution width (RDW): a measure of size variability of the sampled population of red cells
- Total white-cell count with differential
- Platelet count

Red cell parameters and the description terms used to describe abnormalities of the full blood count are given in Table 2.3. When interpreting results, be aware that the normal range will usually vary slightly depending on the population subgroup and the assessing laboratory.

Table 2.3 Red cell parameters: diagnostic inference

Parameter	Normal range (adult male)	Elevation/ reduction nomenclature
Red cell count	$4.4–5.8 \times 10^{12}$/L	↑ Polycythaemia ↓ Anaemia
Haemoglobin concentration	13–17 g/dL	↑ Polycythaemia ↓ Anaemia
Haematocrit (packed cell volume; Hct)	40%–51%	↑ Polycythaemia ↓ Anaemia
Mean cell volume (MCV)	80–100 fL	↑ Macrocytic ↓ Microcytic
Mean corpuscular haemoglobin (MCH)	27–32 pg	↓ hypochromic
Reticulocyte count	$10–100 \times 10^{9}$/L 1%–2% of red cell population	↑ reticulocytosis ↓ reticulocytopenia

PERIPHERAL BLOOD FILM

Examination of a peripheral blood film is a simple hae-matological investigation, which can provide an enor-mous amount of diagnostic information (Table 2.4). The blood sample is evenly spread across a glass slide, forming a film of blood on the glass. This is then dried and stained, usually with a Romanowsky stain. The blood film allows assessment of the morphology of blood cells and can show intracellular inclusions. A normal peripheral blood film is shown in Fig 2.11. A film stained with supravital stain (which precipitates intracellular RNA) is used to identify reticulocytes, which retain RNA (in contrast to mature red cells).

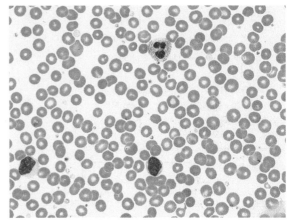

Fig. 2.11 Normal peripheral blood film (Romanowsky stain).

Table 2.4 Description of abnormalities of red cells that may be seen on the blood film

Abnormality	Description	Diagnostic inference
Anisocytosis	Increased variation in size, accompanied by increased RDW	Coexistence of microcytic and macrocytic with normal red cell populations. Combination of >1 disease process, marrow dysplasia
Poikilocytosis	Increased variation in shape	Variable, depending on the specific features of the poikilocyte
Spherocyte	Small, spherical cells (no area of central pallor discernible)	Hereditary spherocytosis, warm autoimmune haemolytic anaemia
Elliptocyte	Elliptically shaped cell	Hereditary elliptocytosis
Echinocyte	Cell with regular long outward projections from the surface	Renal disease
Acanthocyte	Cell with irregular outline	Liver disease, postsplenectomy, abetalipoproteinaemia, pyruvate kinase deficiency
Target cells	Central and peripheral dark staining zones seen separated by a paler area	Thalassaemia, sickle cell disease, iron deficiency (see Chapter 3), liver disease
Teardrop cells	Teardrop-shaped cells	Primary myelofibrosis (see Chapter 5), extramedullary haemopoiesis
Schistocytes	Small fragments of nonintact cells	DIC, microangiopathic haemolytic anaemia (see Chapter 6), mechanical cardiac valve replacement
Polychromasia	Large blueish cells	Reticulocytosis
Rouleaux	Stacks of red cells (similar to piles of coins)	Multiple myeloma, Waldenström macroglobulinaemia (see Chapter 5), any cause of raised globulins
Heinz bodies	Precipitates of oxidized, denatured haemoglobin	Glucose-6-phosphate dehydrogenase deficiency (see Chapter 3)
Howell-Jolly bodies	Small nuclear inclusions	Hyposplenism, post-splenectomy

DIC, disseminated intravascular coagulation; *RDW*, Red cell distribution width.

● **Chapter Summary**

- Red blood cells (erythrocytes) have a biconcave discoid three-dimensional structure.
- This shape increases their surface area, optimizing them for their primary function of gas transfer.
- The protein haemoglobin allows binding of both oxygen and carbon dioxide with release at appropriate locations (peripheral tissues and the lungs respectively).
- Haemoglobin contains haem as a component of its quaternary structure. Haem contains ferrous iron (Fe^{++}) and therefore iron metabolism has important consequences for red cell haemoglobin.
- Anaemia describes the clinical consequences of deficient haemoglobin concentration in the blood. Characteristic manifestations are related to reduced oxygen delivery to tissues, but also include skin, hair and nail abnormalities.
- The binding haemoglobin and oxygen alters at different environmental partial pressures of oxygen. This relationship is described by the oxygen dissociation curve.
- Erythropoiesis (development of erythrocytes from the haemopoietic stem cell) develops via several stages and is promoted by erythropoietin. Disorders of erythropoiesis occur in iron deficiency.
- The full blood count gives information about red cell concentration, size and haemoglobin concentration.
- A peripheral blood film identifies particular structural abnormalities associated with specific disease states and is a key diagnostic investigation in various red cell disorders as well as generalized systemic disorders.
- Red blood cells lack mitochondria, rendering their intracellular milieu anaerobic. They therefore rely on glycolysis as the sole metabolic pathway for ATP generation. Disorders of glycolysis enzymes therefore prominently affect red cell survival.

Red blood cell disorders

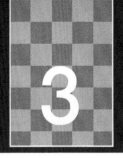

ANAEMIA

Introduction

The term anaemia refers to a low level of haemoglobin (Hb) in the blood. This is defined as <130 g/L (men) or <120g/L (women). As [Hb] falls, additional symptoms appear and become more severe. Symptoms arise due to impaired oxygen delivery to respiring tissues. This is because a reduced [Hb] results in a decrease in the oxygen-carrying capacity of the blood (see Chapter 2: Oxygen transport). Anaemia is caused by one or more of the following factors:

- Reduced or impaired red cell production
- Increased or accelerated red cell destruction
- Blood loss (acute or chronic)

CLINICAL NOTES

SYMPTOMS AND SIGNS OF ANAEMIA

Symptoms include fatigue, exertional breathlessness, palpitations, presyncope/syncope and headache. Signs include skin, conjunctival and mucous membrane pallor. A hyperdynamic cardiovascular response develops in response to the impaired oxygen delivery imposed by the overall reduction in oxygen carriage, typically seen in cases of a resting tachycardia and a new cardiac flow murmur.

Anaemia affects up to one-third of the global population. Specific underlying causes reflect local disease patterns, but the most common cause of anaemia (worldwide and in the UK) is iron deficiency. However, in the UK hospital population, anaemia secondary to chronic disease predominates. In developing countries, hookworm infestation-induced iron deficiency, malaria, human immunodeficiency virus (HIV), and tuberculosis (TB) are the most important causes.

Classification of anaemia

Mean cell volume

Types of anaemia are classified by the mean cell volume (MCV) of red cells, which is an important parameter within the full blood count. The MCV may be:

- Microcytic (MCV <80 fL) (Table 3.1)
- Normocytic (MCV 80–100 fL)
- Macrocytic (MCV >100 fL)

Mean cell haemoglobin

The mean cell haemoglobin (MCH) parameter quantifies the average mass (per red cell) of haemoglobin. It is calculated by dividing the total sample mass of Hb by the number of red cells in the sample. The normal range is 27–31 pg (per cell). Note that the value is usually given in pg, assuming that 'per cell' is intuitively understood.

The MCH usually correlates to the MCV, since a low volume (microcytic cell) typically contains a lower mass of Hb. The suffix 'chromic' is a semi-quantitative descriptive term referring to the MCH. <27 pg/cell is hypochromic, 27–31 pg/cell is normochromic and >31 pg/cell is hyperchromic.

Table 3.1 Diagnostic features of microcytic anaemia

FBC parameter	Iron deficiency	Anaemia of chronic disease	Thalassaemia	Sideroblastic anaemia
MCV	Reduced	Normal (2/3) Reduced (1/3)	Reduced (often disproportionately to the degree of ↓[Hb])	Low (congenital) Raised (acquired)
MCH	Reduced	Normal/mildly reduced	Normal	Raised
TIBC	Raised	Reduced/Normal	Normal	Normal
Serum [ferritin]	Low	Normal/raised	Normal	Raised
Transferrin saturation	Reduced	Reduced	Increased	Increased
Serum [transferrin]	Raised	Normal/low	Variable	Normal
Bone marrow iron stores	Absent	Present	Present	Increased

FBC, Full blood count; *MCH*, mean cell haemoglobin; *MCV*, mean cell volume; *TIBC*, total iron binding capacity.

ANAEMIA SECONDARY TO HAEMATINIC DEFICIENCY

Haematinics is the descriptive term for nutrients required for normal synthesis and development of blood cells. Iron, folate and B12 are the most clinically significant haematinics; deficiency of any of these micronutrients results in anaemia. Common causes of haematinic deficiency are discussed in the following sections.

Iron-deficiency anaemia

Iron deficiency occurs most frequently in women of reproductive age, due to menstrual blood loss. If iron loss/utilization exceeds iron intake, iron stores are ultimately depleted, resulting in a microcytic (MCV <80 fL), hypochromic (MCH <27 pg) anaemia.

Iron deficiency may be caused by:

- Inadequate dietary iron intake (see Chapter 2: Iron metabolism)
- Impaired iron absorption (e.g., high intake of dietary iron-absorption inhibitors or a loss of parietal cell mass, e.g., postgastrectomy; see Chapter 2: Iron absorption)

A relative iron deficiency may develop with normal iron intake and intact absorption when iron requirements are increased, e.g.:

- Growth (childhood and adolescence)
- Pregnancy
- Lactation

The other very important cause of iron deficiency is chronic blood loss, e.g., heavy menstrual bleeding or gastrointestinal (GI) blood loss. Since 1 mL blood contains ~0.5 mg iron, it is easy to appreciate how an iron-deficient state could swiftly develop.

The symptoms and signs of iron-deficiency anaemia are those of anaemia (see Clinical notes: Symptoms and signs of anaemia). Anaemia due to iron deficiency, however, is often accompanied by some additional specific nonhaematological symptoms and signs.

> **RED FLAG**
>
> **IRON DEFICIENCY AS A FEATURE OF MALIGNANCY**
>
> When identified, iron deficiency anaemia is an important indication that chronic blood loss may be occurring. The most vital diagnosis not to miss in this context is gastrointestinal tract neoplasia, e.g., stomach or colon cancer.

> **CLINICAL NOTES**
>
> **SYMPTOMS AND SIGNS ASSOCIATED WITH IRON DEFICIENCY**
>
> These include: angular stomatitis, diffuse hair loss/thinning, nail abnormalities (classically koilonychias: concavity of the nail plate), neurocognitive and/or neuropsychiatric impairment, e.g., depression.

Haematological findings of iron deficiency

- [Hb] <130 g/L (male) or <120 g/L (female)
- Microcytic (↓ MCV), hypochromic (↓ MCH) red cells (Fig. 3.1)
- ↓ serum [iron] and [ferritin]
- ↑ serum [transferrin] and total iron-binding capacity
- ↓ plasma transferrin saturation
- Bone-marrow smear shows absent iron stores
- Microcytic, hypochromic cells will be seen on a blood film. Pencil cells, elliptocytes and target cells may also be present (Fig. 3.1).

Management of iron deficiency anaemia

The underlying cause must be identified and treated in addition to providing iron supplementation. Oral administration of iron is in the form of ferrous sulphate, fumarate or gluconate tablets. These must be taken for ≥3 months to replenish fully the body iron stores. Common side-effects of oral iron supplementation include constipation, diarrhoea, abdominal cramps and dark faeces. Parenteral iron may be used if the patient has impaired gastrointestinal absorption or is very intolerant to oral iron.

Megaloblastic anaemia

In megaloblastic anaemia, impaired DNA synthesis in erythroblasts manifests with abnormal maturation of the developing red cell precursors. These abnormal

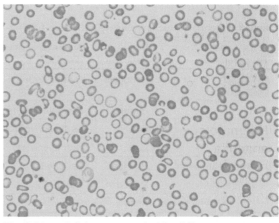

Fig. 3.1 Iron deficiency anaemia: blood film appearance.

erythroblasts, situated in the bone marrow, are called megaloblasts. They are very large cells with retarded nuclear maturation. Megaloblasts are:

- Unable to generate sufficient mature red cell progeny (like normal erythroblasts)
- Destroyed by bone marrow macrophages

Overall, this results in ineffective erythropoiesis. The red cell progeny they do manage to create are macrocytic.

COMMON PITFALLS

MEGALOBLASTIC VERSUS MACROCYTIC ANAEMIA

Although megaloblastic anaemia is macrocytic (MCV > 100 fL), the two terms have different meaning. Macrocytes are red cells with volume >100 fL. Megaloblasts are abnormal, giant red cell precursors with disproportionately large, immature nuclei, located in the bone marrow. All causes of megaloblastic anaemia will cause macrocytosis, but not all causes of macrocytic anaemia are due to megaloblastosis.

RED FLAG

FOLATE AND B12 COSUPPLEMENTATION

Folate and B12 supplements are coadministered. This is because without B12, all tetrahydrofolate eventually becomes trapped as a nonfunctional methylated compound. This compound cannot participate in the usual reactions and thus symptoms of folate deficiency manifest, even where folate intake and absorption are adequate! All B12 deficiency will therefore cause a functional folate deficiency, even if folate intake is sufficient. Replacement of folate in isolation without B12 coadministration will correct the megaloblastic anaemia but will allow neurological damage secondary to B12 deficiency to progress and become irreversible.

Haematological findings of megaloblastic anaemia

Haematological findings particular to megaloblastic anaemia include:

- Macrocytic anaemia (MCV >100 fL)
- Hypersegmentation of neutrophil nuclei (right shift)
- Megaloblasts visible on a bone marrow smear

- Coexisting leucopoenia +/- thrombocytopenia in severe cases
- Low red cell [folate] (in both B12 and folate deficiencies)
- Lowered serum [B12] and/or [folate], depending on which deficiency has provoked the megaloblastic anaemia

Megaloblastic anaemia is most commonly due to vitamin B12 and/or folate deficiency. Both these micronutrients are required for normal DNA synthesis. An example diagnostic approach to differentiate between the respective causes of macrocytic anaemia is given in Fig. 3.2.

Folate deficiency

Folate is required for normal DNA and RNA synthesis. Tetrahydrofolate (THF), the bioactive form of folate, is formed by two sequential reduction reactions (catalyzed by dihydrofolate reductase). THF is required for purine and pyrimidine synthesis and thus for RNA and DNA synthesis. Since the requirement for THF is greatest in rapidly dividing cells, where the greatest rate of DNA replication and protein synthesis occurs, this population of cells is the first to manifest the consequences of deficiency.

Early symptoms of folate deficiency are related to the macrocytic anaemia, which is also megaloblastic. In addition, angular stomatitis, glossitis and neuropsychiatric deficits are reported in severe, prolonged deficiency. Serum [folate] or red cell [folate] are used as biomarkers of folate status, the latter being more representative of long-term status. However, serum [folate] is the more discriminating investigation, since red cell [folate] is lowered in B12 deficiency even if folate stores are replete. Folate deficiency is treated with oral folate supplementation accompanied by B12 supplements.

Folate metabolism

Folate (vitamin B9) is a water-soluble vitamin that is abundant in a wide variety of foods. It is stored in the liver and absorption occurs in the duodenum and jejunum. Unlike vitamin B12, vitamin B9 stores are small relative to daily requirements. Megaloblastic anaemia therefore develops more rapidly (within a few months) of sustained inadequate folate intake.

Causes of folate deficiency can be grouped into: insufficient intake, excessive loss, abnormal THF activation or increased folate demand (rendering a normally sufficient intake insufficient) (Table 3.2). Alcohol excess is particularly effective at inducing folate deficiency since all the risk factors for deficiency typically coexist in alcoholics.

Vitamin B12 deficiency

The bioactive vitamin B12 derivatives are 5′-deoxyadenosylcobalamin and methylcobalamin.

Methylcobalamin

In B12 deficiency, there will always be a functional folate deficiency, even if total body folate stores are replete. This phenomenon arises because the regeneration of THF, the

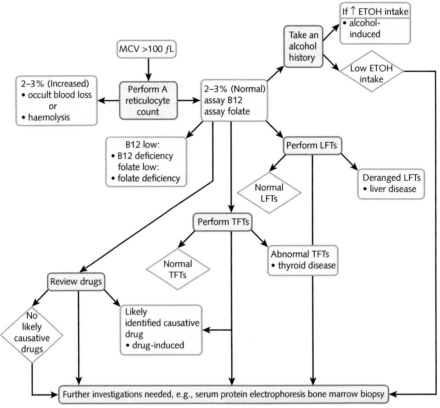

Fig. 3.2 Diagnostic approach to macrocytic anaemia (MCV >100 fL). *ETOH*, Ethanol; *LFTs*, liver function tests; *MCV*, mean cell volume; *TFTs*, thyroid function tests.

bioactive form of folate, is reliant on a B12-dependent enzyme (methionine synthase). This means that even in an individual consuming and absorbing an adequate amount of folate, it is unavailable for participation in metabolism as it is trapped in a biologically inert form (methylfolate). THF availability is mandatory for maintenance of genomic stability, since it is required for normal nucleoside synthesis.

5′-deoxyadenosylcobalamin

Vitamin B12 is also essential for normal fatty acid synthesis. Odd-chain fatty acid synthesis requires 5′-deoxyadenosylcobalamin as a cofactor. Neuronal myelination demands a continuous supply of fatty acids to maintain the myelin sheath integrity (due to constant myelin turnover). Disintegration of the myelin sheath therefore occurs in the context of reduced availability of 5′-deoxyadenosylcobalamin (secondary to B12 deficiency). This mechanism accounts for the neurological symptoms associated with B12 deficiency. These neurological features usually manifest insidiously and much later than the symptoms and signs of the megaloblastic anaemia. They include:

- Peripheral paraesthesia and numbness
- Myelopathy: ascending distal motor weakness, gait disturbance
- Progressive cognitive deficit, depression

Table 3.2 Folate deficiency: causative mechanisms

Mechanism	Examples
Decreased folate intake	Decreased dietary intake of folate (usually due to generalized malnutrition) Impaired GI absorption due to diseases of malabsorption Impaired GI absorption due to drugs (e.g., phenytoin)
Increased loss	Haemodialysis
Increased folate requirement due to high rates of cell division: a usually adequate intake is insufficient in these contexts.	Growth (childhood and adolescence) Pregnancy and lactation Cancer Haemolytic anaemia
Abnormal bioactivation of folate: despite adequate intake/absorption, THF formation is impaired with all the functional consequences of folate deficiency	Vitamin B12 deficiency Dihydrofolate reductase inhibitors: trimethoprim, methotrexate Antifolate metabolites: sulphasalazine

GI, Gastrointestinal; *THF*, tetrahydrofolate.

Nonneurological symptoms include anorexia, glossitis, angular stomatitis and constipation. Treatment is with oral or parenteral vitamin B12.

B12: metabolism

Dietary vitamin B12 is almost exclusively obtained from animal-derived food products, thus veganism confers a risk of deficiency if appropriate supplements are not taken regularly. Absorption of vitamin B12 involves the following steps:

1. Dietary vitamin B12 released from proteins (pepsin-mediated hydrolysis) within the gastric lumen.
2. Free B12 then binds to saliva-secreted R-protein (haptocorrin).
3. R-protein/B12 complex is then cleaved by a pancreatic protease (trypsin) in the duodenum, liberating B12.
4. Intrinsic factor (IF; secreted by the gastric parietal cells) then binds the freed B12 and dimerizes with another B12/IF.
5. IF-bound B12 dimers bind to specific enterocyte receptors (cubilin) in the terminal ileum and are internalized into enterocytes.
6. Within the enterocyte, B12 binds to transcobalamin proteins: I, II or III.
7. B12/transcobalamin complexes are extruded into the portal circulation.
8. B12 may be stored in the liver or delivered to peripheral tissues (liver, bone marrow) where intracellular conversion to the bioactive forms (deoxyadenosylcobalamin and methylcobalamin) takes place.

Abnormalities or defects of any of the above steps will eventually lead to B12 deficiency. Because endogenous B12 stores are sizable and urinary/faecal daily loss is small, the symptoms/signs of deficiency may occur up to 2 years after dietary intake becomes inadequate. Causes of B12 deficiency include:

- Inadequate dietary intake
- Inability to separate B12 from its protein-bound dietary form (food cobalamin malabsorption)
- IF deficiency (congenital, pernicious anaemia or postgastrectomy)
- Intestinal malabsorption, particularly if affecting the terminal ileum (where the bulk of IF-bound B12 is absorbed)
- Blind loop or diverticulae in the small bowel, which breed bacteria that avidly consume B12

Pernicious anaemia

Pernicious anaemia is the most common cause of nondietary B12 deficiency. It is an autoimmune phenomenon, typically secondary to antibody-mediated gastric parietal cell destruction (causing failure of IF secretion), but the cellular B12 transporter (cubilin) or transcobalamin-bound B12 are also potential auto-antibody targets.

Classically, in addition to the anaemic, neurological and mucosal symptoms, premature greying/whitening of the hair

is seen when B12 deficiency arises due to pernicious anaemia and a lemon-yellow pallor is used to describe the combination of mild jaundice (ineffective erythropoiesis→increased red cell fragility and haemolysis) and anaemia-induced pallor.

Schilling test—In the past, this test was performed to confirm/exclude pernicious anaemia as a cause for B12 deficiency. Stages are as follows:

1. Intramuscular injection of nonradioactive B12 (1 mg) is given. This megadose saturates the body's B12 binding sites, ensuring that any subsequent absorbed oral B12 will be completely excreted via the urine.
2. The patient drinks an oral solution of radiolabelled B12.
3. The urine is collected and quantity of the radiolabelled B12 is assayed.

If no (or reduced) radiolabelled B12 is present in the urine, steps 2 and 3 are repeated after providing oral intrinsic factor. A typical patient (with normal levels of endogenous intrinsic factor) will have radiolabelled urine after the first test. In pernicious anaemia, a positive test is demonstrated by appearance in the urine of radiolabelled B12 only after the provision of oral intrinsic factor; in the absence of exogenous intrinsic factor, the radiolabelled B12 is not absorbed into the bloodstream from the GI tract and thus cannot enter the urine. The hazards of using radioactive materials mean that the Schilling test is rarely used nowadays, but it is mentioned here due to its ubiquity on examination syllabuses.

Current diagnosis of pernicious anaemia—In clinical practice, the diagnosis is made if specific autoantibodies (anti-IF or anti-parietal cell antibodies) are present where serum [B12] is reduced. Be aware, however, that despite high specificity, the sensitivity of the IF autoantibody test is only ~70%. Anti-parietal cell autoantibodies have even lower sensitivity and are also poorly specific since they are often raised in gastritis.

Food cobalamin malabsorption

This is a common cause of B12 deficiency in the elderly. Many varied causes leading to achlorhydria such as drugs (antacids, H2 receptor blockers, proton pump inhibitors), *Helicobacter pylori* infection or atrophic gastritis render the gastric luminal pH too high for effective protease action. Dietary B12 thus remains complexed with dietary protein and cannot be absorbed. Pancreatic insufficiency of any cause leads to failure of protease secretion, with the same effect. Note that oral B12 supplementation corrects B12 deficiency secondary to food cobalamin malabsorption, since the downstream processes following protease-mediated separation of B12 from dietary protein are intact.

Metformin use

Chronic biguanide (e.g., metformin) use in type 2 diabetics is a known cause of B12 deficiency. Biguanides interfere with the calcium-dependent absorption of the B12-IF complex at terminal ileal enterocytes.

ANAEMIA OF CHRONIC DISEASE

This is the most common type of anaemia seen in hospital patients and in the elderly. It is associated with chronic inflammatory and malignant disease. The mechanism underlying the anaemia of chronic disease is complex, but it is believed to include:

- Inflammatory cytokine-induced (e.g., interleukin 1, TNF) suppression of erythropoietin (EPO)-mediated erythropoiesis.
- Inflammatory increase in hepcidin. Hepcidin decreases iron exporter expression, impairing the release of iron stores (necessary for erythropoiesis) by bone marrow macrophages.

Whatever the mechanism, anaemia of chronic disease results in reduced red cell production. Two-thirds of cases are normocytic and normochromic, although ~1/3 of cases exhibit instead a microcytic hypochromic anaemia. The anaemia is unresponsive to iron therapy and is corrected only by treatment of the underlying cause. EPO can in some cases help to increase erythrocyte production (but it is rarely used).

Chronic renal failure

Chronic renal failure is almost always associated with anaemia. A decrease in functional renal tissue results in reduced EPO synthesis. The anaemia is typically normochromic and normocytic. It is treated with regular EPO injections.

ANAEMIA DUE TO BLOOD LOSS

Like the anaemia of chronic disease, anaemia secondary to blood loss may be normocytic or microcytic.

Acute blood loss

Common causes of acute blood loss include trauma, surgery, obstetric haemorrhage and gastrointestinal, urinary or pulmonary tract loss.

The plasma lost during haemorrhage is typically restored within ~48 hours. Initially, restoration is due to redistribution of extracellular fluid intravascularly and later increased fluid intake and endocrine homeostasis. However, it takes several weeks for the lost red cells (and therefore the [Hb]) to be replaced to normal levels.

Haematological findings in acute blood loss include:

- Normocytic, normochromic anaemia
- Reticulocytosis, peaking 1–2 weeks post haemorrhage
- ↑ platelet and neutrophil counts
- Following significant haemorrhage, neutrophil precursors are seen in peripheral blood (left shift)

It is important to appreciate that during or immediately after blood loss, parameters such as the red cell count (which is expressed as a concentration) will be normal. This is because both plasma and red cells have been lost in the same proportions as they are present in the blood. Do not be falsely reassured by a normal [Hb] in the context of known or likely blood loss. The levels will not fall until significant early intravascular volume restoration occurs, since the readings show actual concentrations rather than absolute levels.

Chronic blood loss

The most common causes of chronic blood loss are gastrointestinal lesions (such as ulcers or neoplasms) and menorrhagia. Chronic blood loss leads to iron deficiency and symptoms and signs accompanying the anaemia will usually support this. The anaemia of chronic blood loss is microcytic, since it develops secondary to iron deficiency.

MICROCYTIC ANAEMIA: OTHER CAUSES

Fig. 3.3 provides a diagnostic approach to microcytic anaemia. Rare causes of microcytic anaemia include:

- Thalassaemia. These defects of globin synthesis are discussed in the later sections on types of thalassaemia.
- Sideroblastic anaemia (hereditary or acquired). This is a hypochromic anaemia characterized by the presence of ring sideroblasts and increased iron stores in the bone marrow. Ring sideroblasts are abnormal red-cell precursors with a halo of iron granules around the nucleus. Some subtypes respond to vitamin B6 supplementation (B6 is a cofactor for ferrochelatase, which mediates the final iron-incorporation reaction of haem synthesis).
- Lead poisoning, which inhibits both haem and globin synthesis. It may cause a baffling array of diverse symptoms and signs accompanied by a microcytic anaemia. Basophilic stippling of red cells on the peripheral blood film is seen in lead poisoning.

HAEMOLYTIC ANAEMIA

Haemolytic anaemia occurs when red cell lifespan is shortened due to accelerated destruction. Low [Hb] leads to tissue hypoxia, provoking an increase in EPO synthesis (up to sevenfold!). This promotes a compensatory accelerated erythropoiesis. This may succeed in restoring and maintaining a normal [Hb]; as long as the increased destruction is matched by the increased synthesis, anaemia is prevented and symptoms do not develop.

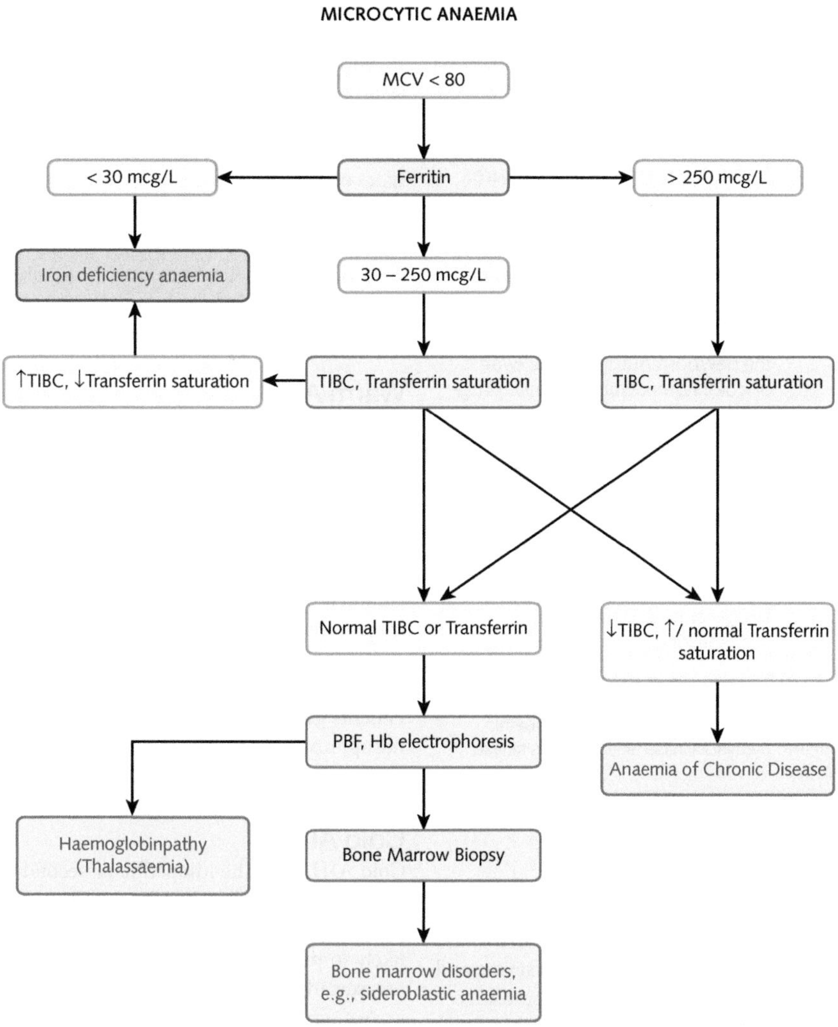

MICROCYTIC ANAEMIA

```
                        MICROCYTIC ANAEMIA

                         ┌─────────────┐
                         │   MCV < 80  │
                         └─────────────┘
                               │
    ┌──────────────┐    ┌─────────────┐    ┌──────────────┐
    │  < 30 mcg/L  │◄───│   Ferritin  │───►│  > 250 mcg/L │
    └──────────────┘    └─────────────┘    └──────────────┘
           │                   │                   │
 ┌────────────────────┐  ┌──────────────┐
 │ Iron deficiency    │  │ 30 – 250     │
 │ anaemia            │  │ mcg/L        │
 └────────────────────┘  └──────────────┘
           │                   │                   │
 ┌──────────────────────┐ ┌──────────────┐  ┌──────────────────┐
 │ ↑TIBC, ↓Transferrin  │◄│ TIBC,        │  │ TIBC, Transferrin│
 │ saturation           │ │ Transferrin  │  │ saturation       │
 └──────────────────────┘ │ saturation   │  └──────────────────┘
                          └──────────────┘
                            (crossing arrows)
               ┌────────────────────┐  ┌──────────────────────┐
               │ Normal TIBC or     │  │ ↓TIBC, ↑/ normal     │
               │ Transferrin        │  │ Transferrin          │
               └────────────────────┘  │ saturation           │
                       │               └──────────────────────┘
               ┌────────────────────┐           │
               │ PBF, Hb            │  ┌──────────────────────┐
               │ electrophoresis    │  │ Anaemia of Chronic   │
               └────────────────────┘  │ Disease              │
                       │               └──────────────────────┘
   ┌──────────────────┐ ┌──────────────────┐
   │ Haemoglobinpathy │ │ Bone Marrow      │
   │ (Thalassaemia)   │ │ Biopsy           │
   └──────────────────┘ └──────────────────┘
                             │
                     ┌──────────────────────┐
                     │ Bone marrow disorders,│
                     │ e.g., sideroblastic   │
                     │ anaemia               │
                     └──────────────────────┘
```

Fig. 3.3 Diagnostic approach to microcytic anaemia (MCV <80 fL). *MCV*, Mean cell volume; *TIBC,* total iron binding capacity.

Causes of haemolysis

A shortened lifespan (<120 days) may arise due to intrinsic defects (typically hereditary) of erythrocyte structure or function. Alternatively, several particular environmental conditions (extracorpuscular features) may result in premature destruction of the red cells. Table 3.3 gives various examples, categorized by underlying causative mechanisms, i.e., intrinsic or extracorpuscular.

Laboratory findings in haemolysis

Haemolysis is suggested by:

- ↑ serum bilirubin (unconjugated)
- ↑ urinary urinobilinogen and faecal stercobilinogen
- ↑ serum lactate dehydrogenase

- ↓ or absent haptoglobins
- Reticulocytosis on blood film (apparent ↑ MCV on full blood count). The film may also show polychromasia (in keeping with reticulocytosis), spherocytes (in immune mediated haemolysis) or schistocytes (in microangiopathic haemolysis).
- Folate deficiency (excessive folate consumption due to DNA synthesis during rapid cell division of upregulated erythropoiesis)
- Erythroid hyperplasia (within bone marrow) → marrow cavity expansion

Classification of haemolysis

Haemolysis is typically classified into intravascular and extravascular, depending on the physiological location of the haemolysis.

Table 3.3 Examples of specific causes of haemolytic anaemia classified by underlying mechanism

Main mechanism	Submechanism
Intrinsic erythrocyte defects	**Defective metabolism:** G6PD deficiency, PK deficiency **Defective membrane structure:** Hereditary spherocytosis, hereditary elliptocytosis **Defective haemoglobin structure:** Sickle cell disease, thalassaemia
Environmental (extracorpuscular) causes	**Immune:** Haemolytic transfusion reactions, haemolytic disease of the newborn Autoimmune: (warm or cold) haemolytic anaemia, drug-induced immune haemolysis **Infectious:** Falciparum malaria, clostridia species, generalized septicaemia **Mechanical:** Mechanical cardiac valves, MAHA, extreme repetitive impact exercise Hypersplenism: (see Chapter 1: Hypersplenism) **Drug-related:** Dapsone, sulfasalazine

G6PD, Glucose-6-phosphate dehydrogenase (see Glucose-6-phosphate dehydrogenase deficiency section); *MAHA,* microangiopathic haemolytic anaemia (see Microangiopathic haemolysis section); *PK,* pyruvate kinase (see Pyruvate kinase deficiency section).

Extravascular haemolysis

Extravascular haemolysis refers to an enhanced rate of the normal red cell breakdown process, i.e., by reticuloendothelial macrophages (in the spleen, bone marrow and liver). Extravascular haemolysis tends to be less severe and progress more gradually than intravascular haemolysis.

Intravascular haemolysis

Intravascular haemolysis is the destruction of red cells within the circulatory system. Intravascular haemolysis exhibits all the laboratory findings listed above (in common with extravascular haemolysis), but in addition:

- Free serum Hb is elevated (haemoglobinaemia) with the following clinical consequences:
  - Hb appears in the urine once serum Hb exceeds renal tubular resorption capacity
  - Haemosiderin (an iron storage protein) appears in the urine
- Methaemalbuminaemia: free Hb is oxidized ($\rightarrow$MetHb) and binds to serum albumin

ANTIBODY-MEDIATED HAEMOLYSIS

The following sections describe antibody-mediated mechanisms responsible for haemolytic anaemia.

Autoimmune haemolytic anaemia

In autoimmune haemolytic anaemia (AIHA), antibodies against red cell antigens result in the haemolytic destruction of red cells bearing the relevant antigen. A positive direct antigen test (DAT or Coombs test) is seen. There are three types of AIHA:

1. Warm AIHA, where haemolysis usually occurs at body temperature
2. Cold AIHA, where haemolysis usually occurs below core body temperature
3. Paroxysmal cold haemoglobinuria

Warm AIHA

Warm AIHA may be idiopathic or secondary to autoimmune disease or malignancy. Particular diseases carrying a high probability of secondary warm AIHA include systemic lupus erythematosus (SLE), leukaemia and lymphomas. Certain drugs are known to provoke warm AIHA (e.g., mefenamic acid). In addition to the usual anaemia and jaundice associated with haemolysis, mild splenomegaly frequently occurs.

The underlying cause (if identified) should be treated, in addition to the management of the haemolysis itself. Patients generally respond well to steroids but other immunosuppressive therapies (e.g., azothiaprine), rituximab (see Chapter 5, Table 5.6) or splenectomy may be beneficial.

Cold AIHA

Cold AIHA may be idiopathic or secondary to lymphoma, leukaemia or infection. Certain infections (e.g., mycoplasma pneumonia, Epstein-Barr virus) are particularly likely to provoke a cold AIHA. The clinical features, which are exacerbated by cold temperatures, include:

- Raynaud phenomenon (peripheral localized vasospasm, which may lead to ischaemic damage of tissues)
- Acrocyanosis (purplish discolouration of the skin) due to vascular sludging secondary to red-cell agglutination

Treatment involves avoidance of cold environments, as well as aggressive management of the underlying provoking disease (if identified). As for warm AIHA, rituximab is effective in idiopathic cold AIHA and cold AIHA associated with B-lymphoproliferative diseases.

Paroxysmal cold haemoglobinuria

Paroxysmal cold haemoglobinuria (PCH) is a rare condition, usually presenting with acute haemolysis in childhood following a viral infection. It is a subset of cold AIHA. However, while haemolysis occurs at body temperature, the antibody–red cell interaction only occurs at cold temperatures in vitro. This antibody behaviour is diagnostic (the Donath-Landsteiner test). PCH is usually self-limiting, but in cases of life-threatening haemolysis supportive red cell transfusion (via a blood warmer) is employed. The patient should be kept warm, preferably at an ambient temperature

Table 3.4 Laboratory findings in autoimmune haemolytic anaemia

	Warm AIHA	Cold AIHA	PCH
Antibody type	IgG	IgM	IgG
Antigen targeted	Rh factor	L or I antigens	P antigen
Antibody binding temperature	37°C	<32°C	<32°C
Red cell agglutination	No	Yes	Yes
Complement fixation	No	Yes	Yes
Haemolysis mechanism	Mainly extravascular	Mainly intravascular	Mainly intravascular
Direct antigen test (Coomb test)	+ve for IgG and complement	+ve for complement	+ve for IgG and complement

AIHA, Autoimmune haemolytic anaemia; *Ig,* immunoglobulin; *PCH,* paroxysmal cold haemoglobinuria; *Rh,* Rhesus.

of 37°C. Table 3.4 details the laboratory findings associated with the various AIHAs.

Drug-induced immune haemolytic anaemia

Certain drugs (e.g., penicillin, cephalosporin and fludarabine) are established precipitants of haemolysis. Individual specific mechanisms vary with the precipitant.

Alloimmune haemolytic anaemia

Alloimmune haemolytic anaemia is caused by a reaction between the patient's antibodies and donor blood cells following transfusion or transplant, e.g.:

- Transfusion of ABO-incompatible blood (typically IgM-mediated)
- Transfer of maternal antibodies across the placenta to the fetus (haemolytic disease in newborn)
- Allogeneic transplantation (including stem cell or organ transplants)

INTRINSIC RED CELL DEFECTS CAUSING HAEMOLYSIS

Defects intrinsic to red cell structure or metabolism can lead to haemolysis and characteristic morphological abnormalities are often apparent on the blood film.

Cytoskeletal defects

Hereditary spherocytosis

Hereditary spherocytosis (HS) is an autosomal dominant disorder with variable penetrance. Clinical presentation ranges from asymptomatic to significant jaundice at birth. A typical disease course would be a low-grade anaemia with fluctuating haemolysis and jaundice. Splenomegaly may be present.

HS is relatively common (prevalence 1:2000 in Northern Europeans). A defective cytoskeletal protein, most commonly spectrin, impairs membrane integrity. This causes progressive spherification of the red cell, with marked reduction in flexibility. The spherocytes are visible on a blood film (Fig. 3.4) and classically demonstrate increased osmotic fragility in hypotonic solutions (the historical osmotic fragility membrane test). The haemolysis of HS is defined as extravascular, since premature removal of spherocytic red cells occurs in the spleen, where the microcirculation is too tortuous for poorly flexible cells to successfully pass through.

Hereditary elliptocytosis

This autosomal dominant disorder arises as a result of an abnormality of the spectrin protein, which impedes normal tetramer formation from spectrin dimers. Clinical and laboratory findings are as for HS, however the film appearance differs (elliptocytes have a more elongated appearance). However, patients with elliptocytosis typically experience less severe symptoms. Membrane disorders are now diagnosed with EMA (eosin 5′ maleimide) binding test.

Enzyme defects

Pyruvate kinase deficiency

This rare autosomal recessive condition impairs glycolysis, which represents the sole source of adenosine triphosphate (ATP) synthesis in red cells. The earliest manifestation of

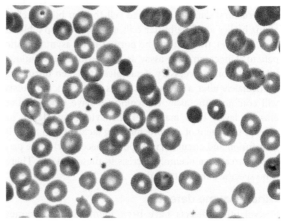

Fig. 3.4 Blood film appearance of hereditary spherocytosis. Note that the spherocytes are smaller and thicker than normal cells but are rarely completely spherical.

insufficient ATP is structural rigidity, which significantly increases the probability of red cell removal by the spleen as they traverse the splenic filtration beds. The haemolysis of pyruvate kinase (PK) is thus designated as extravascular. Splenectomy improves the anaemia by removing the main mechanism of red cell destruction. PK-induced anaemia varies widely in severity and thus depending upon the severity, affected individuals may be asymptomatic or present with jaundice at birth. Diagnosis is suggested by the film appearance (poikilocytosis and acanthocytes are seen) and confirmed by direct enzyme assay.

Glucose-6-phosphate dehydrogenase deficiency

Glucose-6-phosphate dehydrogenase (G6PD) deficiency is an X-linked disorder affecting the pentose phosphate pathway. There are numerous variants of G6PD deficiency, two of which account for the vast majority of cases: the African and Mediterranean subtypes. Of these two, the Mediterranean type is clinically more serious, because the abnormal enzyme's functional impairment is more extreme. Patients with G6PD deficiency usually remain asymptomatic unless exposed to oxidative stress, e.g.:

- Infection
- Acidosis, e.g., critical illness, diabetic ketoacidosis
- Drugs, e.g., dapsone, primaquine, sulphonamides
- Broad (fava) beans: favism (Mediterranean subtype only)

Such oxidant stresses increase red cell reliance on NADPH+H$^+$ to ensure adequate glutathione regeneration. However, in G6PD deficiency intracellular [NADPH+H$^+$] is reduced, as a result of failure of the pentose phosphate pathway. Oxidative damage accumulates more rapidly, shortening the lifespan of the cell.

Haemolysis of G6PD deficiency is primarily intravascular. During oxidative-stress induced haemolysis, Heinz bodies (precipitates of oxidized, denatured Hb) form intracellularly. The spleen usually removes Heinz bodies, leaving structural damage to the red cell (bite or blister cells). Heinz bodies and bite/blister cells are apparent on a blood film; however, the film can be normal in an asymptomatic patient. Direct enzyme assay is diagnostic, but cautious interpretation is necessary if samples are taken during or immediately after a haemolytic crisis when reticulocytosis will confound the assay (reticulocytes have much higher enzyme levels than mature erythrocytes). Avoidance or prompt treatment of any precipitating factors (with red cell transfusion and circulatory support if necessary) is the priority in treating a haemolytic crisis in these patients. There is no specific curative treatment.

Other enzyme defects

Several other defects have been identified in enzymes involved in erythrocyte metabolism. They are very rare and include hexokinase and glutathione synthetase deficiencies.

OTHER CAUSES OF HAEMOLYSIS

Various additional causes of haemolysis exist. A useful diagnostic approach to haemolysis is given in Fig. 3.5.

Microangiopathic haemolysis

Microangiopathic haemolytic anaemia (MAHA) occurs when fibrin is deposited in small vessels. Red cell haemolysis occurs due to shearing and collision with obstructing fibrin strands. The traumatic red cell destruction provides a pathognomonic blood film appearance with red cell fragments (schistocytes). Occurrence of MAHA usually indicates a serious underlying disorder. Common causes include Haemolytic Uraemic syndrome (HUS), Thrombotic Thrombocytopenic Purpura (TTP), Disseminated Intravascular Coagulation (DIC) of any cause (septicaemia, disseminated carcinoma), malignant hypertension and pre-eclampsia/eclampsia microangiopathic haemolytic anaemia later in this chapter. Rarely, MAHA is seen in patients with metallic heart valves, where it may indicate valvular dysfunction.

Infections

Falciparum malaria may cause both intravascular and extravascular haemolysis, because parasitized red cells are both destroyed within the circulation and removed by the spleen. Blackwater fever is the term used to describe acute kidney injury secondary to haemoglobinaemia in the context of falciparum malaria. The term refers to passing of very dark/black urine secondary to haemoglobinuria.

Mechanical

Physical trauma to red cells within the circulation may cause traumatic destruction of red cells. Mechanical cardiac valves are the classic cause.

Toxins

Copper toxicity in Wilson disease may provoke haemolytic anaemia. Lead, chloral and arsine cause severe haemolysis. Certain drugs (e.g., dapsone and sulphasalazine) cause oxidative damage resulting in haemolysis.

Burns

Severe, extensive burns lead to red cell damage in the disrupted burn zone microvasculature. Acanthosis and spherocytosis may be seen on the blood film.

Exercise

March haemoglobinuria is caused by damage to red cells in the feet during long periods of repetitive weight-bearing exercise, e.g., walking or running. The blood film does not show fragments, spherocytes or pathognomonic abnormalities.

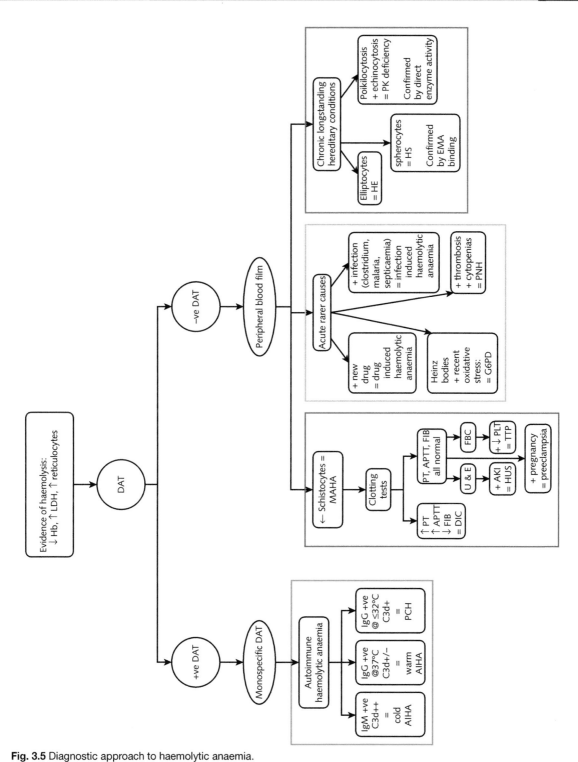

Fig. 3.5 Diagnostic approach to haemolytic anaemia.
AIHA, Autoimmune haemolytic anaemia; *DAT,* direct antigen test; *EMA* binding, eosin 5′ maleimide binding; *G6PD,* glucose-6-phosphate dehydrogenase; *HE,* hereditary elliptocytosis; *HS,* hereditary spherocytosis; *Ig,* immunoglobulin; *PCH,* paroxysmal cold haemoglobinuria; *PK,* pyruvate kinase (all discussed earlier in this chapter).
APTT, Activated partial thromboplastin time; *DIC,* disseminated intravascular coagulation; *FIB,* fibrinogen (see Chapter 6: Fibrinogen); *HUS,* haemolytic uraemic syndrome; *MAHA,* microangiopathic haemolytic anaemia (see Chapter 6: Platelet consumption by microthrombi); *PT,* prothrombin time; *TTP,* thrombotic thrombocytopenic purpura.

Paroxysmal nocturnal haemoglobinuria

Paroxysmal nocturnal haemoglobinuria (PNH) is an acquired bone marrow stem cell disorder caused by expansion of an abnormal haemopoietic stem cell clone harbouring the phosphatidylinositol glycan protein A (PIG-A) mutation on the X chromosome. Mutant PIG-A leads to absent/deficient glycosyl phosphatidylinositol (GPI) synthesis. GPI plays an important role: it anchors immunoprotective proteins (e.g., CD55 and CD59 proteins) to the cell membrane. These proteins normally protect the red cell from complement-induced cell lysis. Absence of surface CD55 and CD59 results in a chronic, intravascular red cell haemolysis with constant haemosiderinuria, anaemia, jaundice and fatigue. Secondary iron deficiency requiring supplementation often occurs.

Since the abnormality is present in a haemopoietic cell, complications related to cytopenia of other cell lineages derived from the same clone (e.g., leucopoenia and thrombocytopenia, pancytopenia, aplastic anaemia) may also occur in addition to the haemolytic anaemia.

Several other features also characterize PNH:

- Recurrent thrombosis: both arterial and venous (despite a typically low platelet count). This warrants lifelong anticoagulation and is a key feature of the disease.
- Renal impairment: this may be due to renal vein thrombosis or acute tubular necrosis (secondary to haemoglobinuria).
- Smooth muscle abnormalities: the presence of free haemoglobin in the circulation depletes nitric oxide, dysregulating normal smooth muscle tone, which manifests as dysphagia, odynophagia, erectile dysfunction and ileus.
- Pulmonary hypertension: likely secondary to nitric oxide depletion.

HAEMOGLOBINOPATHIES

Abnormalities of haemoglobin (haemoglobinopathies) may result from:

- Abnormal haemoglobin (e.g., sickle cell anaemia). Abnormal structure leads to abnormal function and behaviour, resulting in disease.
- Reduced synthesis of normal haemoglobin (thalassaemia)

Reviewing structural features of the haemoglobin molecule (see Chapter 2: Structure) may facilitate understanding of this section.

Sickle cell disease

In sickle variant haemoglobin, a single base-pair substitution in the gene coding for the β globin results in a valine substitution for glutamic acid. This single amino acid substitution has immense structural and functional consequences for haemoglobin incorporating this abnormal beta globin (βS), which is known as HbS (sickle variant haemoglobin). At low pO$_2$, de-oxy HbS polymerizes into long intracellular fibres (tactoids). This elongation deforms the red cell into an inflexible sickle shape (Fig. 3.6). Initially, reoxygenation in conditions of high pO$_2$ will reverse the sickle deformation, but after several recurrences the shape becomes irreversibly sickled. This inflexibility of sickled red cells causes capillary occlusion with distal tissue hypoxia. Chronically, recurrent hypoxic injury and structural vascular damage accumulate with time and cause irreparable damage to organs such as the spleen, accounting for the bulk of the long-term morbidity of sickle cell anaemia. Acute episodes (sickle cell crises) are due to the same underlying mechanisms. Sickle cell crises manifest with severe pain from ischaemic tissue distal to vessels occluded by sickled cells.

Persistence of the sickle gene

The HbS gene is prevalent in tropical Africa and parts of the Mediterranean, Middle East and India. In some areas, up to 40% of the population are heterozygous (HbA/HbS). Sickle-cell heterozygosity confers protection against *Plasmodium falciparum* (the protozoan responsible for severe malaria) parasitization of red cells, perhaps accounting for the persistence of the genotype in malaria-endemic areas.

Sickle cell anaemia

If an individual possesses two copies of the β^S gene (i.e., a homozygous genotype: β^S/β^S), their phenotype is sickle cell anaemia. This disease carries significant morbidity due to the extensive complications it presents to sufferers. Table 3.5 lists the main complications with discussion of the underlying mechanisms.

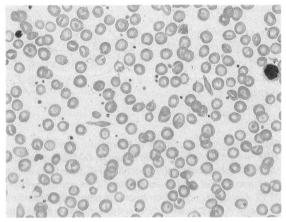

Fig. 3.6 Blood film in sickle cell anaemia

Table 3.5 Complications of sickle cell disease

Clinical feature	Causative mechanism
Chronic haemolytic anaemia	Poorly deformable red cells are removed from the circulation, shortening their lifespan to 10–20 days (compared with the normal 120-day red cell lifespan).
Haemolytic crises	Often accompanying an infarctive crisis, an acute worsening of haemolysis is accompanied by an acute fall in Hb and red cell count. Reticulocytosis increases in an attempt to compensate.
Painful infarctive crises	Vaso-occlusive crises are the hallmark of sickle cell disease. These are acute episodes of pain, usually in the lower back, pelvis, legs but also sometimes abdomen and chest. Painful infarctive crises are the most common reason for hospital admissions in this patient population. Infection, acidosis, dehydration, cold and hypoxia predispose to infarcts in areas of complete ischaemia distal to occluded microvasculature. In many cases, no specific precipitating factor can be identified. Any organ or tissue may be affected, sometimes irreversibly.
Aplastic crises	These may be provoked by folate deficiency or parvovirus B19 infections. The abrupt fall in Hb of an aplastic crisis is differentiated from that in an acute haemolytic crisis by absence of reticulocytes.
Splenic complications	The tortuous microvasculature of the splenic filtration beds is a prime zone of susceptibility for sickling vaso-occlusion. Repeated micro-infarctions lead to destruction and atrophy of splenic tissue (hyposplenism). Acute splenic sequestration refers to sudden, rapid spleen engorgement with trapped blood. It presents with abdominal pain, acute splenomegaly and a falling Hb level.
Infection susceptibility	Hyposplenic patients are susceptible to infections, which may be catastrophic. Susceptibility to encapsulated microorganisms is particularly high.
Acute chest syndrome	This diagnosis is defined by dyspnoea, low arterial pO_2, chest pain and clinical and radiographic evidence of pulmonary oedema.
Cerebrovascular ischaemia	Intracerebral vaso-occlusion of brain microvasculature may cause complications ranging from transient (TIA) to irreversible ischaemic events (stroke).
Other complications	Other phenomena (secondary to microvasculature occlusion) particularly associated with sickle cell anaemia include priapism (prolonged and painful erections), skin ulceration and proliferative retinopathy.

Hb, Haemoglobin; *TIA,* transient ischaemic attack.

Diagnosis

Hb is typically 60–90 g/L. It is typically a normochromic, normocytic anaemia with reticulocytosis (due to the chronic haemolytic anaemia). Sickle cells and target cells are seen on blood film. Hb electrophoresis shows HbS, variable amounts of HbF and absent HbA in homozygous patients.

Long-term management

These patients are managed by haematologists, who oversee outpatient management and inpatient crises. Treatment goals include maintaining a stable Hb, prompt management of acute crises, preventing infections and trying to minimize the numerous long-term complications of the disease.

- Haemoglobin levels may be maintained with top-up transfusions as needed or exchange transfusions. Iron status must be monitored to avoid iron overload.
- Influenza, pneumococcal, meningococcal and *Haemophilus influenzae* type B (Hib) vaccination is mandatory, as is oral daily antibiotic prophylaxis (due to functional hyposplenism or asplenia if the spleen has been resected). Prompt, aggressive treatment of infection is essential.
- Folate supplements reduce the likelihood of a folate deficiency-induced aplastic crisis.
- Patients must be effectively counselled as to lifestyle habits to minimize their exposure to factors known to provoke infarctive crises (dehydration, cold, etc.). It is also very important to ensure they understand how to self-care appropriately in mild self-limiting crises scenarios as well as providing a clear escalation plan for medical intervention if self-care is not sufficient.
- Hydroxyurea stimulates the production of HbF ($\alpha2\gamma2$), which can limit the impact of sickle cell disease for patients with moderate-to-severe recurrent episodes of vaso-occlusive crises. Unfortunately, not all patients respond to hydroxyurea.
- Bone marrow transplantation is the only potential cure. Due to the high risk of this procedure, it is only performed for selected individuals.

Acute management of sickle crises

Prompt treatment of any reversible precipitating factors is a priority. Aggressive rehydration and antibiotics (intravenous if necessary), adequate analgesia, supplemental oxygen (to increase oxygen saturation and thus delivery capacity of intact haemoglobin) and warming are important components of supportive treatment. Simple transfusion or exchange transfusion may be necessary. A haematologist should be consulted when possible for guidance as to target Hb parameters.

Acute chest crisis

For symptoms/signs, please refer to Table 3.5. An acute chest crisis is a life-threatening complication and remains the most common cause of death in young patients with sickle cell anaemia. It can be triggered by infection or simply vaso-occlusion of the pulmonary vasculature. It should be managed with sufficient intravenous analgesia, antibiotics (including antivirals if influenza suspected) and rehydration. Particular caution is needed to avoid exacerbating pulmonary oedema while attempting to restore intravascular volume. A bronchodilator should be used if there is evidence of bronchospasm or coexisting asthma. Early haematology advice regarding therapeutic simple (see earlier Clinical Notes: Transfusion in sickle cell anaemia) or exchange transfusion (see earlier Clinical Notes: Exchange transfusions) is necessary because appropriate transfusion reduces the chance of progressive deterioration. Continuous oximetry as a minimum is appropriate and regular blood gases advisable. Rapid respiratory decompensation is not unusual and this requires involvement of the critical care team and mechanical ventilation if indicated.

Sickle cell trait

This heterozygous (genotype β^S/β) condition is typically benign and asymptomatic, even though up to 45% of Hb may be HbS. Sickling in this context occurs only at extremely low pO_2 and rarely occurs in vivo. Pregnancy, labour, altitude and anaesthesia may, however, cause increased risk. Both HbA and HbS are present on electrophoresis. Heterozygous patients are carriers and can pass the HbS gene on to their children.

Sickle cell/haemoglobin C disease

This condition is defined by heterozygosity of the β globin gene; one copy is the β^S and the other is β^C (forming haemoglobin C). β^C has an amino acid substitution (GLU→LYS) at the same site as the responsible substitution in the β^S mutant gene with similar abnormal aggregation under conditions of low pO_2. Both HbC and HbS are present on electrophoresis. Compared with sickle cell anaemia (β^S/β^S), these patients typically have milder anaemia and complications with greater life expectancy. However, they have a greater risk of thrombotic complications, particularly during pregnancy.

Sickle cell beta thalassaemia

This condition is also defined by heterozygosity of the β globin gene; one copy is the β^S, while the other copy carries the β thalassaemia variant of the globin gene. The MCV and MCH are significantly lower than the relatively normal values seen in sickle cell anaemia (β^S/β^S).

Thalassaemia

Thalassaemia arises from mutations in the genes coding for the α or β globin protein component of haemoglobin. They are accordingly classified as α or β thalassaemia, depending on which gene is mutated. The mutation gives rise to abnormality of the corresponding globin in terms of both structure and function. Each type of thalassaemia results in a surfeit of unpaired normal globins (α globins in β thalassaemia, β globins in α thalassaemia). These unpartnered globins precipitate within red cell precursors, causing ineffective or abortive erythropoiesis and predisposing precursors to phagocytosis by bone marrow macrophages. Red cells that reach the circulation haemolyze easily and therefore have a shortened lifespan.

HINTS AND TIPS

DIFFERENCE BETWEEN THALASSAEMIA AND SICKLE CELL SYNDROMES

Thalassaemia is characterized by a deficiency of either α- or β-globins. Sickle-cell syndromes are due to abnormal β-globin chains only.

Beta thalassaemia

β-Thalassaemia is much more frequent in individuals originating within a broad geographical band starting in the Iberian Peninsula and ending in the Philippines in south-east Asia.

A partial (β⁻) or complete (β°) failure of β globin synthesis arises from a wide array of possible mutations, ranging from single base changes to deletions, aberrant splicing, premature truncations and frameshifts. The severity of disease depends on the particular mutation and whether one or both copies of the β globin gene are affected.

If both copies of the β globin gene are affected (homozygosity), the disease is called β thalassaemia major. A single affected copy (heterozygosity) is called β thalassaemia trait.

CLINICAL NOTES

β THALASSAEMIA TRAIT

Also known as β thalassaemia minor, this is where the patient has one abnormal copy of the β globin gene and one normal copy (β⁻/β). It is usually asymptomatic, although a microcytic and hypochromic appearance is seen on blood film. Anaemia is usually mild due to a higher than normal red cell count. It is diagnosed when an increased proportion of HbA2 is demonstrated by electrophoresis. Recognition of this syndrome is important as it has implications for genetic counselling and may otherwise be misdiagnosed as iron-deficiency anaemia, leading to inappropriate iron therapy.

Reduction or lack of β chains leads to unpaired α chains precipitating.

- Developing erythroblasts (→ ineffective erythropoiesis and reduced red cell synthesis)

- Mature red cells (→ premature haemolysis and shortened red cell lifespan).

The ineffective erythropoiesis and haemolysis are proportionate to the relative excess of α globins. Severe anaemia manifests at 3–6 months when the developmental switch from γ globin to β globins occurs. Extramedullary haemopoiesis causes hepatosplenomegaly and expansion of marrow cavities into cortical bone. This impairs structural integrity, predisposing to fractures and causing a characteristic appearance of the skull X-ray (Fig 3.7).

A severe microcytic (low MCV), hypochromic (low MCH) anaemia is present, with elevated reticulocytes and the presence of normoblasts, target cells and red cell basophilic stippling on the peripheral blood film. DNA analysis will define the responsible genetic mutation. Haemoglobin electrophoresis is also diagnostic and reveals partial (β thalassaemia trait) or complete (β thalassaemia major) absence of HbA (HbF is present instead).

Regular red cell transfusions are life-sustaining, but these patients are highly vulnerable to iron overload and require chelation therapy and vigilant monitoring of iron status. This susceptibility is exacerbated by enhanced absorption of dietary iron, probably in response to anaemia-induced tissue hypoxia.

Alpha thalassaemia

α-Thalassaemia is most common in people of South-East Asian and West African origin. There are four (rather than two) copies of the α globin gene and α thalassaemia typically results from deletion of one or more of these genes. Clinical severity is proportional to the number of lost (deleted) genes. Deletion of all four genes sadly results in

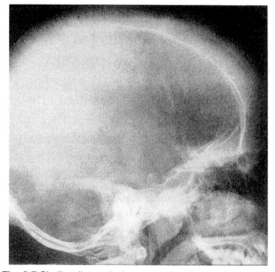

Fig. 3.7 Skull radiograph demonstrating the hair-on-end appearance due to expansion of marrow cavity into cortical bone.

Table 3.6 Features of alpha thalassaemia

Condition	Alpha genes deleted	Functional alpha genes	Electrophoresis
Normal	0	4	HbA (minimal HbF)
Alpha thalassaemia trait	1	3	HbA (minimal HbF) Clinically normal Electrophoresis normal Microcytosis MCV 70–80 fL
Alpha thalassaemia minor	2	2	HbA 90% + Mild anaemia Hb 90–120 g/L Microcytosis MCV 70–80 fL
Haemoglobin H disease	3	1	Haemoglobin H (β tetramer) 5%–30% HbA 70% + Marked anaemia Hb 60–100 g/L Marked microcytosis MCV 60–70 fL
Alpha thalassaemia major	4	0	Incompatible with life; death in utero from hydrops fetalis

Hb, Haemoglobin; *HbA*, adult haemoglobin; *HbF*, fetal haemoglobin; *MCV*, mean cell volume.

death in utero, while the deletion of three gene results in a moderately severe anaemia with microcytic, hypochromic red cells and splenomegaly. The abnormal tetramer of unpaired β globins is called haemoglobin H, hence the name haemoglobin H disease. A reduced amount of (normal) HbA and an increased amount of haemoglobin H is seen on electrophoresis.

One deletion (three functional alpha globin genes) is referred to as α thalassaemia trait (Table 3.6). Two deletions (two functional alpha genes) is referred to as alpha thalassaemia minor. This is typically associated with mild anaemia (Hb is normal), although MCV and MCH are reduced and red cell count proportionally elevated. Haemoglobin electrophoresis in α thalassaemia trait is normal.

ELECTROPHORESIS: INVESTIGATION OF HAEMOGLOBINOPATHIES

Electrophoresis is a method used to discriminate biological molecules by molecular weight. Samples of interest are processed to isolate chemically the molecule of interest (haemoglobin, in this context).

A detergent denatures the protein samples so that elements of tertiary/quaternary structure cannot confound the outcome and to confer each protein with a uniform negative charge. Each sample is loaded into a depression (loading well) in a gel-phase matrix (typically sodium dodecyl sulphate). The molecular structure of the gel matrix is a network of crisscrossing polymers forming a uniform mesh. When an electric current is applied across the gel, the denatured proteins migrate through the gel. The larger a protein, the less it can travel in a given time, due to more ob-

struction by the meshwork. The smallest proteins therefore travel the furthest. Since all molecules being analyzed have been conferring with the same negative charge, electrostatic influence is negligible and the distance travelled is inversely related to molecular size alone.

The gel with the migrated proteins is then stained, to allow visualization of each sample's end-position. Every electrophoretic gel also has a control lane that has a mixture of proteins of known molecular size loaded into the corresponding well. This ladder calibrates migration distance of the test protein in terms of molecular size. Then each protein is compared against the control lane to infer its molecular size.

Each type of haemoglobin, e.g., HbA, HbF, HbS, will migrate a different difference on gel electrophoresis. The control lane will include examples of each of the abnormal Hb types to allow identification.

MARROW DEFECTS CAUSING ANAEMIA

Aplastic anaemia

Aplastic anaemia is a misleading name because, as it affects haemopoietic stems cells, it reduces all cell counts in all cell lines (pancytopenia), causing leucopoenia and thrombocytopenia as well as anaemia. It is also characterized by aplasia (hypocellularity) of the bone marrow with a reduction in haemopoietic stem cells. Those that are present are defective and unable to repopulate the depleted marrow. ~75% of cases are idiopathic (no cause can be identified); the remaining ~25% cases are due to various factors listed in Table 3.7.

Treatment involves supportive actions: prompt antibiotic treatment in infection, transfusions as needed (red cells

Table 3.7 Causes of aplastic anaemia with specific examples

Causative mechanism	Examples
Drugs	Antibiotics: chloramphenicol, nitrofurantoin, sulphonamides, ribavarin Antimalarials: quinacrine, chloroquine Rheumatoid arthritis treatment: gold salts, NSAIDs Metal chelators: Penicillamine Antiepileptics: phenytoin, carbamazepine
Viral infection	HIV, parvovirus B19, hepatitis B and C, EBV, Varicella-zoster virus
Cytotoxic drugs	Chemotherapeutic agents
Chemical toxins	Benzene, chemical solvents, glue vapour (solvent abuse)
Ionizing radiation	Radiation therapy (cancer treatment) or accidental exposure to ionizing radiation
Pregnancy	—
Autoimmune disease	Any autoimmune disease where immune sensitization develops towards haemopoietic stem cells
Rare genetic conditions	Diamond-Blackfan anaemia Shwachman-Diamond syndrome Fanconi anaemia

EBV, Epstein-Barr virus; *HIV,* human immunodeficiency virus; *NSAIDS,* nonsteroidal antiinflammatory drugs.

or platelets), growth factors and immunosuppression. Most patients are treated with anti-thymocyte globulin (ATG) as first-line. This product is derived from horses or rabbits and consists of antibodies directed against human T cells. The T cell destruction results in intense immunosuppression. Although some patients achieve lasting remission, others relapse. Stem cell transplant offers a cure for carefully selected patients with this disease, but it is a high-risk intervention.

Pure red-cell aplasia

This is a rare condition. A severe normocytic anaemia with <1% reticulocytes is present, but white cell and platelet counts are normal. It may be triggered by certain drugs, infections and autoantibody formation. Parvovirus B19 infection may cause a transient pure red cell aplasia. Red-cell precursors in the bone marrow are absent, but aside from erythroblast absence, the bone marrow cellularity is normal. Treatment is supportive, focusing on red cell transfusion. Stem cell transplantation may be considered in appropriate candidates.

Other causes

In terms of haematological disease, leukaemia and lymphomas may cause anaemia due to marrow infiltration. Myelodysplasia (see Chapter 5: Myelodysplasia) may present with a macrocytic anaemia.

Any space-occupying lesions that occupy an area of normal bone marrow territory large enough to disrupt the normal architecture may cause anaemia. Metastases or primary neoplasms affecting the bone marrow may have this effect. However, it is more likely that all cell lines would be affected: isolated anaemia in these cases due to bone marrow infiltration would be unusual.

POLYCYTHAEMIA

Polycythaemia (erythrocytosis) is the term used to describe an increase in red cell count above normal levels. It may be primary or secondary.

Primary polycythaemia

Primary polycythaemia arises from an abnormal clone of cells (see Chapter 5: Polycythaemia rubra vera).

Secondary polycythaemia

Secondary polycythaemia is a normal physiological reaction to tissue hypoxia. Renal cells detect hypoxia and in response increase EPO synthesis, upregulating erythropoiesis. The oxygen-carrying capacity of the blood increases. The hypoxia provoking this response may or may not be due to insufficient Hb, but the body is unable to identify the cause and responds with an increase in red cell count. As an example: chronic mild hypoxia seen in heavy smokers is usually indicated by an increased haematocrit. If a reasonable cause of the provocative hypoxia is not clearly apparent, serum EPO can differentiate secondary polycythaemia from primary; EPO is elevated in secondary but not primary polycythaemia.

Secondary polycythaemia is much more common than primary polycythaemia. Since secondary polycythaemia is an appropriate physiological response, treatment is not necessary just to normalize red cell counts. Complications may arise due to increased viscosity; in this instance, venesection to reduce the haematocrit to ≤0.55 may be considered.

Apparent polycythaemia is due to a decrease in intravascular volume unaccompanied by the loss of red cells; this contraction of intravascular volume usually results from dehydration or inappropriate third space redistribution.

Chronic excessive vasoconstriction, as seen in long-term hypertension, results in such a contracted intravascular volume. This specific scenario, known as Gaisbock syndrome, is typically seen in obese men with hypertension and is a favourite in exams as an example of secondary polycythaemia.

● Chapter Summary

- Anaemia (defined as reduced Hb) gives rise to a common set of symptoms but can result from many different underlying causes.
- Symptoms common to anaemia (no matter what underlying cause) include fatigue, exertional breathlessness, palpitations, presyncope/syncope and headache.
- Common causes of anaemia include haematinics deficiency, chronic disease, blood loss or haemolysis.
- Haemolysis may be subclassified by its primary location: intravascular (e.g., all causes of microangiopathic haemolysis) or extravascular (e.g., hereditary enzyme deficiencies).
- Rarer causes of anaemia are hereditary abnormalities of haemoglobin structure such as sickle cell anaemia and thalassaemia or bone marrow disorders such as aplastic anaemia and pure red cell aplasia.
- Enzyme deficiencies affecting glycolysis such as pyruvate kinase or glucose-6-phosphate dehydrogenase lead to shortened red cell survival due to red cell reliance on glycolysis for ATP generation.
- Polycythaemia (an abnormally raised Hb and red cell count) is usually due to various states resulting chronic tissue hypoxia, but rarely may be due to pathological mutations of red cell precursors (polycythaemia rubra vera, also called primary polycythaemia).

LEUCOCYTE STRUCTURE

'Leucocytes' is the term used to describe *white* blood cells. The immunological functions of each type of leucocyte are explained in detail in Chapter 9.

Lymphocytes

Appearance and structure
Lymphocytes (Fig. 4.1) are the smallest of the leucocytes (~6–8 μm diameter). The term 'lymphocytes' includes T cells, B cells and natural killer (NK) cells. They all derive from lymphoid lineage. Each population expresses characteristic molecular surface markers. Their shape varies from spherical to pleomorphic. Lymphocyte nuclei are large, round, densely staining and may be situated off-centre ('eccentrically'). Basophilic (blue-staining) cytoplasm is sparse, so the nucleus:cytoplasm ratio is high. However, this ratio falls on lymphocyte activation, since cytoplasmic volume increases with intracellular synthetic activity.

Location
Lymphocytes usually represent ~20%–25% of the blood population of leucocytes. They circulate in blood and the lymphatic system when travelling between bone marrow and lymphoid tissue such as the spleen or lymph nodes.

Function
Lymphocytes produce antibodies (B cells) or kill foreign or infected cells (T cells and NK cells). Their lifespan is variable, according to antigenic interaction. Memory B or T cells, for example, survive for decades.

Granulocytes: Neutrophils

Appearance and structure
Neutrophils, also known as 'polymorphonuclear leucocytes,' measure 12–14 μm in diameter (Fig. 4.2). Nuclei are segmented, with 2–5 lobes connected by thin chromatin threads. Cytoplasm stains pink and contains glycogen and numerous granules.

Location
Neutrophils circulate in blood for up to 10 hours and represent the majority (~60%) of the leucocyte blood population. They migrate into tissues in response to chemotactic agents, where they survive for a further 1–3 days.

Function
Neutrophils are the first cells to arrive at a zone of inflammation, comprising a prominent aspect of the innate immune system. They recruit further immune cells with chemotactic mediators. Neutrophils destroy microorganisms by:

- Release of hydrolytic enzymes from their granules
- Phagocytosis

Dead neutrophils are the major constituent of pus.

Granulocytes: Eosinophils

Appearance and structure
Eosinophils (Fig. 4.3) are larger than neutrophils (~12–17 μm diameter). Their nucleus is bilobed or reniform (kidney-shaped). Cytoplasm stains brick-red and contains numerous cationic granules with cytotoxic contents including major basic protein and eosinophil-derived neurotoxin, peroxidase and cationic protein.

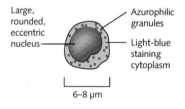

Large, rounded, eccentric nucleus

Azurophilic granules

Light-blue staining cytoplasm

6–8 μm

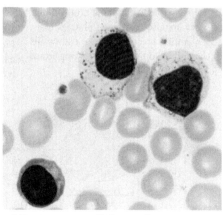

Fig. 4.1 Lymphocyte structure. Line diagram (left panel) and film appearance (right panel).

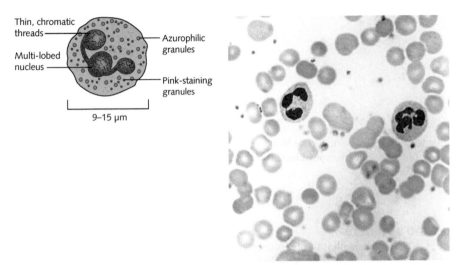

Fig. 4.2 Neutrophil structure. Line diagram (left panel) and film appearance (right panel). Note that only the azurophilic granules are visible in the film view of the neutrophil (right hand panel). Other granules present (but not visible on the film) include glycogen, tertiary and specific granules.

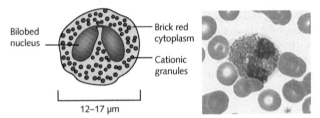

Fig. 4.3 Eosinophil structure. Line diagram (left panel) and film appearance (right panel).

Location

The vast majority of eosinophils reside the tissues (mainly at epithelial barriers including lungs, skin and gastrointestinal tract). They circulate in blood for 1–2 days, where they represent ~1%–6% of the circulating leucocyte population.

Function

Eosinophils play the primary role in attacking multicellular parasitic organisms. They are also capable of phagocytosis, particularly of antigen–antibody complexes. Eosinophils (similarly to mast cells and basophils) are also important mediators of allergic reactions.

Basophils

Appearance and structure

Basophils (Fig. 4.4) are ~14–16 µm in diameter with an 'S-shaped' nucleus. Cytoplasm is densely packed with large blue-staining (basophilic) granules that may obscure the nucleus and cause bulging outward of the cell membrane, giving a 'roughened' appearance to the perimeter. These granules contain heparin, histamine, chemotactic factors and peroxidase.

Location

Basophils are scarce (<1% of circulating leucocytes), with a lifespan in the circulation of 1–2 days (whilst travelling to lymphoid and nonlymphoid tissues).

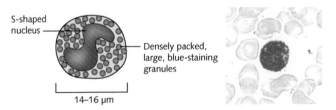

Fig. 4.4 Basophil structure. Line diagram (left panel) and film appearance (right panel).

Function

Basophils are functionally very similar to mast cells, although their lineages differ and mast cells are restricted to tissues and thus do not appear in the blood. They both release a similar array of mediators in response to immunoglobulin E (IgE) cross-linking and thus are thought to participate in type 1 hypersensitivity reactions.

Monocytes

Appearance and structure

Monocytes (Fig. 4.5) are the largest leucocytes (≤25 μm diameter). They have a large, eccentric, reniform nucleus. Nucleoli are often visible, giving the nucleus a 'moth-eaten' appearance. Basophilic cytoplasm contains numerous lysosomes and vacuole-like spaces, producing a 'ground-glass' appearance. Microtubules, microfilaments, pinocytotic vesicles and filopodia/pseudopodia are present at the cell periphery.

Location

Monocytes spend 1–3 days in blood, where they represent ~2%–10% of bloodstream leucocytes. They then enter the tissues, where they differentiate further and become macrophages. Macrophages survive within tissues for months to years.

Function

Macrophages make up the reticuloendothelial system and are found in tissues throughout the body. They phagocytose elderly/damaged red cells, pathogens and cellular debris. They also process and present antigen to lymphocytes as part of the adaptive immune response (see Chapter 10). Macrophages also have a pro-inflammatory function, releasing a variety of cytokines.

LEUCOCYTE DIFFERENTIATION

Please refer to Fig. 1.2 for a detailed overview of white cell differentiation. In brief:

- Lymphocytes (T cells, B cells and NK cells) are lymphoid lineage leucocytes derived from the lymphoid lineage progenitor cell.
- Eosinophils and basophils develop from the myeloid lineage progenitor cells Colony forming unit eosinophil progenitor (CFU-Eos) and Colony forming unit basophil progenitor (CFU-Baso), respectively. These progenitors are themselves derived from the Colony forming unit common myeloid progenitor (CFU-GEMM) multipotent progenitor.
- Neutrophils and monocytes develop from the myeloid lineage progenitor cell (Colony forming unit granulocyte-myeloid precursor (the neutrophil/monocyte precursor) [CFU-GM]) which may differentiate into the Colony forming unit granulocyte precursor (CFU-G) progenitor (which ultimately develops into a neutrophil) or the CFU-M progenitor (which ultimately develops into a monocyte). The CFU-GM progenitor is itself derived from the CFU-GEMM multipotent progenitor.

LEFT AND RIGHT SHIFT

'Left shift' describes the phenomenon where an increased proportion of immature neutrophils are released from the bone marrow into peripheral blood. This accelerated release is triggered by inflammatory cytokines produced in response to (usually) inflammation or infection. Left shift can also be seen in certain diseases, including bone

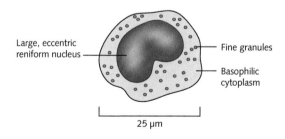

Large, eccentric reniform nucleus — Fine granules — Basophilic cytoplasm

25 μm

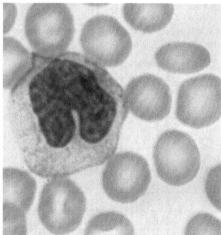

Fig. 4.5 Monocyte structure. Line diagram (left panel) and film appearance (right panel). The monocyte is surrounded by red cells, giving a good relative indication of the size. Note that the pointed extrusion is due to the 'squashing' between the adjacent cells on the slide rather than a specific feature of monocyte structure.

marrow disorders. For example, in bacterial infection, the physiological response is a rise in neutrophils. Initially, the demand for mature neutrophils temporarily outstrips the supply available in the bone marrow, so immature neutrophils are also released into blood. Band cells are most common, but earlier versions may be released also in response to increasingly severe inflammatory stimuli.

'Right shift' refers to the converse scenario, where leucocytes persist longer than normal in the circulation and acquire morphological characteristics of 'hypermaturity' (e.g., hypersegmented and enlarged 'giant' neutrophils). This occurs in noninfectious inflammatory processes such as malignancy and bone marrow synthesis disorders such as megaloblastic or iron-deficiency anaemia.

WHITE COUNT DIFFERENTIAL

The white count differential breaks down the leucocyte count into components: neutrophils, lymphocytes, monocytes, eosinophils and basophils. This process is automated and uses stains, cell size and light scatter to differentiate among different cell types. Normal leucocyte parameters and nomenclature of abnormalities are given in Table 4.1. Abnormal leucocyte appearances on blood film may suggest specific disease processes. Table 4.2 details some common morphological abnormalities with corresponding diagnostic inferences.

LEUCOCYTOSIS

'Leucocytosis' describes an increased total white cell count (i.e., $>11 \times 10^9$/L). One particular type of leucocyte, most commonly neutrophils, usually predominates, with smaller increases in the other types of leucocyte. Many things can lead to a leucocytosis, not all of which are pathological. The nature

of the predominant population is mandatory for forming any diagnosis (see Table 4.3 for examples of particular diseases associated with elevation of specific populations of leucocytes).

CLINICAL NOTES

REACTIVE LEUCOCYTOSIS

An acute rise in total white cell count is usually in response to infection, particularly if it occurs rapidly. This is termed a 'reactive leucocytosis.'

CLINICAL NOTES

BENIGN CAUSES OF NEUTROPHILIA

These include pregnancy or recent delivery, vigorous exercise, post-antibiotic diarrhoea, and vaccination. Exogenous factors such as cigarette smoking (possibly the most common cause of mild neutrophilia) or a chronic state of anxiety may also cause a neutrophilia.

LEUCOPENIA

'Leucopenia' describes a *total* white blood count of less than 4×10^9/L (see Table 4.1 for definitions).

Causes of neutropenia ($<2 \times 10^9$/L) and agranulocytosis ($<0.5 \times 10^9$/L)

Reduced neutrophil count may arise due to inadequate granulopoiesis or an accelerated removal of granulocytes.

Inadequate granulopoiesis

Reduced or ineffective neutrophil production by bone marrow causes neutropenia. Such inadequate granulopoiesis may be secondary to generalized bone marrow failure, which may be primary [myelodysplastic syndrome (MDS),

CLINICAL NOTES

IATROGENIC NEUTROPENIA

In all instances, drugs are the most common cause of neutropenia. Always review the patient's medications and consider if a known culprit (Table 4.4) could be responsible for a new neutropenia.

Table 4.1 White cell count parameters and nomenclature of abnormalities

Parameter	Normal range (× 10⁹/L)ᵃ	Abnormality
Total white cell count	4.0–11	↑ : 'leucocytosis' ↓ : 'leucopenia'
Lymphocytes	1.3–4.5	↑ : 'lymphocytosis' ↓ : 'lymphopenia'
Neutrophils	2–7.5	↑ : 'neutrophilia' ↓: 'neutropenia' (aka 'granulocytopenia')
Eosinophils	0.04–0.4	↑ : 'eosinophilia'
Basophils	0–0.1	↑ : 'basophilia'
Monocytes	0.2–0.8	↑ : 'monocytosis'

ᵃ *Ranges given represent normal parameters in 95% of the normal population.*

Table 4.2 Blood film abnormalities of leucocyte morphology and their diagnostic inferences

Abnormality	Description	Diagnostic inference
Hypersegmentation of neutrophils	≥5 lobes per nucleus	Megaloblastic anaemia Renal failure Iron-deficiency anaemia
Left shift of neutrophils	Various earlier developmental stages of neutrophil Band cells are the most common, but all stages are possible	Severe infection CML Pregnancy Use of G-CSF
Blast cells	The most immature form of the blood cell lineage (e.g., myeloblast or a lymphoblast could be seen in the peripheral blood in AML and ALL, respectively	Acute leukaemias (AML and ALL: see Chapter 5) Occasional blast seen with leucoerythroblastic reaction (see below)
Auer rods	Rod-like accretions of granular material which may appear in the cytoplasm of leukaemic blast cells in AML	AML
Smear cells (also known as 'smudge' cells or 'basket'. cells)	Remnants of a cell, lacking a clearly identifiable cell membrane or nucleus These are seen when abnormally fragile cells are abundant in the blood	Reactive lymphocytosis CLL
Leucoerythroblastic change	Presence of immature leucocytes including occasional blast *and* immature (still nucleated) red cells	Severe haemorrhage Severe haemolysis Sepsis Myelofibrosis (either primary or secondary to metastatic disease in bone marrow) DIC

ALL, Acute lymphoblastic leukaemia; *AML,* acute myeloid leukaemia; *CLL,* chronic lymphocytic leukaemia; *CML,* chronic myeloid leukaemia; *DIC,* Disseminated intravascular coagulation; *G-CSF,* Granulocyte-colony stimulating factor.

Table 4.3 Diseases associated with increases in particular leucocyte population

Leucocyte population	General causative mechanism	Specific examples
Neutrophil (neutrophilia)	Bacterial infection (acute and chronic)	
	Acute inflammation and/or tissue necrosis	Infarction, surgery, rhabdomyolysis, myositis, burns, trauma, vasculitis, RA
	Myeloproliferative disorders	CML, primary myelofibrosis
	Metabolic or endocrine disease	DKA, thyrotoxicosis, gout, eclampsia
	Drugs	G-CSF, steroids, adrenaline
Lymphocytes (lymphocytosis)	Viral infection	EBV, CMV, rubella
	Bacterial infection	TB, brucellosis, syphilis, pertussis
	Parasitic infections	Toxoplasmosis, rickettsial infections
	Neoplastic	CLL, ALL, lymphoma
	Other	Postsplenectomy, postadrenaline
Eosinophils (eosinophilia)	Parasitic infection	Helminth (worm) infections, schistosomiasis, malaria
	Hypersensitivity	Asthma, hay fever

Continued

Table 4.3 Diseases associated with increases in particular leucocyte population—cont'd

Leucocyte population	General causative mechanism	Specific examples
	Drugs	Drug-related eosinophilia, DRESS
	Skin disease	Eczema, psoriasis, urticaria, pemphigus, dermatitis herpetiformis
	Neoplastic	Hodgkin lymphoma, T cell non-Hodgkin lymphoma, CML, hypereosinophilic syndrome, solid tumours
	Post-infectious	Convalescence phase following any infection
Basophils (basophilia)	Myeloproliferative disorders	Classically CML, although basophilia may be seen in PRV, PMF and ET
	IgE-mediated hypersensitivity reactions	Anaphylaxis
	Infection	Viral, helminths, mycobacterial
	Endocrine	Hypothyroidism, diabetes, oestrogen treatment
	Autoimmune	UC, RA
Monocytes (monocytosis)	Neoplastic	Most commonly in CMML, CML and AML May be seen in some lymphoma and myelodysplastic syndromes
	Bacterial infection	TB, bacterial endocarditis, syphilis, typhoid, brucellosis
	Viral infection	Varicella zoster
	Parasitic infection	Malaria, trypanosomiasis, leishmaniasis

ALL, Acute lymphoblastic leukaemia; *AML*, acute myeloid leukaemia; *CLL*, chronic lymphocytic leukaemia; *CML*, chronic myeloid leukaemia; *CMML*, chronic myelomonocytic leukaemia; *CMV*, cytomegalovirus; *DIC*, disseminated intravascular coagulation; *DKA*, diabetic ketoacidosis; *DRESS*, drug-related eosinophilia with systemic symptoms; *EBV*, Epstein-Barr virus; *ET*, essential thrombocytosis; *G-CSF*, Granulocyte-colony stimulating factor; *PMF*, primary myelofibrosis; *PRV*, polycythaemia rubra vera; *RA*, rheumatoid arthritis; *TB*, tuberculosis; *UC*, ulcerative colitis.

lymphomas, leukaemias (see Chapter 5) or aplastic anaemias (see Chapter 3: Aplastic anaemia)] or secondary (chemotherapy, megaloblastic anaemia, metastatic infiltration or drugs such as methotrexate or azathioprine).

Alternatively, inadequate granulopoiesis may be due to a specific failure of neutrophil production. This may be:

- A dose-related drug exposure phenomenon (Table 4.4)
- Rare congenital diseases (e.g., Kostmann syndrome, cyclical neutropenia, Schwachman syndrome)

Accelerated removal of granulocytes

Neutropenia due to increased destruction/distribution may be secondary to several mechanisms:

- Drug-induced immune-mediated destruction (Table 4.4): note that drug-induced neutropenia operating via an immune mechanism is *not* dose-dependent
- Immune-mediated destruction (idiopathic or related to co-existing autoimmune disease-related)

Table 4.4 Drugs known to cause neutropenia by therapeutic class (not exhaustive)

Anticonvulsants	Phenytoin, carbamazepine, lamotrigine
Antithyroid	Carbimazole, propylthiouracil
Immunomodulatory	NSAIDS, sulphasalazine, gold, phenylbutazone, penicillamine
Antibiotic	Cephalosporins, co-trimoxazole, chloramphenicol, dapsone, vancomycin
Psychotropic	Clozapine, tricyclic antidepressants, phenothiazines
Gastrointestinal	H2-receptor antagonists (cimetidine, ranitidine)
Antiarrhythmic	Propanolol, digoxin, flecainide, procainamide
Diuretic	Thiazide, furosemide, spironolactone, acetazolamide
Antiplatelet	Dipyramidole, ticlodipine
Oral hypoglycaemics (sulphonylureas)	Tolbutamide, chlorpropamide

NSAIDs, Nonsteroidal antiinflammatory drugs.

- Hypersplenism (i.e., splenic neutrophil sequestration, typically accompanied by pancytopenia)
- Severe infection, resulting in rapid exit from the circulation to the site of sepsis

CLINICAL NOTES

FELTY SYNDROME

This term refers to the triad of rheumatoid arthritis (RA), splenomegaly and neutropenia. It arises as a complication of severe, long-standing RA. With improvements in treatment for RA, this is rarely seen nowadays.

Causes of lymphopenia

Lymphopenia is most commonly secondary to minor, community-acquired viral infections. Other important causes of lymphopenia are shown below.

CLINICAL NOTES

CAUSES OF LYMPHOPENIA

HIV infection, corticosteroid or other immunosuppressive drugs treatment, chemotherapy, Cushing syndrome, autoimmune disease (e.g., systemic lupus erythematosus, rheumatoid arthritis, sarcoidosis), Hodgkin lymphoma, MDS, trauma or surgery, liver or renal failure.

Mild lymphopenia has little in the way of clinical consequences. Prolonged severe lymphopenia, however, such as that seen in human immunodeficiency virus (HIV)-positive patients, carries with it the significant clinical consequences of immunodeficiency, primarily recurrent, severe and opportunistic infections.

● **Chapter Summary**

- Leucocytes are white blood cells. This group encompasses lymphocytes, neutrophils, eosinophils, basophils and monocytes. Each is differentiated by structure and function.
- Increased counts of particular groups of white cells are seen with particular infections, disease states and/or malignancies.
- Decreased counts ('leucopenia') of white blood cells overall (i.e., $\leq 4 \times 10^9$/L) place the patient at increased rate of infection.
- A decrease in the count of a specific white cell type (e.g., neutrophils: 'neutropenia') allow narrowing of the differential diagnosis, because the identity of the cell type with the decreased count will usually be associated with a particular set of conditions.
- Leucopenia may also suggest disorder of the bone marrow or immune system.
- The blood film, as for red cells, provides extremely useful diagnostic information for various acute and chronic disease states. For example, presence of immature neutrophils in peripheral blood may indicate acute infection.

Haematological malignancies

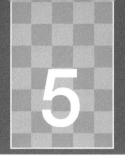

INTRODUCTION

Haematological malignancies can affect the bone marrow, lymph nodes, spleen and blood components. As with all neoplasias, the process begins with an abnormal DNA mutation. The pathological change may occur at any stage in haematopoietic development in any of the cell lineages. The change may occur due to genetic and/or environmental factors, often specific to each malignancy, but always results in:

- Unregulated, increased proliferation producing large numbers of identical daughter cells (clones) and
- Cellular 'immortalisation; resistance to normal apoptosis signals

CLINICAL NOTES

CONSTITUTIONAL SYMPTOMS ('B SYMPTOMS')

These include unexplained weight loss, low-grade fever and drenching night sweats. This is clarified early in this chapter as they are a feature at some point in nearly all haematological malignancies.

Classification of haematological malignancies is complex and has often varied with the categorising organisation, although the World Health Organization (WHO) classification is now considered standard and is widely accepted. Broadly, this is based on the cell of origin, the tissue location and the molecular change(s) resulting from the causative DNA mutation. In this chapter, we will classify them as follows:

- Myeloproliferative disorders: defined by excessive proliferation of one or more specific cell line(s) derived from a myeloid progenitor. These cells retain the ability to mature and differentiate normally. The myeloproliferative disorders typically follow an indolent course.
- Myelodysplastic disorders: a diverse group of bone marrow disorders characterised by clonal proliferation of myeloid cells that mature abnormally and incompletely ('dysplastic' cells). The most immature of these cells are known as 'blasts.'
- Leukaemias (acute and chronic): abnormal clonal proliferation of white blood cells.
- Lymphomas: pathological clonal proliferation of lymphoid cells, usually located in lymph nodes, spleen or extranodal lymphoid tissues.

- Plasma cell dyscrasias: abnormal clonal proliferation of plasma cells, which can secrete detectable levels of paraproteins (monoclonal immunoglobulins or immunoglobulin fragments).

MYELOPROLIFERATIVE NEOPLASMS

Myeloproliferative disorders arise from neoplastic transformation of a cellular precursor of myeloid lineage. The neoplastic cell proliferates, and the cells produced may follow one or more differentiation pathways. Myeloproliferative disorders differ from myelodysplasia and leukaemia in that these neoplastic cells are capable of differentiation and maturing. Myeloproliferative disorders are nonmalignant neoplasms but have the potential to further evolve into acute myeloid leukaemia. Clinically important myeloproliferative disorders are discussed in the following sections.

JAK2 gene mutation

JAK2 gene mutations are now seen as one of the defining features of myeloproliferative disorders. This gain-of-function mutation leads to a constitutively active (i.e., active response in absence of cytokine stimulus) proliferation scenario. Testing for the JAK2 mutation (performed on peripheral blood samples) is widely available and has become an integral test in the diagnosis of myeloproliferative disorders.

Polycythaemia rubra vera (primary polycythaemia)

This disorder is characterised by excessively high red cell numbers, resulting from a red cell precursor mutating and acquiring invulnerability to apoptosis. One of the established mechanisms leading to immortalisation in polycythaemia rubra vera (PRV) is an increase in sensitivity to antiapoptotic growth factor insulin-like growth factor. The pathologically elevated red cell levels are often accompanied by neutrophilia (in ~66% of cases) and thrombocytosis (in ~50% of cases). Transformation to acute leukaemia (probability of ~5% after 10 years) or myelofibrosis (probability of 20% after 10 years) can occur even if adequately treated. Treated patients have a median survival of at least 10–15 years. Thrombosis is the main cause of death in untreated patients.

Clinical features

PRV often presents insidiously at a median age of 60 years. Symptoms arise secondary to blood hyperviscosity due to increased cell numbers (Box 5.2). Around 40% of patients also have elevated histamine levels, resulting in gastroduodenal ulcers and pruritus exacerbated by warm baths/showers. On examination patients are plethoric and 30%–50% will have palpable splenomegaly or hepatosplenomegaly due to extramedullary haematopoiesis. The most serious complication of PRV is thrombosis, which may be arterial (myocardial infarction, cerebrovascular accident) or venous (deep venous thrombosis, pulmonary embolism).

CLINICAL NOTES

HYPERVISCOSITY SYNDROME

This may be due to increased cell numbers, as in PRV, or paraproteins, as in Waldenstrom macroglobulinaemia. Symptoms include headache, dizziness, tinnitus, vertigo, blurred vision, paraesthesia, oronasal bleeding, stupor and coma. Cerebral, coronary and peripheral vascular insufficiency (resulting from thromboses or flow disturbances) may lead to stroke, myocardial infarction and claudication, respectively.

Diagnostic tests

Full blood count (FBC) demonstrates raised red cell count, red cell mass, haemoglobin and haematocrit (>0.52 in men, >0.48 in women). There may be elevated neutrophil and/or platelet counts. Serum erythropoietin is low whilst plasma urate and lactate dehydrogenase (LDH) are often elevated. Bone marrow biopsy exhibits trilineage hyperplasia of erythroid, granulocytic and megakaryocytic cells and iron store depletion. Most patients can now be diagnosed on the basis of a raised haematocrit together with the presence of the JAK2 mutation, which is present in >90% of the patients, but there is still value in the above tests, particularly for complicated cases.

COMMON PITFALLS

EXCLUSION OF PHYSIOLOGICAL POLYCYTHAEMIA

Before diagnosing polycythaemia rubra vera, one must first exclude both *secondary* and *apparent* *polycythaemia*. Secondary polycythaemia is a predictable and appropriate rise in red cell numbers in response to factors such as chronic hypoxia

---

(e.g., chronic obstructive pulmonary disease, sleep apnoea or cyanotic heart disease) or excessively high erythropoietin (as in some hepatic, endocrine or renal disease). Red cell mass is increased in this subtype but there is no primary pathology in haematopoiesis. *Apparent polycythaemia* refers to conditions where the red cell mass is not increased but there is a reduced plasma volume. This is often seen in obesity, smoking, diuretic use, alcohol abuse and hypertension. Secondary and apparent polycythaemia are vastly more common than myeloproliferative disease and do not share the same risks or complications with the primary form of this disorder

Treatment

First-line treatment is venesection, lowering the haematocrit to ≤0.45. Aspirin reduces the risk of thrombosis, the major complication of PRV. Cytoreductive drugs such as hydroxycarbamide can be used. Radioactive phosphate (^{32}P) is restricted to elderly patients as it increases the chance of leukaemic transformation.

Primary (essential) thrombocythaemia

Also known as essential thrombocytosis (ET), this is a rare chronic disorder characterised by excessive production of platelets and thus elevated levels of platelets in the blood.

Clinical features

Nearly 50% of individuals with primary thrombocythaemia are asymptomatic at diagnosis, the elevated platelets being identified incidentally on a routine FBC performed for other reasons. Primary thrombocythaemia usually presents in patients older than 50 years but may occur at any age. In symptomatic individuals, the clinical presentation usually relates to complications of thrombus formation in blood vessels. Like PRV, ET can manifest with thrombosis in arteries, veins or the microvasculature. Microvascular thromboses may cause erythromelalgia (red, painful fingers and toes), gangrene and transient ischaemic attacks. Abnormal bleeding may also occur, particularly with platelet counts >1500 × 10^9/L, which can cause acquired von Willebrand disease (see Chapter 6: von Willebrand Disease) but is rarely severe. Around 5% of patients will have palpable splenomegaly. The risk of transformation to acute leukaemia (~1%–2% at 10 years) or myelofibrosis (~10% at 10 years) is less than that observed in PRV.

Diagnostic tests

A sustained, unexplained elevated platelet count (>450 × 10^9/L) suggests the diagnosis. This prompts bone marrow biopsy, which in ET exhibits a large number of abnormal megakaryocytes and hypercellularity. Cytogenetic studies may also identify chromosomal abnormalities associated with the diagnosis. Nearly 90% of patients will have an identifiable mutation. In 60% of patients with an identifiable mutation, it is the JAK2 mutation. CALR and MPL mutations are the next most common. Identification of JAK2, CALR or MPL mutations can obviate the need for a bone marrow biopsy.

COMMON PITFALLS

EXCLUSION OF REACTIVE THROMBOCYTOSIS

Before diagnosing essential thrombocytosis, one must first exclude *reactive thrombocytosis* as a cause of the raised platelet count which is much more common. Factors such as bleeding, infection, inflammation and iron deficiency anaemia must be first ruled out before considering myeloproliferative disease as the cause. Of particular note, elevated platelet counts are commonly seen postoperatively, especially following splenectomy. Importantly, all types of cancer may lead to thrombocytosis, which is thought to be mediated by increased interleukin-6.

Treatment

Initial management should address common vascular risk factors (i.e., hypertension, hypercholesterolaemia, smoking, diabetes, etc.). As ET has a generally favourable survival, only patients with a high risk of complications undergo treatment. A high risk of complications is conferred by:

- age older than 60 years
- platelet count >1500 × 10^9/L
- history of thrombosis.

Cytoreductive drugs are used to reduce platelet numbers to normal limits. These include hydroxycarbamide (first line), anagrelide, busulphan and interferon alpha (second-line). Daily low-dose aspirin is also given to reduce the risk of thrombosis.

Primary myelofibrosis

Primary myelofibrosis (PMF) is caused by clonal proliferation of a pluripotent stem cell. Fibrous tissue invades and replaces bone marrow territory. This occurs secondary to fibroblast proliferation and extracellular matrix formation, resulting from an abnormally high cytokine secretion (platelet-derived growth factor, transforming growth factor β) from abnormal megakaryocytes. Extramedullary haematopoiesis is a prominent feature, leading to massive splenomegaly and sometimes also hepatomegaly. Myelofibrosis may present de novo or evolve from other myeloproliferative conditions (e.g., PRV or ET). PMF has the worst prognosis of the myeloproliferative disorders. Median survival is just 5 years, and ~25% of cases transform further into acute myeloid leukaemia.

Clinical features

Patients, usually aged between 50 and 60 years, present with constitutional symptoms secondary to a hypermetabolic state. They may also complain of anaemic symptoms (fatigue, shortness of breath, palpitations) or abdominal pain (due to massive splenomegaly).

Diagnostic tests

Elevated white cell and platelet counts and reduced red cell counts are features of the FBC. The film is often diagnostic, revealing poikilocytosis (see Table 2.4), nucleated red cell precursors and granulocyte precursors. Bone marrow aspirate often results in a 'dry tap' where no aspirate is obtained due to fibrosis of the usual bone marrow territory. Trephine biopsy reveals patchily hypercellular marrow with prominent reticulin fibrosis: this finding is mandatory for diagnosis.

Cytogenetic analysis reveals karyotypic abnormalities in ~50% of patients. These are associated with a poorer prognosis. Approximately 50% exhibit the same JAK2 mutation that is seen in PRV and ET.

Treatment

Supportive transfusion of red cells, androgens, erythropoietin, thalidomide, lenalidomide or splenectomy are all options to controls the anaemia. Ruxolitinib is the first approved JAK2 inhibitor and is the treatment of choice for severe constitutional symptoms or symptomatic splenomegaly. The only curative treatment for PMF is bone marrow transplantation, but this is only appropriate for a small proportion of young patients and represents a very high-risk treatment strategy.

MYELODYSPLASTIC SYNDROMES

A heterogeneous array of disorders; myelodysplastic syndromes (MDS) are defined as a clonal disorder of haematopoietic stem cells where there is replacement of normal marrow by dysplastic, abnormal and immature ('blast') cells. Although the stem cells otherwise retain the capacity to differentiate into mature cells, they fail to mature normally and are functionally suboptimal. The cell counts of any cell line may be reduced. Often more than one cell line is affected. MDS may further develop into acute myeloid leukaemia.

Clinical features

Usually a disease of the elderly, the symptoms depend on the affected cell lines (e.g., neutropenia→recurrent infections, thrombocytopenia→easy bruising). Isolated anaemia is the most common presentation. However, MDS often presents nonspecifically or is discovered incidentally when unexplained cytopenias are further investigated in asymptomatic patients. MDS can develop in patients who have received chemotherapy and/or radiotherapy for another condition

Diagnostic tests

FBC usually reveals cytopenia(s) and blood film demonstrates characteristic morphological abnormalities in the affected cell lines. Red cell macrocytosis is a common finding in MDS, and in one of the subtypes peripheral monocytosis is an additional common feature. Bone marrow examination, together with cytogenetic analysis, are diagnostic and facilitates classification (Table 5.1), prognostication and treatment decision-making.

Treatment

Treatment (and prognosis) is guided by a prognostic scoring system. In elderly or less fit patients, treatment is essentially supportive. Anaemia can sometimes be managed with erythropoietin or lenalidomide but more commonly regular red cell transfusions are required. Thrombocytopenia (if associated with abnormal bleeding) is managed with regular platelet transfusions. Neutropenic patients require appropriate antimicrobial prophylaxis and may benefit from G-CSF. Regular clinical supervision is essential to monitor for development of acute myeloid leukaemia (AML).

In fitter patients, more intensive treatment can be used. Azacytidine, a hypomethylating agent, may induce remissions but is not curative. Chemotherapy (as for AML) followed by stem cell transplant is the only curative option.

LEUKAEMIAS

Leukaemias are characterised by an accumulation of leukaemic cells in bone marrow and often also peripheral blood.

Table 5.1 The 2016 World Health Organization myelodysplastic syndrome subtypes (simplified)

Name	Dysplastic lineages	Cytopenias[a]	BM and PB blasts
MDS with single lineage dysplasia	1	1 or 2	BM <5%, PB <1%, no Auer rods
MDS with multilineage dysplasia	2 or 3	1 to 3	BM <5%, PB <1%, no Auer rods
MDS with ring sideroblasts	1–3	1–3	BM <5%, PB <1%, no Auer rods *and* ring sideroblasts ≥15% (or ≥5% if *SF3B1* mutation positive)
MDS with isolated del(5q)	1–3	1–2	BM <5%, PB <1%, no Auer rods with del (5q) mutation alone *or* with 1 additional abnormality (excluding -7 or del (7q))
MDS with excess blasts: MDS-EB-1	0–3	1–3	BM 5 to 9% or PB 2%–4%, no Auer rods
MDS with excess blasts: MDS-EB-2	0–3	1–3	BM 10%–19% or PB 5%–19% or Auer rods
MDS-U with 1% blood blasts	1–3	1–3	BM <5%, PB = 1%, no Auer rods
MDS-U with single lineage dysplasia and pancytopenia	1	3	BM <5%, PB <1%, no Auer rods
MDS-U based on defining cytogenetic abnormality	0	1 to 3	BM <5%, PB <1%, no Auer rods

[a] *In this context, cytopenias are defined as haemoglobin <100 g/L, platelet count <100 × 10⁹/L and neutrophil count <1.8 × 10⁹/L. Rarely, MDS may present with mild anaemia or thrombocytopenia above these levels. Peripheral blood monocytes must be <1 × 10⁹/L.*
BM, Bone marrow; MDS, myelodysplastic syndrome; MDS-U, myelodysplastic syndrome unclassifiable; PB, peripheral blood.

Leukaemic cells are 'clonal' (i.e., identical to the original neoplastic cell) and nonfunctional. However, they occupy marrow territory, impairing normal haematopoiesis. This leads to cytopenia in all cell lines. Leukaemias are classified according to:

- Cell lineage – lymphoid or myeloid
- Maturity of the abnormal cell population: this defines whether the leukaemia is classified as 'acute' or 'chronic,' rather than purely by the clinical course and presentation as one might expect from the name.

Acute leukaemias are defined by proliferation of an immature 'blast' cell, and untreated are rapidly fatal. Chronic leukaemias are defined by proliferation of a more mature cell, and the clinical course is more prolonged. Treatment for leukaemias, particularly acute leukaemias, can lead to tumour lysis syndrome.

ACUTE LEUKAEMIAS

Clinical features

Patients are usually very unwell at presentation. Immediate admission and acute resuscitation including intravenous antibiotics, appropriate transfusion and correction of any metabolic abnormalities (these are particularly associated with a high tumour burden) comprise acute management. Intensive chemotherapy is urgently required or death occurs rapidly from sepsis or bleeding. Constitutional and leucostatic symptoms are common. Symptoms may also relate to the cytopenias and include:

- severe fatigue, pallor and breathlessness (anaemia)
- easy bruising or abnormal bleeding (thrombocytopenia, disseminated intravascular coagulation (DIC))
- fever and recurrent infections (neutropenia)

Other symptoms include:

- Deposition of leukaemic cells in tissue (e.g., gum hypertrophy in AML)
- Lymphadenopathy and hepatosplenomegaly in acute lymphoblastic leukaemia (ALL)
- Infiltration of leukaemic cells in the cerebrospinal fluid (CSF) and central nervous system (CNS; most commonly seen in ALL)

There is usually no particular cause identified, but AML and ALL may be associated with radiation, toxins or drug exposure and certain chromosomal disorders (e.g., trisomy 21).

Diagnostic tests

FBC exhibits anaemia and thrombocytopenia. The white cell count may be very high or very low. Blood film demonstrates the abnormal morphology of blast cells. Bone marrow biopsy exhibiting blasts is diagnostic, and cytogenetics is mandatory as the leukaemic cell karyotype is the strongest prognostic factor regarding survival and response to treatment. Molecular genetics are also important as particular mutations carry prognostic significance. Levels of LDH and uric acid may offer an indication of the tumour burden.

Acute myeloid leukaemia

Acute myeloid leukaemia (AML) is the most common adult acute leukaemia. The original neoplastic blast cell is a myeloid precursor cell. Particular chromosomal rearrangements, such as t(15:17), t(8:21) and inversion of 16 have better prognoses than others (e.g., monosomy 7). Importantly, AML can evolve from existing myeloproliferative or myelodysplastic disorders or chronic myeloid leukaemia (CML). As well as accumulation of blasts in marrow and peripheral blood, skin, gum and organ infiltration may occur. The current WHO classification of AML is complex and based on cytogenetic re-arrangements and molecular mutations present in the neoplastic clone. The old FAB classification was based on degree of maturation and differentiation of the myeloid lineage (M1 to M7). These subtypes impact on prognosis and crucially whether a patient requires a stem cell transplant. Overall cure rates vary from 30%–80% depending on the subtype.

CLINICAL NOTES

INDUCTION TREATMENT

'Induction treatment' aims to reduce or eradicate the leukaemic cell population and restore normal bone marrow haemopoiesis (i.e., 'induce' remission). 'Consolidation' treatment aims to destroy lingering but undetectable leukaemic cells.

CLINICAL NOTES

ALLOGENEIC STEM CELL TRANSPLANTATION (SCT)

SCT aims to replace cancerous marrow cells with disease-free haematopoietic stem cells from donor marrow ('bone marrow transplant') or donor peripheral blood ('peripheral blood stem cell transplant'). Prior to donation, chemotherapy and/or radiotherapy is employed to destroy the native cancerous cells before replacing with the healthy donor cells. Ideally the donor is HLA-matched to reduce the probability of graft-versus-host disease (GVHD), which is when the donor (graft) cells recognize patient (host) cells as foreign, thereby initiating an immune reaction in the transplant recipient. This is primarily a T cell mediated disease and a major cause of morbidity and mortality. Immunosuppressive therapy is also used to reduce the chances of GVHD. In addition to GVHD, graft failure (immune rejection of donor cells by the recipient) and organ damage may complicate SCT. This is thus a high-risk procedure with treatment-related mortality of 20%–30% (death due to the procedure rather that the underlying condition).

HINTS AND TIPS

REMISSION

The term 'remission' describes an absence of disease signs and symptoms. It may be permanent or temporary, ending with reappearance of signs and symptoms ('relapse'). 'Complete remission' describes clinical absence as well as normalised histology and function.

Acute promyelocytic leukaemia

Acute promyelocytic leukaemia (APML) is a particular subtype of AML (M3 in the previous FAB classification). It is characterised by the t(15:17) translocation and (in addition to the findings listed above) often shows features of DIC. It carries a high risk of fatal haemorrhage during the early phase of treatment. However, after the initial phase, it has the best prognosis of all subtypes with cure rates of >80%.

Treatment of AML

This comprises two phases: induction and consolidation. In AML, induction treatment usually comprises cytarabine plus an anthracycline such as daunorubicin. Postinduction treatment usually comprises further chemotherapy, allogeneic stem cell transplantation or a combination of the two. Certain specific mutations respond to specific treatments; for example, t(15:17), associated with acute promyelocytic leukaemia responds to all-trans retinoic acid.

HINTS AND TIPS

STEM CELL SOURCES

Stem cells may be sourced from the patient themselves (autologous transplant) as opposed to a different person (allogeneic transplant). Autologous SCT is often used as consolidation in treatment of myeloma and lymphoma but not for leukaemias.

Acute lymphoblastic leukaemia

The most common childhood cancer, acute lymphoblastic leukaemia (ALL) accounts for 80% of all childhood leukaemias. The leukaemic blast cells may be of B cell (~80%) or T cell origin. Of note, the Philadelphia chromosome (see subsequent CML section), when seen in ALL (up to 20% of ALL cases), carries a poorer prognosis. As well as the clinical features of acute leukaemias described earlier, hepatosplenomegaly is often present at diagnosis.

Treatment

Fortunately, childhood ALL is more responsive to treatment than AML, with cure rates of >80%. However, adult cure rates are only ~40%. Unlike AML, treatment comprises four phases: induction, consolidation, CNS prophylaxis and continuing then on with maintenance treatment which lasts 2–3 years. In high-risk ALL, stem cell transplant (SCT) is used in place of maintenance treatment.

Induction treatment usually comprises daunorubicin, vincristine, corticosteroids and asparaginase, and if the Philadelphia chromosome is present, tyrosine kinase inhibitors are added (see CML). Allopurinol or rasburicase are used as prophylaxis against tumour lysis syndrome. Consolidation treatment, followed by maintenance treatment, may include cytarabine, methotrexate, mercaptopurine, anthracyclines (e.g., daunorubicin), alkylating agents (e.g., cyclophosphamide), vincristine and epipodophyllotoxins (e.g., etoposide).

ALL has a very high propensity to spread to the CNS and thus a specific treatment phase for CNS prophylaxis is included. This is further boosted by intrathecal chemotherapy i.e., chemotherapy injected directly into the CSF.

CHRONIC LEUKAEMIAS

Chronic leukaemias are often detected incidentally in asymptomatic patients when an elevated white count is noted on FBC. Large numbers of leukaemic cells exist, due to both proliferation and decreased apoptosis. Symptoms develop insidiously and are often secondary to cytopenias (as with the acute leukaemias), which arise due to marrow displacement by leukaemic cells. Similarly, constitutional or leucostatic symptoms often occur. They differ from acute leukaemias in that:

- the marrow is not infiltrated with immature blasts
- near-normal maturation and differentiation of nonclonal 'normal' cell lines continue in parallel with the neoplastic clone.

Chronic myeloid leukaemia

The original neoplastic cell is a myeloid cell precursor that undergoes uncontrolled proliferation as well reduced apoptosis. This proliferation causes an increase in all cells of myeloid lineage (i.e., granulocytes and their precursors [neutrophils, myelocytes, metamyelocytes, eosinophils, basophils, etc.]). Granulocyte hyperplasia is apparent in the blood, bone marrow and spleen. These cells all display the original neoplastic abnormality, a translocation known as the Philadelphia chromosome. Chronic myeloid leukaemia (CML) cells all possess the potential to transform to AML.

However, unlike the acute leukaemias, the actual leukaemic cell ('blast') population is not dramatically increased in peripheral blood. If the blast population does increase, this may represent the 'accelerated' phase in the disease progression, or above a certain level the transition to acute myeloid leukaemia.

The Philadelphia chromosome

The chromosomal translocation t(9:22) results in movement of the proto-oncogene ABL (normally located on chromosome 9) adjacent to the BCR gene on chromosome 22. This leads to a shortened chromosome 22, which is termed the Philadelphia chromosome and is a hallmark of CML, diagnostic when present in a patient with clinical manifestations of CML. The BCR/ABL fusion gene encodes a constitutively active tyrosine kinase. Expression of this protein leads to development of CML.

Clinical features

CML evolves following a predictable course, consisting of three stages: chronic, accelerated and blast crisis. Ninety percent of CML is diagnosed in the earliest chronic stage, when asymptomatic patients are further investigated after markedly elevated granulocytic counts are noted on a FBC. When CML is symptomatic, the symptoms result from splenomegaly, leucostasis or they may be constitutional in nature. Dramatic splenomegaly is present in >50% patients at diagnosis.

Diagnostic tests

White cell count, attributable to leukaemic granulocytes, is significantly ($>20 \times 10^9$/L) and often dramatically elevated. Basophil, eosinophils and myeloid precursor cells are elevated, and anaemia may be present. Appearance of blasts on film and thrombocytopenia signals progression to the accelerated disease stage. Serum PCR identifies and quantifies the amount of the BCR-ABL fusion gene transcript, thus allowing diagnosis with a simple blood sample. Bone marrow biopsy assists with staging and confirmation of the disease, and cytogenetics confirms presence of the Philadelphia chromosome.

Treatment

Because the chromosomal hallmark of CML results in abnormal tyrosine kinase activity, CML treatments centre around tyrosine kinase inhibitors (TKI). Imatinib was the first of the TKI inhibitors and has become a paradigm for targeted therapies; this has completely changed the landscape of first-line treatment for CML. While in the past, without an SCT, most patients would transform to acute leukaemia, today imatinib and other TKIs can induce complete haematological, cytogenetic and molecular remission. Since its initial development, several other TKIs have been developed which appear to be even more effective that imatinib (see Table 5.6).

If diagnosed in the blast crisis stage, treatment resembles that of the acute leukaemias. Severe leucostatic symptoms may be managed with leucopheresis. However even at this stage, one of the TKI drugs is added to the treatment.

Chronic lymphocytic leukaemia

The original neoplastic cell is usually a lymphoid B cell precursor, arrested in development. The resulting leukaemic cell population resemble mature (but nonfunctional) B cells. They infiltrate bone marrow, lymph nodes, spleen and liver. Those in peripheral blood may appear normal or as 'smear cells.' As with other haematological malignancies, chromosomal mutations are common and have an important bearing on the prognosis and response to treatment. Clinical progression is widely variable depending on the stage of the disease at diagnosis. Staging is determined according to number of lymphadenopathy sites, anaemia and thrombocytopenia and presence of various biomarkers. Significantly, up to 5% of cases of chronic lymphocytic leukaemia (CLL) can evolve further into high-grade lymphomas. This evolution is termed Richter's transformation.

Clinical features

CLL is the most common adult leukaemia, is nearly twice as common in males and usually occurs in the elderly (median age at presentation, 72 years). In addition to the features common to the chronic leukaemias listed above, painless generalised lymphadenopathy is the most common presenting symptom. Cytopenias are the other common finding. Patients with CLL are particularly prone to infections even in the absence of cytopenias as they often have hypogammaglobulinaemia with poor antibody response to infections. Patients with CLL also have a high incidence of autoimmune cytopenias, in particular immune thrombocytopenia and autoimmune haemolytic anaemia.

Diagnostic tests

The initial finding is usually a mild to marked elevation in total white cell count due to the leukemic cell population. Unusually, bone marrow examination is not mandatory for CLL diagnosis: diagnosis is instead based on characteristic morphology of leukaemic cells ('smear cells') on blood film, a sustained count $>5 \times 10^9$/L clonal B cells and presence of a diagnostic immunophenotype. Lymphocyte doubling time (LDT) as an index of disease progression can be established with serial measurements.

Treatment

'Early' CLL is simply monitored with regular review because the risk:benefit ratio favours this approach in inactive disease. Treatment is commenced when the disease is deemed 'active.' This is defined by:

- progressive failure of bone marrow haematopoiesis (indicated by worsening cytopenias)
- massive, progressive or symptomatic splenomegaly or lymphadenopathy
- an LDT <6 months
- presence of constitutional symptoms

Treatment is not to cure but to achieve remission, which can last years. The disease tends to recur, requiring additional treatment strategies. The treatment usually involves various combinations of chemotherapy and immunotherapy drugs. Common chemotherapy drugs used include fludarabine (F), cyclophosphamide (C), bendamustine (B) and chlorambucil (Chl). Commonly used monoclonal antibodies used include rituximab (R), obinutuzumab (O) and ofatumumab (Of). Depending on the fitness of the patient, various combinations are used (e.g., FCR, BR and OChl).

Treatment of CLL has undergone a revolution in the last few years with 'chemotherapy free' treatments becoming available. These targeted drugs act on the cellular pathways in the B lymphocytes, are orally active and used as continuous daily treatment as long as the disease remains responsive. Ibrutinib, idelalisib and venetoclax are three such drugs all available for the second-line treatments, although they will soon most probably be recategorized as first-line treatments.

MALIGNANT LYMPHOMAS

Lymphomas are characterised by accumulation of clonal neoplastic cells in lymph nodes and extranodal lymphoid tissue (e.g., lungs). The original mutated cell a primitive lymphoid cell. They are nonfunctional and occupy lymph node territory, impairing normal development of immune cells. Lymphomas are categorised as:

- Non-Hodgkin lymphoma (NHL; ~90%)
- Hodgkin lymphoma (HL; ~10%)

Clinical features of lymphomas

Presentation varies enormously among individuals. Common clinical features shared by most lymphomas include:

- Painless, nontender lymphadenopathy (most common sites cervical, then axillary)
- Constitutional, aka B symptoms (fever, night sweats, weight loss)
- Pruritus
- Mild/moderate splenomegaly

- Superior vena cava obstruction or respiratory symptoms in cases with mediastinal lymphadenopathy
- Human immunodeficiency virus infection significantly increases the risk of developing many high-grade B cell NHL as well as HL.

COMMON PITFALLS

DIFFERENTIATING LEUKAEMIAS AND LYMPHOMAS

Avoid the common pitfall of oversimplifying leukaemias as being bone marrow diseases and lymphomas being lymph node diseases. Both leukaemic and lymphoma cells are also present in the blood and lymphoma cells may invade marrow too.

Differentiating clinical and aetiological features differentiating HL and NHL are shown in Table 5.2

Lymphoma staging is predominantly clinical, traditionally via the Ann Arbor staging system, shown in Table 5.3. Stages I and II are described as 'limited stage' and III and IV as 'advanced stage.'

Diagnostic tests in lymphomas

Serum uric acid and LDH are often elevated. FBC may show cytopenias. An enlarged lymph node is surgically resected and examined by a histopathologist for histology, immunophenotype and molecular genetics. Bone marrow examination will identify presence and extent of invasion by lymphoma cells. Computed tomography (CT) scanning identifies clinically impalpable or unnoticed areas of lymphadenopathy. A positron emission tomography-CT (PET-CT) scan can give further information regarding the extent of the disease and has become mandatory in all high-grade NHL and HL.

Non-Hodgkin lymphomas

These consist of around 60 subtypes with heterogeneous characteristics. Incidence rises with age (median age being 60) and is higher in males. In ~85% the original neoplastic cell is a mature B cell or a B-cell progenitor. The remainder are of T or natural killer (NK) cell origin. They are characterised by grade. Tumour lysis syndrome is a dangerous complication that is not uncommon in NHL patients undergoing treatment.

Table 5.2 Features differentiating Hodgkin lymphoma from non-Hodgkin lymphoma

Non-Hodgkin lymphoma	Hodgkin lymphoma
Median age of presentation for most NHL tends to be >50 years of age	Presentations peak at ages in both 20s and 60s
Alcohol-induced pain in lymph nodes is not seen in NHL	A small fraction of HL patients may experience alcohol-induced pain of enlarged lymph nodes – a classical pathognomic feature
Cyclical fever not a feature	Patients may experience cyclical fever, known as Pel-Ebstein fever
Tends to involve extranodal lymphoid tissue more than HL Spleen, liver, thymus and mucosally associated lymphoid tissue in the gastrointestinal tract are predilection zones	Less likely to involve extranodal lymphoid tissue
Distant lymph node involvement with the intermediate lymph nodes 'skipped' is common	Lymph node involvement is typically contiguous
May be associated with: • Infection (e.g., EBV or HTLV) • Immunodeficiency (e.g., HIV) • Autoimmune disease • Exposure to radiation therapy or carcinogens • Certain inherited diseases such as ataxia telangiectasia, Fanconi syndrome, etc.	May also associated with: • Infection (e.g., EBV) • Immunodeficiency (e.g., HIV)
Patients more likely to experience cytopenias due to increased likelihood of marrow invasion	Patients less likely to experience marrow invasion and cytopenias
Tumour lysis syndrome occurs more commonly in NHL patients undergoing treatment	Tumour lysis syndrome is very rare in HL patients

EBV, Epstein–Barr virus; HIV, human immunodeficiency virus; HL, Hodgkin lymphoma; HTLV, human T cell lymphoma virus; NHL, non-Hodgkin lymphoma.

Table 5.3 Cotswold-modified Ann Arbor lymphoma staging system

Stage[a]	Sites of involvement
I	Single lymph node region or one contiguous extranodal lymphatic site (e.g., liver)
II	Two or more lymph node regions on the *same* side of the diaphragm
III	Lymph node regions on *both* sides of the diaphragm, which may involve extralymphatic extension
IV	Diffuse involvement of more than one extranodal lymphatic site (e.g., bone marrow, gut, lung, liver)

[a] *Each stage is further subclassified to indicate absence (A) or presence (B) or one or more of the following three systemic symptoms: unexplained fever (≥38.3°C), night sweats and/or unexplained weight loss ≥10% body weight in the 6 months preceding diagnosis.*

RED FLAG

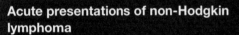

Acute presentations of non-Hodgkin lymphoma

Features may include hypercalcemia, tumour lysis syndrome, spinal cord compression, superior or inferior vena cava compression, autoimmune haemolytic anaemia, intestinal or ureteral compression, central nervous system mass lesions or lymphomatous meningitis.

High-grade non-Hodgkin lymphomas

These are aggressive and progress rapidly. The rapid division means they are susceptible to chemotherapy and a significant proportion are curable. They often present

---

RED FLAG

Tumour lysis syndrome

This a dangerous complication of chemotherapy for leukaemias and lymphomas with a high neoplastic cell load. As these are destroyed they release intracellular components into the circulation, manifesting as hyperkalaemia, hyperuricaemia and hyperphosphataemia, the latter causing secondary hypocalcaemia. This can cause fatal arrhythmias and acute kidney injury, as well as acute gout. As prophylaxis, all patients receive uric acid reducing drugs (allopurinol or rasburicase) as well as intravenous hydration and vigilant monitoring for evidence of hyperkalaemia.

---

acutely. Examples include diffuse large B cell lymphoma, mantle cell lymphoma and Burkitt lymphoma. T-cell NHL can also manifest cutaneously, which may be localised (Mycosis fungoides) or widespread (Sézary syndrome).

Low-grade NHL

These are 'indolent,' with clinical signs (e.g., lymphadenopathy/organomegaly) developing slowly. They have a longer median survival but are usually incurable. Examples include follicular lymphoma, small lymphocytic lymphoma and splenic marginal zone lymphoma.

One particular indolent NHL is called mucosa associated lymphoid tissue (MALT) lymphoma, which usually arises due to persistent chronic inflammation at these sites. Gastric MALT lymphoma is the most common form and is preceded by *Helicobacter pylori* infection. When localised to the gastric mucosa, it often responds to antibiotic therapy aimed at eliminating the bacteria.

Treatment of NHL

The R-CHOP regimen is one of the most commonly employed regimens. This consists of rituximab, cyclophosphamide, doxorubicin, vincristine and prednisolone. Radiation may additionally be utilised. However, there are various regimes used for particular subtypes.

Hodgkin lymphoma

Previously known as Hodgkin disease, HL typically has bimodal age distribution with a first peak in the 20s and the second peak in the 60s, with a slight male preponderance. The original neoplastic cell is a B cell derivative with a dysfunctional immunoglobulin gene, termed a Reed-Sternberg (RS) cell. Microscopically the RS cell has an 'owl's eye' appearance, with prominent multinucleated nuclei and eosinophilic cytoplasm. The RS cells usually make up 1%–2% of the lymph node cellularity with surrounding reactive macrophages, lymphocytes, plasma cells and eosinophils. Ninety-five percent of HL is 'classical' and classified histologically as follows:

- Nodular sclerosing: the most common subtype. Collagen bands divide affected nodes into nodules.
- Lymphocyte-rich: large numbers of lymphocytes are seen, relative to RS cells. This carries a more favourable prognosis.
- Mixed cellularity: more RS cells are present relative to lymphocytes.
- Lymphocyte-depleted: RS cells are present in the highest proportion relative to lymphocytes. This subtype has the poorest prognosis of all HL subtypes.

The remaining 5% of HL is termed nodular lymphocyte – predominant Hodgkin lymphoma (NLPHL). Clinical staging is the most accurate indicator of long-term prognosis in HL, and as for NHL the revised Ann Arbor system is used. The histological subtypes, on the other hand, have very little prognostic value. In classical HL, the most common lymph nodes involved are the cervical lymph nodes (~75% of patients) followed by mediastinal, axillary and the para-aortic lymph nodes (see Fig. 1.3).

Treatment

Treatment strategy is chosen according to stage. Many patients require dual treatment with both combination chemotherapy and radiotherapy. With current treatment protocols cure rates vary from ~60 to ≥90%, depending upon the stage at diagnosis.

AGE-SPECIFIC HAEMATOLOGICAL MALIGNANCY RISK

Certain haematological malignancies are more common in different age groups. The *most* common haematological malignancies for each of the following age groups are as follows:

- Childhood: acute lymphoblastic leukaemia
- Adult leukaemia: chronic lymphocyte leukaemia
- Adult lymphoma: diffuse large-cell B cell lymphoma
- Teenagers/young adults: Hodgkin lymphoma

PLASMA CELL DYSCRASI AS

These are malignant monoclonal proliferations of a neoplastic plasma cell, which synthesise an abnormal immunoglobulin (paraprotein) and/or abnormal light chain. Paraproteins and light chains can be identified in the serum while the light chains can also be found in the urine (Bence-Jones proteins). The most common dyscrasia is monoclonal gammopathy of undetermined significance (MGUS), but multiple myeloma, solitary plasmacytoma and Waldenstrom macroglobulinaemia are also clinically important entities.

Multiple myeloma

This is a disease of late middle age onwards with incidence ~5/100,000 annually. Aetiology is unclear, although there is an increased incidence in patients with previous exposure to ionising radiation. Staging according to International Staging System is from stages I to III according to age, laboratory and cytogenetic findings.

Clinical features

These are legion but the four most common are abbreviated as 'CRAB' symptoms.

- Calcium. Hypercalcaemia (due to increased bone resorption)
- Renal. The kidneys are particularly affected, leading to renal impairment in ~25% of patients and severe renal failure in ~5%. This may be secondary to dehydration, nonsteroidal antiinflammatory drug use (for bone pain), recurrent sepsis, hypercalcaemia, renal tubular obstruction from proteinaceous casts and light chain proximal tubular toxicity to proximal tubules.
- Anaemia (normochromic and normocytic) due to plasma cell infiltration of the bone marrow.
- Bone. Lytic lesions (Fig. 5.1) resulting from bone destruction, predominantly affecting the axial skeleton, are a hallmark of the disease, with back pain being a very common symptom. Diffuse osteoporosis results in pathological fractures. Bone pain is the most common symptom of multiple myeloma, present in ~60% of patients.

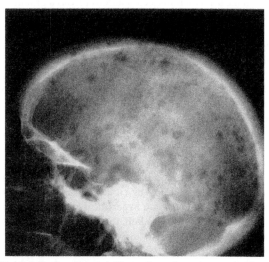

Fig. 5.1 Skull radiograph illustrating a 'pepper-pot skull' in a patient with multiple myeloma. The appearance is of multiple osteolytic bone lesions. Courtesy Dr M. Makris.

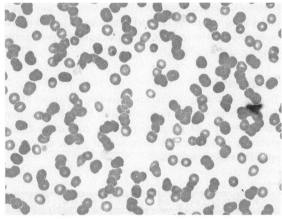

Fig. 5.2 Blood film showing red cell rouleaux (stacked, overlapping cells). These arise due to excessive levels of high-molecular-weight proteins in blood. This is seen in multiple myeloma, but also in other nonhaematological inflammatory conditions.

Other symptoms include:

- Immune. Neutropenia and lack of functional immunoglobulins results in high susceptibility to persistent and recurrent infections.
- Neurological. Symptoms secondary to spinal cord or nerve root compression by collapse of the vertebrae due to lytic bone lesions.
- Amyloidosis. ~10% of patients with myeloma will develop AL amyloidosis.

Diagnostic tests

The erythrocyte sedimentation rate (ESR) is raised and blood film demonstrates rouleaux (Fig. 5.2). Bence-Jones proteins (which are essentially light chains) are often present in the urine. Serum electrophoresis reveals a prominent discrete band (Fig. 5.3, lane 4) representing the paraprotein (immunoglobulin) in 80% of patients. (IgG > IgA > IgD: IgM paraproteins are associated with Waldenstrom rather than multiple myeloma.)

In the remaining 20% only *free* light chains are produced; since the clonal plasma cells produce only *one* type of light chain (kappa or lambda), it leads to a very abnormal κ:λ ratio. This is called light chain myeloma.

In a very small percentage the malignant plasma cell *does not* secrete a paraprotein *or* light chains – this rare variant is referred to as nonsecretory myeloma.

Bone marrow examination in multiple myeloma shows >10% occupation by clonal plasma cells. There may be renal impairment, hypercalcaemia and anaemia (CRAB signs). X-rays of skull, thorax, pelvis and proximal long bones comprises a skeletal survey, looking for lytic lesions. Such skeletal assessments are more often being replaced by magnetic resonance imaging and PET scans.

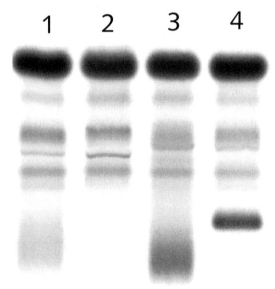

Fig. 5.3 Serum electrophoresis. Electrophoresis uses an electric field to separate proteins across a gel matrix according to various properties including molecular size. Each band, which is visible when stained appropriately, represents a protein of a specific molecular weight. Lane 1: normal serum. Lane 2: antibody-deficient serum. Lane 3: serum from an infected patient, illustrating polyclonal immunoglobulins. Lane 4: myeloma patient serum illustrating prominent band representing monoclonal immunoglobulin.

Treatment

Without effective treatment, median survival is 6 months. Patients are risk stratified according to presence/absence of specific genetic abnormalities in their neoplastic clone. Induction therapy is commenced in all patients regardless of suitability for SCT. This usually consists of various combinations of traditional chemotherapy drugs (cyclophosphamide, melphalan), immunomodulatory drugs (thalidomide, lenalidomide), proteasome inhibitors (bortezomib, carfilzomib) and a steroid. Fitter patients then receive consolidation treatment with autologous stem cell transplantation, while others may remain on a single agent as maintenance therapy. Although such treatments can achieve complete remissions, relapse is inevitable and further lines of treatments are necessary. Supportive management includes adequate analgesia, sufficient hydration and bisphosphonates.

Solitary plasmacytoma

A solitary plasmacytoma is a solid tumour consisting of a neoplastic proliferation of plasma cells. They may be osseous (develop in bone) or extraosseous (develop in soft tissue). The former usually progresses to multiple myeloma, but the latter responds well to surgical resection and radiotherapy, thus it has an excellent prognosis.

Monoclonal gammopathy of uncertain significance

When a paraprotein is present, but the neoplastic plasma cells occupy <10% of the marrow, and clinical features of myeloma are absent, the condition is termed monoclonal gammopathy of uncertain significance (MGUS). This is present in ~3% of people older than 50 years and the incidence rises to >7% by age 80 years. Only ~1% of patients with MGUS will progress to symptomatic myeloma (if IgG or IgA) or NHL/ Waldenstrom (if IgM) annually. There are various prognostic factors and scoring systems that more accurately quantify this risk.

Differentiation between MGUS and MM

Both are plasma cell dyscrasias, but MGUS is benign and asymptomatic, in particular lacking any of the CRAB signs (hypercalcaemia, renal impairment, anaemia and bone lesions) and does not warrant treatment.

Amyloidosis

Amyloidosis refers to the extracellular deposition of abnormal protein variants. These variants restructure into fibrils with a beta-pleated sheet secondary structure. Various soluble serum proteins have the potential to restructure abnormally and deposit in this manner (e.g., immunoglobulin light chains). This subtype is referred to as Amyloid light-chain (AL) amyloidosis and may occur in association with plasma cell dyscrasias. Amyloidosis is also a feature of other unrelated disorders such as chronic inflammatory illnesses (amyloid A protein (AA) amyloidosis). The hereditary form is referred to as amyloid transthyretin (ATTR) amyloidosis. It may be multi-system, or rarely, localised.

Clinical features

An enormous range of clinical manifestations may occur, determined by the location, precursor protein type and the extent of deposits. Marked proteinuria in the nephrotic range (renal disease), peripheral and autonomic neuropathies and restrictive cardiomyopathy form the classic triad of symptoms. Other symptoms include organomegaly, CNS disease, skin manifestations and musculoskeletal and pulmonary disease.

Diagnosis

Diagnosis is made when biopsied subcutaneous fat stained with Congo red show green birefringence on exposure to polarised light. In AL amyloidosis, an abnormal light chain ratio can often be demonstrated in the blood, and bone marrow examination may show evidence of clonal plasma cells. A serum amyloid P component scan allows detection and localisation of amyloid deposits and is available at the NHS National Amyloidosis Centre, London.

Treatment

In AL amyloidosis, management focuses on treatment of the underlying plasma cell dyscrasia, which is similar to the treatment for myeloma, but with additional aggressive supportive treatment for the renal and cardiac disease.

Waldenstrom macroglobulinaemia

This rare disorder (incidence: 3/million/year) usually presents around age 50–70 years, more frequently in males. It is characterised by a B-cell lymphoproliferative marrow-based process, IgM paraprotein and elevated blood viscosity. If hyperviscosity occurs, plasmapheresis may be necessary. Constitutional symptoms, cytopenias and paraneoplastic neuropathy may occur. As with multiple myeloma, the paraprotein interferes with normal platelet function and coagulation factors, increasing bleeding tendency. Treatment aims to control symptoms and minimise end-organ damage.

INVESTIGATIONS IN HAEMATOLOGICAL MALIGNANCY

Erythrocyte sedimentation rate and plasma viscosity

ESR is the rate at which red cells sediment in 1 hour. The 'normal' rate varies with age, gender and pregnancy. The major variable affecting ESR is the concentration of plasma proteins; the higher the concentration, the higher the ESR. ESR corresponds with plasma viscosity, an automated test. It is raised in inflammation (infectious and noninfectious) and, importantly, in malignancy.

Serum lactate dehydrogenase

In malignancy, normal tissues damaged by the neoplastic process experience increased cell death, releasing their intracellular LDH. In addition, the increased metabolic rate of rapidly dividing neoplastic cells enforces increased reliance on glycolysis, resulting in very high intracellular LDH. When these cells die, this LDH is released. Elevated levels are thus used as a serum marker of cellular damage. Malignancies with a particularly large malignant cell load (i.e., many haematological malignancies) can exhibit dramatically elevated LDH. Likewise, haemolysis results in raised LDH. It is useful in approximating disease load in lymphomas and leukaemias, particularly in quantifying response to treatment and prognosis.

Serum urate

Elevated uric acid (which at physiological pH exists as the urate anion) is known as 'hyperuricaemia'. More commonly clinically associated with gout, renal failure or genetic errors in purine metabolism, hyperuricaemia very important in the context of haematological malignancy. This is because hyperuricaemia is associated with high rates of cell death and nucleoprotein destruction, as occurs in chemotherapy, and sometimes as a feature of the malignancy itself.

> **RED FLAG**
>
> **Hyperuricaemia**
>
> This results in painful urate crystal deposition in joints, renal stones and renal failure. To avoid hyperuricaemia, xanthine oxidase inhibitors such as allopurinol or recombinant urate oxidase (e.g., rasburicase) are coadministered prophylactically during chemotherapy.

Bone marrow biopsies

Biopsies of bone marrow are used to diagnose and/or stage haematological diseases, including malignancies. It is an ambulatory procedure with low morbidity performed under local anaesthesia. Two techniques are employed: bone marrow aspiration and trephine biopsy.

Trephine biopsy

A trephine biopsy is obtained via a large-bore needle, inserted into the iliac crest. This yields a core of bone and marrow, which is examined as a histological specimen. These are useful for assessing marrow cellularity and architecture. Table 5.4 describes the appearance of bone marrow in particular haematological diseases.

Bone marrow aspiration

A fine-bore needle is inserted into the iliac crest. The material aspirated makes individual cells available for microscopy and analysis. A 'smear' is performed, allowing for examination of the stages of haemopoiesis using specialist stains (e.g., MGG dye). The aspirate is also subjected to immunophenotyping and cytogenetic analysis.

Table 5.4 Bone marrow appearance in specific conditions

Disease/disorder	Bone marrow appearance
Iron-deficiency anaemia	Macrophage iron stores absent
Megaloblastic anaemia	Hypercellular marrow with megaloblasts ± giant metamyelocytes
Haemolytic anaemia	Hypercellular marrow with erythroid hyperplasia and reduced ratio of myeloid to erythroid precursors
Aplastic anaemia	Hypocellular marrow
Polycythaemia rubra vera	Hypercellular marrow with hyperplasia of all cell lineages
Essential thrombocythaemia	Hypercellular marrow with a marked increase in megakaryocytes, distributed in clusters
Myelofibrosis	Reduced haemopoiesis Hypercellularity in early disease or reactive fibrosis in late disease
Acute leukaemias	Hypercellular marrow with blast infiltration
CLL	Hypercellular marrow with lymphocytic infiltration
CML	Hypercellular marrow with granulocyte and megakaryocyte hyperplasia
Multiple myeloma	Increased presence of clonal plasma cells

CLL, Chronic lymphocytic leukaemia; CML, chronic myeloid leukaemia.

A 'Dry tap'

When bone marrow aspiration fails to produce marrow cells, this is a 'dry tap.' Rather than due to technical failure, this is indicative of certain marrow pathologies and is useful in diagnosis in of itself. Patients with CML, PMF and metastases will often yield a 'dry tap' on aspiration.

Cytogenetic analysis

Conventional cytogenetic analysis includes visual assessment of chromosomal size and structure on microscopy of metaphase chromosome preparation. Expert analysis may detect abnormalities of ~4–6 MB size or greater using this approach. Molecular cytogenetic analysis, also known as fluorescence in-situ hybridisation (FISH), can identify particular deletions or duplications associated with particular diseases. This approach identifies if a particular clinical suspicion is correct, since appropriate DNA probes must be used to detect if the particular suspected abnormality is present. Important translocation examples relevant to haematological malignancies are shown in Table 5.5.

Lymph node biopsy

A suspicious enlarged lymph node is biopsied under local or general anaesthesia. Ideally, a superficial site is chosen to limit surgical/anaesthetic morbidity. This investigation is particularly important in lymphomas. Although 'core' biopsies can provide diagnostic material, wherever possible excision biopsy must be performed.

Lymphadenopathy 'red flags'

Painless, nontender lymphadenopathy that is generalised (i.e., involves several noncontiguous areas and feels hard or matted on palpation) suggests a noninfectious cause (i.e., a pathological manifestation of a disease rather than normal physiological reactive lymphadenopathy in response to infection in the drainage territory (see Chapter 1: Lymphadenopathy). Further red flags are raised by features such as hepatic/splenic enlargement and a history of constitutional symptoms (see p. 5-1) accompanying the lymphadenopathy.

Immunophenotyping

This technique detects if particular antigenic protein structures are present on analysed leucocytes. Normal leucocytes possess a standard array of individual antigens, whilst characteristically different arrays are present on the abnormal leucocytes seen in leukaemias and lymphomas. This allows diagnosis and classification of the malignancy. Immunophenotyping may be performed on any cell sample (e.g., marrow, blood, tissue). Flow cytometry is the technique most often employed with liquid samples, and immunocytochemistry is used with solid samples.

CHEMOTHERAPY AND TARGETED TREATMENTS

Treatment of haematological malignancies is immensely complex and must always be managed by appropriate specialists. In the past, chemotherapy was the only pharmacological strategy available to treat haematological cancers; however, new 'targeted' agents continue to be developed, allowing the haematologist's therapeutic arsenal to evolve and improve. Examples of targeted agents are shown in Table 5.6.

Table 5.6 Examples of new targeted agents

Agent(s)	Target	Condition treated
Imatinib, dasatinib, nilotinib	BCR-ABL fusion protein	CML
Rituximab, ofatumumab, obinutuzumab	CD20	CD20-positive B-cell non-Hodgkin lymphomas
Brentuximab	CD30	CD30-positive lymphomas (e.g., Hodgkin lymphoma)
Ruxolitinib	JAK2	PMF
Ibrutinib, idelalisib, venetoclax	B-cell receptor pathways	CLL
Nivolumab, pembrolizumab	PD-1 pathway	Hodgkin lymphoma

CLL, Chronic lymphocytic leukaemia; CML, chronic myeloid leukaemia; PMF, primary myelofibrosis.

Table 5.5 Translocations associated with specific malignancy

Translocation	Malignancy
t(9:22)	Pathognomic of CML but also may occur in small percentage of ALL The altered chromosome 22 is known as the Philadelphia chromosome
t(14:18)	Follicular lymphoma (NHL)
t(8:14)	Burkitt lymphoma (NHL)
t(15:17)	Acute promyelocytic leukaemia (AML M3)

ALL, Acute lymphoblastic leukaemia; AML, acute myeloid leukaemia; CML, chronic myeloid leukaemia; NHL, non-Hodgkin lymphoma.

CLINICAL NOTES

CHEMOTHERAPY

Traditional chemotherapeutic agents arrest cell division and thus nonselectively damage/destroy *all* dividing cells, not just the cancerous cells. Neoplastic cells are more likely to be undergoing division due their abnormally rapid proliferation than normal cells, so are more likely to be damaged by the chemotherapy drug, but 'innocent bystanders' that appropriately undergo rapid division, such as cells regenerating the constantly shedding gastrointestinal tract lining and mucosal surfaces, and hair too, are similarly affected. This accounts for symptoms commonly seen in patients undergoing chemotherapy.

CLINICAL NOTES

TARGETED TREATMENTS

In contrast, targeted treatments damage *only* the specific cell type associated with the neoplastic disease. For example, Rituximab is a monoclonal antibody that binds CD20-positive B cells; thus it selectively recruits the immune system to destroy only B cells, which makes it effective at malignancies of B-cell origin.

● Chapter Summary

- Myeloproliferative syndromes include PRV, ET and PMF. These result in overproduction of specific cell lines, and often evolve further into other types of haematological malignancy.
- Myelodysplastic syndromes usually lead to reduction in counts and functionality of one or more cell lines. They arise from a clonal disorder of the haematopoietic stem cell and may progress to AML.
- Leukaemias are subclassified by the cell progenitor affected (myeloid or lymphocytic) and are termed 'acute' or 'chronic' according to a combination of acuity of presentations, marrow blast infiltration and persistence of normal cell manufacture alongside the neoplastic clone proliferation. Important leukaemias to be aware of include acute and chronic myeloid leukaemias and acute and chronic lymphocytic leukaemias.
- Lymphomas (non-Hodgkin or Hodgkin) present heterogeneously, but symptoms may include painless lymphadenopathy, pruritus, splenomegaly and constitutional symptoms. They arise due to occupation of lymph node territory by abnormal primitive lymphoid cells, which impair normal immune cell maturation.
- Neutropenic sepsis may arise due to haematological malignancy or chemotherapy treatment. It is a medical emergency, presenting with low neutrophil count and typically septic shock. Sepsis must be treated urgently as neutropenic sepsis carries a high mortality
- Tumour lysis syndrome, a complication of chemotherapy where the neoplastic cell load is very high. Release of intracellular components from the dying cells causes electrolyte derangement, the most acute consequence being hyperkalaemic cardiac arrhythmias.
- Multiple myeloma is most commonly characterised by multifactorial renal impairment, hypercalcaemia, anaemia and lytic lesions of bone. Immune impairment, neurological issues and secondary amyloidosis are also often problematic.
- Important investigations in suspected haematological malignancy include serum ESR, LDH and urate, the FBC, bone marrow or lymph node biopsy, cytogenetics and immunophenotyping
- Stem cell transplantation involves therapeutic obliteration of diseased bone marrow and recolonization with disease-free donor haematopoietic stem cells. Along with chemotherapy and 'targeted treatments,' SCT represents a key weapon in the haematologist's antimalignancy arsenal

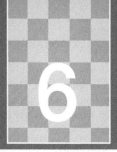
INTRODUCTION

Haemostasis, defined as the processes occurring to arrest bleeding, is necessary to limit blood loss from damaged blood vessels. Unchecked, blood loss reduces circulating volume which compromises tissue perfusion. A complex myriad of cellular and biochemical interactions underpins the process of haemostasis. However; it is based on simple principles as follows:

- Vasoconstriction: an increase in vascular tone reduces the diameter of proximal vessels, reducing blood flow to the damaged area. This minimises blood loss, and maximizes interaction between the platelets, coagulation factors and the endothelium. Vasoconstriction occurs in response to factors released by endothelial cells local to the injured area.
- Formation of a primary platelet plug: this initial structure forms a framework for the developing clot and temporarily seals the vessel wall, stopping blood loss. Platelets adhere to underlying tissue exposed by the vessel wall injury and each other with the help of von Willebrand factor (vWF). This step is termed 'primary haemostasis'. This can be measured clinically as 'bleeding time'.
- Reinforcement of the primary plug: circulating coagulation factors undergo a cascade of reactions, ultimately generating fibrin. Fibrin forms a mesh, stabilising platelets in the developing clot and recruiting passing platelets. This allows the clot to remain until the underlying damage is repaired. This step is termed 'secondary haemostasis'.

CLINICAL NOTES

BLEEDING TIME

This is the time taken for a small cut to stop bleeding, correlating approximately to the time taken for a platelet plug to form (primary haemostasis). It assesses platelet function and is increased in the context of platelet disorders. It is rarely used these days as it is affected by too many variables, and there is controversy regarding its clinical utility.

PLATELETS

Platelets are nonnucleated, granular cells. The usual lifespan is 7–10 days. At any time, up to one-third of circulating platelets are sequestered within the spleen.

Structure

Platelets exhibit a biconvex discoid shape, which is maintained by a circumferential bundle of microtubules. There are two tubule systems: the dense tubular system and the surface-opening canalicular system. The cytoplasm contains numerous granules (α, δ and lysosomal) which contain an array of bioactive molecules.

Platelet synthesis ('thrombopoiesis')

Platelets are synthesised from megakaryocytes in the bone marrow. These are large (50–100 µm) precursor cells that originate from pluripotent stem cells under the influence of thrombopoietin (TPO), a hormone produced mainly by the liver. Megakaryocytes develop lobulated, polyploid nuclei and an expanded cytoplasm volume via endomitosis (deoxyribonucleic acid [DNA] replication without cellular division). They mature by distributing their cytoplasm into 10–20 processes ('proplatelets') that first radiate outwards then elongate, narrow and branch. Platelets develop at the tips of proplatelets and disperse into the circulation. Each megakaryocyte may spawn up to 7000 platelets. Multiple factors influence platelet synthesis, including:

Platelet functions

The main functions fulfilled by platelets are primary haemostasis and tissue repair.

Sequence of primary haemostasis

Vessel injury
Endothelial damage exposes underlying subendothelium, causing release of endothelin. Endothelin induces vasoconstriction, reducing blood flow to the damage zone. Circulating vWF binds to exposed collagen myofibrils in the subendothelium.

Transient tethering
Transient tethering of platelets to the damage zone is mediated by a binding interaction between platelet glycoprotein (GP) Ib receptors and collagen-bound vWF in exposed

subendothelium. The vWF functions as anchor for platelets to bind to the vessel wall. This bond is short-lived but allows an initial monolayer of platelets to cover the damage zone (Fig. 6.1).

Adhesion

Adhesion describes permanent adherence of platelets to the damage zone following transient tethering recruitment of platelets to the damage zone. In this step, platelet receptors (GP Ia, GP IIa and GP VI) bind directly to the subendothelial collagen. This also leads to cytoskeletal alterations making the platelets flatter and lead to formation of podia thus increasing the available surface area for interactions with other platelets.

Platelet activation and release reaction

The 'release reaction' occurs within 2 seconds of adhesion. This describes the release of bioactive contents from platelet storage granules into the local environment via the surface-opening canalicular system. The release reaction is triggered by calcium ion $[Ca^{++}]$ influx and consequent intracellular $[Ca^{++}]$ elevation.

Bioactive granule contents 'activate' additional platelets for incorporation in the platelet plug. 'Activation' in this context refers to a concert of intracellular signalling cascades that impose multiple changes promoting platelet aggregation, including conformational change of the platelet itself (lens-shape → spiny sphere) and the GP IIb/IIIa receptor. The GP IIb/IIIa receptor activation allows it to bind vWF and fibrinogen.

Aggregation

Aggregation describes the process of cross-linking between platelets, which stabilizes the developing clot and allows additional recruitment of passing platelets to expand the volume of the clot. Aggregation can only occur following activation, since the GP IIb/IIIA receptor conformation must be competent to bind vWF and fibrinogen. Aggregation is promoted by raised intraplatelet $[Ca^{++}]$ concentration.

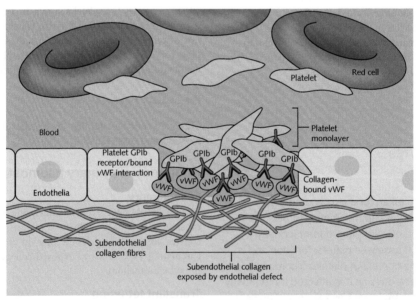

Fig. 6.1 Transient tethering. Circulating von Willebrand factor (vWF) binds exposed subendothelial collagen and is immobilized in an endothelial defect. Platelet GPIb receptors then bind the immobilized vWF. This allows a monolayer of platelets to form over endothelial defects. The tethered platelets are then able to interact with the damage zone in a more permanent way (via platelet receptors GP Ia, GP IIa and GP VI) by binding directly to subendothelial collagen.

Permanent aggregation

Aggregation is rendered irreversible by insoluble fibrin formation. Recruited fibrinogen (bound to activated GP IIb/IIIA receptors) is cleaved to fibrin by thrombin. Thrombin may be:

- Derived from platelets
- Generated by activation of the coagulation cascade (see see later in this chapter Coagulation cascade)

Fibrin creates a reinforcing network between platelets in the primary platelet plug, as well as polymerising to form a mesh-like network which traps additional platelets and blood cells for integration into the clot. Factor XIIIa, activated in the coagulation pathway, further stabilizes the clot by covalently cross-linking fibrin polymers.

Prevention of inappropriate primary haemostasis

In the absence of vessel injury, endothelial cells exert an antiplatelet influence to prevent unnecessary thrombus formation in healthy vessels. Important mechanisms include:

- Endothelial synthesis and release of prostacyclin (PGI2; Fig. 6.2) and nitric oxide, both of which inhibit platelet aggregation.
- Electrostatic repulsion between the negative electrostatic charges of endothelial and platelet surface membranes limits physical interaction.

Tissue repair

Platelets stimulate wound healing by secretion of platelet-derived growth factor, which stimulates mitogenesis of vascular smooth muscle cells and fibroblasts.

ANTIPLATELET DRUGS

Given the pivotal role of platelets in thrombosis, platelets are pharmacologically targeted to reduce disease risk arising from inappropriate thrombosis, e.g., myocardial infarction (MI) and ischaemic stroke. The following sections discuss antiplatelet drug mechanisms, which are illustrated in Fig. 6.3.

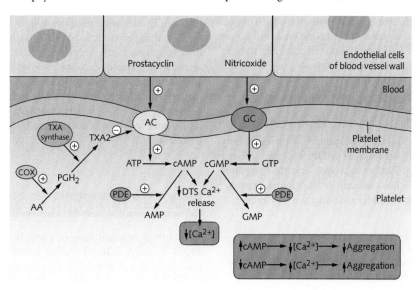

Fig. 6.2 Mechanisms of endothelial prostacyclin/nitric oxide impairment of aggregation. Membrane bound adenylate cyclase (AC) is stimulated by prostacyclin, whilst guanylate cyclase (GC) is stimulated by nitric oxide (NO). This increases the intracellular cyclic adenosine monophosphate (cAMP) and cyclic guanosine monophosphate (cGMP) respectively. Thromboxane A2 (TXA2) conversely, inhibits AC, whilst phosphodiesterases (PDE) enhance cAMP and cGMP degradation, i.e., TXA2 and PDE both lower intracellular [cAMP] in opposition to prostacyclin and NO. The relevance of intracellular [cAMP] or [cGMP] is that their elevation impairs Ca^{++} release from the dense tubular system (DTS), which lowers the intracellular [Ca^{++}], impairing platelet aggregation. Similarly, reduction in [cAMP] or [cGMP] increases Ca^{++} release from the DTS, elevating intracellular [Ca^{++}] and increasing platelet aggregation. Thus prostacyclin and NO are antiaggregatory factors while TXA2 and PDE are proaggregation. Consequently, drugs that inhibit the latter act as antiplatelet agents. *AA,* arachidonic acid; *ATP,* adenosine triphosphate; *COX,* cyclooxygenase; *PGH2,* prostaglandin H2.

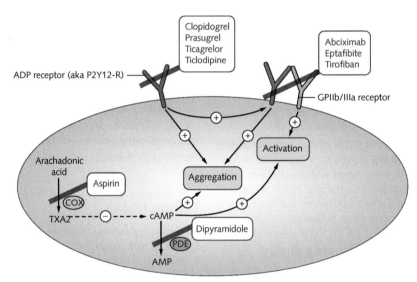

Fig. 6.3 Mechanism of action of antiplatelet drugs. *ADP,* Adenosine diphosphate; *cAMP,* cyclic adenosine monophosphate; *COX,* cyclooxygenase; *PDE,* phosphodiesterases; *TXA2,* thromboxane A2. For detailed explanation of mechanism, see Antiplatelet drugs section.

COX inhibition

Cyclooxygenase (COX) is responsible for thromboxane A2 (TXA2) synthesis. Inhibition of COX reduces TXA2 availability and thus impairs platelets aggregation and clot formation. COX inhibitors may be selective for particular subtypes or nonselective (inhibiting all subtypes). They can be reversible or irreversible. Aspirin is the most well-known example of a COX inhibitor. It is nonselective and irreversible, permanently acetylating the enzyme.

Adenosine diphosphate receptor antagonism

These drugs exerting their antiplatelet effect by occupying the adenosine diphosphate (ADP) receptor, preventing ADP binding. Platelet aggregation is thus impaired. Important drugs in this class include clopidogrel, prasugrel, and ticlodipine (irreversible) and ticagrelor (reversible).

COMMON PITFALLS

The adenosine diphosphate receptor is also known as the 'P2Y12' receptor.

GPIIb/IIIa-R antagonism

Antagonism of the GPIIb/IIIa receptor impairs clot formation by impairing:

- Platelet binding to collagen-bound vWF
- Fibrinogen recruitment and subsequent cross-linking between platelets

Abciximab, epitifibatide and tirofiban are examples of this class of drugs.

Phosphodiesterase inhibition

Inhibition of platelet phosphodiesterase prevents intracellular cyclic adenosine monophosphate (cAMP) degradation, resulting in a high [cAMP]. This disrupts virtually all the changes necessary for platelet activation including degranulation (release reaction), cytoskeletal rearrangement and conformational change of the GPIIb/IIIa receptor. The platelet is unable to undergo adhesion and aggregation, preventing effective primary haemostasis. Dipyramidole is the most commonly encountered antiplatelet drug of this class.

PLATELET DISORDERS

The normal concentration of platelets in blood is 150–400 × 10^9/L. A reduced platelet count (thrombocytopenia) or defects of platelet function both lead to bleeding (Table 6.1). Impaired synthesis, reduced lifespan or excessive consumption of platelets by incorporation into blood clots are the most common abnormalities leading to thrombocytopenia.

Thrombocytopenia: decreased platelet production

The most common explanation for thrombocytopenia is a decrease in platelet production (Table 6.2).

Table 6.1 Platelet count and bleeding tendency

Platelet count ($\times 10^9$/L)	Clinical manifestation
>100	No abnormal bleeding (no spontaneous bleeding and no increase in bleeding associated with surgery or trauma)
50–100	No spontaneous bleeding +/- mild increase in surgical/traumatic bleeding
30–50	Occasional mild spontaneous bleeding (usually limited to petechiae & purpura) Moderately increased surgical/traumatic bleeding
10–30	Spontaneous bleeding including petechiae, purpura and mucocutaneous bleeding Significantly increased surgical/traumatic bleeding
<10	Severe spontaneous bleeding including petechiae, purpura, mucocutaneous bleeding and risk of intracranial haemorrhage Potentially catastrophically increased surgical/traumatic bleeding

Petechiae: small (<3 mm diameter) reddish purple lesions resulting from bleeding into the skin
Purpura: as petechiae, but larger, and may be slightly raised (i.e., palpable).
Mucocutaneous bleeding: bleeding from mucosal or epithelialized surfaces e.g., epistaxis, menorrhagia, haematuria.

Table 6.2 Reduced platelet production: specific causes and their mechanisms

Mechanism of decreased production	Specific causes
Drug-induced (immune and nonimmune)	Alcohol Quinine Antibiotics (Co-trimoxazole, vancomycin, linezolid, daptomycin, penicillin, rifampicin, ceftriaxone) Diuretics (furosemide, thiazides) Valaciclovir Antiepileptics (valproate, carbamazepine) Antipsychotics (mirtazapine) Heparin NSAIDs (ibuprofen) Vaccine (MMR) Chemotherapy
Bone marrow infiltration/failure	Metastatic malignancy Leukaemia Lymphoma Multiple myeloma Myelofibrosis Aplastic anaemia
Viral infection of megakaryoctyes	Measles, HIV
Ineffective/reduced megakaryocyte development	Megaloblastic anaemias Myelodysplasia syndromes Chronic liver disease (reduced thrombopoietin)

HIV, Human immunodeficiency virus; MMR, measles, mumps, rubella; NSAIDs, nonsteroidal antiinflammatory drugs.

Bone marrow disease

Any disease affecting bone marrow synthetic function can reduce platelet production. Primary bone marrow disease (leukaemia, myeloma, lymphoma etc.) and similarly infiltrative disease (where cancerous or pathologic tissue replaces normal marrow) more commonly cause bicytopenia or pancytopenia but can cause isolated thrombocytopenia too.

Drug-induced thrombocytopenia

This is the most common cause of thrombocytopenia. Specific drugs may cause thrombocytopenia by generalized depression of haemopoiesis, specifically impairing megakaryocyte production or by immune destruction.

Ineffective megakaryopoiesis

Generalized impairment of DNA synthesis, as seen in megaloblastic anaemia (see Chapter 3: Megaloblastic anaemia) reduces platelet as well as red cell production.

Thrombocytopenia: shortened platelet lifespan

Reduction in platelet lifespan leads to a reduction in circulating numbers. The following sections discuss the various mechanisms that can lead to shortened platelet survival.

Splenic sequestration

Platelet sequestration by the spleen is seen in functional hypersplenism (see Chapter 1: Hypersplenism).

Immune destruction

Platelet destruction by immune mechanisms is discussed in the following sections.

Immune thrombocytopenic purpura

Immune thrombocytopenic purpura (ITP) has a different cause and clinical features depending on whether it affects children or adults. In both, the platelet count is usually $<20 \times 10^9/L$, and symptoms include easy bruising and mucocutaneous bleeding.

Children—In children, ITP is a usually self-limiting postviral illness. Antibody-viral antigen complexes bind to platelets, resulting in removal of platelets by the reticuloendothelial system.

Adults—In adults, there is usually no association with recent viral infection, but ITP is associated with autoimmune diseases. Incidence is higher in women. Onset is often insidious. Immunoglobulin (Ig) G antibodies bind to platelet glycoproteins, and the resultant IgG–platelet complexes are removed by the liver (if complement interaction occurs) or splenic macrophages. ITP in adults rarely resolves spontaneously and often relapses and remits.

CLINICAL NOTES

MANAGEMENT OF IMMUNE THROMBOCYTOPENIC PURPURA IN ADULTS

This consists of three components.
Immunosuppression; using steroids, ciclosporin or rituximab. Intravenous immunoglobulin or anti-D immunoglobulin is given to saturate splenic macrophages, restricting their platelet destruction. Thrombopoietic (TPO) mimetics (romiplostim and eltrombopag) increase platelet counts by binding to the megakaryocyte TPO receptors, stimulating platelet production.

Drug-induced ITP

In drug-induced ITP, a drug-dependent antibody-mediated destruction of platelets occurs. The platelet count is often $<50 \times 10^9/L$. Note that drugs can also cause thrombocytopenia by impairing platelet production as well as provoking immune destruction.

Posttransfusion purpura

Posttransfusion purpura occurs 5–10 days after a red cell transfusion. The recipient develops antibodies towards platelet antigen 1 (HPA-1a); an antigen present on the donor's platelets, of which a small number will be present in the transfused red cells. In a bizarre phenomenon known as 'bystander destruction,' the recipient's own platelets are then targeted for destruction by their immune system, despite not expressing the HPA-1a antigen themselves.

Neonatal alloimmune thrombocytopenia

Neonatal alloimmune thrombocytopenia arises from transfer of antiplatelet antibodies (from mother to foetus) across the placenta. It is most commonly seen in the setting where maternal platelets lack HPA-1a, but HPA-1a is expressed by foetal platelets. There is a high risk of severe bleeding (e.g., intracranial) and this condition requires transfusion(s) of known HPA-1a negative platelets.

Heparin-induced thrombocytopenia

This life-threatening condition is a complication of heparin therapy. It occurs in up to 5% of patients treated with heparins, including the low-molecular-weight heparins (LMWHs). An antibody is generated against a complex formed between heparin and endogenous platelet factor 4. This antibody activates platelets inappropriately, which manifests clinically as venous and arterial thrombus formation. Critical ischaemia may develop secondary to large vessel occlusion. Bleeding is not a feature, despite thrombocytopenia (resulting from reticuloendothelial clearance of antibody-coated platelets). Immediate discontinuation of heparin products usually allows platelet counts to recover in ~7 days, but lifelong heparin avoidance is essential. Acutely, commencement of a nonheparin anticoagulant to limit venous/arterial thrombosis is essential.

Thrombocytopenia: excessive platelet consumption

Three important conditions hallmarked by excessive platelet consumption are discussed here.

Platelet consumption by microthrombi formation (with associated Microangiopathic haemolytic anaemia)

As well as arising because of inappropriate fibrin deposition, widespread microthrombi formation in small vessels can lead to microangiopathic haemolytic anaemia (MAHA; see Chapter 3: Microangiopathic haemolytic anaemia). In this scenario, microthrombi formation consumes platelets, leading to severe thrombocytopenia. Haemolytic uraemic syndrome (HUS), thrombotic thrombocytopenic purpura (TTP) and disseminated intravascular coagulation (DIC) are three examples of diseases hallmarked by the combination of thrombocytopenia and MAHA.

Thrombotic thrombocytopenic purpura

TTP is a rare disorder, usually affecting adults (3:1 female:male ratio). Although the diagnosis is defined by the classic pentad of fever, transient focal neurologic defects, acute kidney injury (AKI) accompanied by MAHA and thrombocytopenia, only the latter two are essential to make the diagnosis. In TTP, deficiency (usually acquired) of the protease enzyme "a disintegrin and metalloproteinase with thrombospondin motifs" (ADAMTS-13) arises from pathologic antibody formation against the enzyme. TTP is a medical emergency and is fatal if untreated. Treatment is urgent plasmapheresis. This performs dual functions; removing the pathologic ADAMTS-13–directed antibodies and replacing them with functional ADAMTS-13 which is present in the donor plasma.

HINTS AND TIPS

ADAMTS-13

ADAMTS-13 is a protease enzyme which cleaves large multimers of von Willebrand factor (vWF), reducing their activity to normal levels. Deficiency of this enzyme allows persistence of large vWF multimers, which provoke inappropriate primary haemostasis. Platelet-rich microthrombi form in the absence of vessel damage, and occlusion of blood flow leads to distal ischaemia.

Haemolytic-uraemic syndrome

HUS manifests with thrombocytopenia secondary to microthrombi formation and MAHA, similar to TTP. However, in HUS, the microthrombi mainly occur in the glomeruli of the kidney, and AKI develops, resulting in uraemia. HUS is usually provoked by infection with shiga-toxin producing Escherichia coli (specifically the O157:H7 strain) or Shigella. The shiga-toxin directly inhibits ADAMTS-13 enzyme. HUS is the most common cause of AKI in children. The triad of AKI, low platelets and blood film suggestive of MAHA is diagnostic.

Disseminated intravascular coagulation

This life-threatening condition, discussed in detail later in the chapter, DIC, both consumes platelets and shortens their lifespan.

Dilutional thrombocytopenia

Rather than a reduction in the absolute numbers of platelets present, significant expansion of intravascular volume results in a dilutional thrombocytopenia. This adverse effect is most commonly encountered secondary to massive transfusion (see Chapter 7: Massive transfusion).

Defects of platelet function

If the functional ability of the platelets is impaired, there is an increase in bleeding risk despite a normal platelet count. Causes of impaired platelet function include:

- Antiplatelet drugs
- Uraemia
- Congenital platelet disorders
- Myelodysplastic disease
- Plasma cell dyscrasias
- Myeloproliferative disease
- Cardiopulmonary bypass

THE COAGULATION CASCADE

Once a platelet plug (primary haemostasis) has arrested bleeding, the plug is reinforced by products of the coagulation pathway (secondary haemostasis). Coagulation involves a cascade of protein activations, culminating with the conversion of prothrombin to thrombin. Thrombin is the end-product of the complex sequence of interaction. Thrombin converts fibrinogen to fibrin and thus mediates reinforcement and stabilisation of the clot.

The proteins involved are known as clotting or coagulation factors. They exist in the circulation as inactive proenzymes. The activated enzymes are serine proteases (except FXIII) which cleave other inactive proenzymes to their active versions. All coagulation factors are synthesized in the liver.

HINTS AND TIPS

CLOTTING FACTORS (COAGULATION FACTORS)

Clotting factors are usually referred to clinically by Roman numerals. However, some are also referred to by particular names, e.g., factor II is usually referred to by name as prothrombin. Activated factors have the suffix 'a' (e.g., activated factor VIII = FVIIIa).

The surface of activated platelets within the primary platelet plug functions as a catalytic membrane for complexes of coagulation factors. Platelet presence therefore is mandatory for an intact secondary coagulation response; in terms of magnitude and rapidity.

TRADITIONAL PATHWAYS

The traditional pathways represent the historic interpretation of the coagulation process. They are discussed here as they are still examination topics, plus two commonly used clotting parameters (the activated partial thromboplastin time [APTT] and prothrombin time [PT]) each broadly relate to the activity of factors that are differentiated by the concept of each pathway model (Fig. 6.4). They are named according to whether coagulation initiation arises from within (intrinsic) or outside (extrinsic) the circulation.

The extrinsic pathway

The secondary haemostatic response is initiated by tissue factor (TF), a glycoprotein expressed within vessel subendothelium and nonvascular cells. Blood passing through normal, nondamaged blood vessels is not exposed to TF. Following vessel wall damage:

- TF is exposed to the circulation
- Circulating factor VII is activated by TF
- TF then forms a complex with FVIIa plus Ca^{++} ions (TF-FVII- Ca^{++})
- This complex then activates factors IX (in the intrinsic pathway) and X (in the common pathway; but note that the extent of factor X activation is small relative to that generated by the intrinsic pathway)

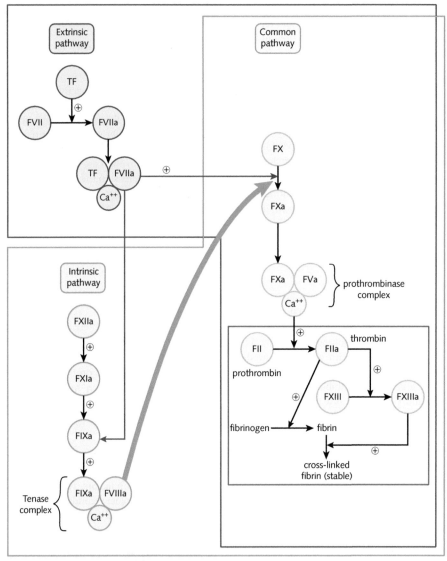

Fig. 6.4 The traditional pathways. See Traditional pathways section for detail of the extrinsic (*shown in red*), intrinsic (*shown in green*) and common (*shown in yellow/mustard*) pathways. Green outline: the processes that together are measured by the activated thromboplastin time (i.e., the intrinsic and common pathways). Red outline: the processes that together are measured by the prothrombin time (i.e., the extrinsic and the common pathways together). *Blue outline,* Processes contributing to the thrombin time.

Intrinsic pathway

The intrinsic pathway commences when FXII comes into contact with a negatively charged surface, such as an activated platelet cell membrane.

- This contact activates FXII
- FXIIa then cleaves FXI → FXIa
- FXIa then cleaves FIX → FIXa. In addition, a small amount of FIX is also activated by TF-FVII from the extrinsic pathway
- Circulating thrombin (FIIa) converts a small amount of FVIII to FVIIIa
- FIXa, FVIIIa and Ca^{++} ions together form the 'tenase' complex
- Tenase (FVIIIa-FIXa-Ca^{++}) powerfully activates FX, forming large quantities of FXa (remember that a small amount of FXa is generated by TF-FVII-Ca^{++} from the extrinsic pathway)
- FXa then enters the common pathway

Common pathway

Factor X may be activated by either:

- The tenase complex (FVIIIa-FIXa- Ca^{++}) from the intrinsic pathway

- The (TF-FVIIa-Ca^{++}) complex from the extrinsic pathway

Either way, FXa then combines with FVa and Ca^{++} to form the 'prothrombinase complex,' which cleaves prothrombin (FII) to generate thrombin (FIIa).

Thrombin has many haemostatic functions, including:

- Conversion of fibrinogen to fibrin (most important role)
- Further activation of factors V, VIII and XI. This forms the basis of the amplification process; i.e., thrombin further activates proteins of the 'intrinsic' and 'common' pathway to produce even more thrombin.
- Activation of factor XIII
- Releasing FVIII from its plasma carrier protein (vWF)
- Further platelet activation
- Binding to thrombomodulin, which then activates protein C. This accounts for the anticoagulant function of thrombin.

Fibrinogen → Fibrin

The ultimate outcome of the common pathway is the thrombin-mediated cleavage of soluble plasma fibrinogen to insoluble fibrin (Fig. 6.5). Fibrin monomers spontaneously polymerize (via hydrogen bonds) into long fibres.

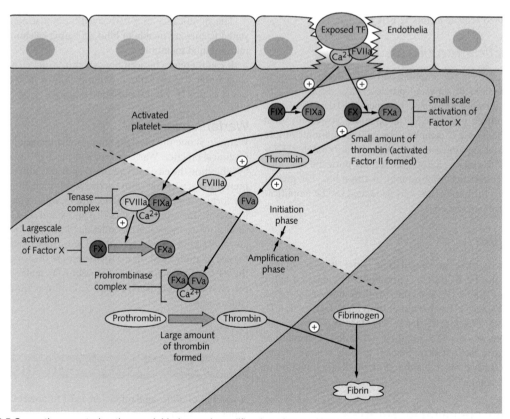

Fig. 6.5 Currently accepted pathways: initiation and amplification phases. Note that the reactions occur at the external surface of activated platelets, an important feature of the clotting cascade incorporated into this more recently accepted version of events.

These create complex networks within the platelet plug. Thrombin-activated FXIIIa further stabilizes the fibrin reinforcement of the clot, mediating covalent cross-linking between fibrin polymers.

CURRENTLY ACCEPTED PATHWAY

The cascades, as explained earlier, have been the accepted interpretations of the clotting system for decades. However, certain clotting factors are important for their own production; the most obvious one being thrombin (FIIa). Thrombin participates in reactions that occur before its own activation, making the cascade approach seem nonsensical. The more recent interpretation of coagulation sees the two 'separate' cascades integrated and delineated by two phases: initiation and amplification.

Initiation phase

Initiation commences with TF binding to activated FVIIa. The resultant FVIIa-TF-Ca^{++} complex then activates factors IX and X. The surface membrane of activated platelets then functions as a catalyst for the conversion of a relatively small amount of prothrombin to thrombin by FXa. Thrombin is then able to activate factors V, VIII and XI.

Amplification phase

The reactions of the amplification phase occur on the external surfaces of activated platelets. FIXa associates with FVIIIa, forming the tenase complex (FVIIIa-FIXa-Ca^{2+}). This complex activates FX much more powerfully than the FVIIa-TF-Ca^{++} complex. These larger amounts of FXa then form large amounts of prothrombinase complex (FXa-FVa-Ca^{2+}), which is 300,000 times more powerful than lone FXa at converting prothrombin to thrombin. Far greater amounts of thrombin are thus generated by the amplification phase (see Fig. 6.5).

Calcium

Calcium is vital for coagulation, since it is a component of the TF-FVIIa-Ca^{2+} complex, the tenase complex (FVIIIa-FIXa-Ca^{2+}) and the prothrombinase complex (FXa-FVa-Ca^{2+}). Furthermore, individual factors II, VII, IX and X (vitamin-K dependent factors) require calcium ions as cofactors for their activation. Coagulation is therefore facilitated by platelet granule release of calcium on activation and is therefore markedly impaired in hypocalcaemia.

Calcium chelation for samples
This calcium-dependency of clotting is exploited to prevent blood clotting when it would be undesirable, for

example storage of donated blood or transfer of samples to the laboratory. Chelation (e.g., with Ethylene diamine tetra acetic acid (EDTA)) or deionisation (e.g., with citrate) of calcium ions is used in these instances. Thus the 'full blood count' sample is collected in vacutainers that contain EDTA, which causes irreversible chelation of the calcium ions. This renders the sample 'unclottable' so it remains in the fluid state necessary for performing cell counts and also blood films. The 'clotting sample' is collected in vacutainers that contain citrate, which causes deionisation of calcium ions, thus again preventing the clotting of blood in the container. However, unlike EDTA, this process is easily reversed by adding calcium in the laboratory, allowing various clotting times to be studied.

Vitamin K

Factors II, VII, IX and X undergo posttranslational γ-carboxylation at glutamic acid residues. This is a mandatory posttranslational modification required to complete the synthesis of a mature and functional factor. Active (reduced) vitamin K is required for this carboxylation. Performing the carboxylation oxidizes (inactivating) vitamin K. The epoxide reductase enzyme mediates reactivation (reduction) of vitamin K, allowing further synthesis of the vitamin K-dependent factors.

The significance of γ-carboxylation is that noncarboxylated factors are unable to bind activating calcium ions or phospholipid membranes.

It can therefore be seen how vitamin K deficiency leads to disordered coagulation resulting from a lack of functional factors II, VII, IX and X.

Warfarin overdose
Warfarin is one the most common oral anticoagulant used in clinical practice. Warfarin exerts its mechanism of action by inhibiting the enzyme vitamin K epoxide reductase. This prevents regeneration of the active form of vitamin K (i.e., the form competent to mediate the essential posttranslational modification of factors II, VII, IX and X). Overdose results in excessive anticoagulation, indicated by a prolonged PT [and raised international normalized ratio (INR), see coagulation tests]. In massive overdose, it also prolongs the APTT. Treatment of this scenario is by replacement of the relevant factors (see Chapter 7: Prothrombin complex concentrate).

REGULATION OF COAGULATION

A number of anticoagulant factors exist to prevent spontaneous activation of coagulation (in the absence of injury) and also to limit the activation of coagulation to within the local area in the context of vessel injury.

Tissue-factor pathway inhibitor

Tissue-factor pathway inhibitor (TFPI) is linked via GPI to endothelial cell surfaces. It exerts a background anticoagulant influence by binding the TF-FVIIa-Ca^{2+} complex, thus preventing TF-mediated initiation of coagulation.

Proteins C and S

Protein C is a serine protease that destroys the activated cofactors Va and VIIIa (both factors form part of the amplification process). Protein C is activated when thrombin binds to thrombomodulin, itself located at the surface of endothelial cells. Protein S is a required cofactor for protein C. Both proteins C and S are vitamin K-dependent.

Deficiencies of protein C or S

Hereditary or acquired deficiencies of these anticoagulant proteins places patients at risk for inappropriate thrombosis. This may result in venous thrombosis and thromboembolism.

Thrombomodulin

Thrombomodulin, a glycosaminoglycan produced by uninjured endothelial cells, binds thrombin, sequestering it and preventing its participation in coagulation. Immobilized thrombin is then able to activate protein C, which in turn exerts an anticoagulant action.

Antithrombin

Antithrombin (AT), also known as antithrombin III, is a potent inhibitor of both thrombin, FIXa, FXa and FXIIa. AT binds to the active site of these factors. The inhibitory effect of AT is potentiated by heparin.

FIBRINOLYSIS

Breakdown of stable fibrin polymers is termed 'fibrinolysis.' The fibrinolytic system degrades fibrin and thus enables clot breakdown. Fibrinolysis also acts to dismantle any inappropriate fibrin networks obstructing vessel lumens in the absence of injury. Important components of the fibrinolytic system are discussed here.

Plasmin

Plasmin (cleaved from plasminogen) is a serine protease that cleaves peptide bonds within fibrin polymers, degrading fibrin networks and destroying the architecture and stability

CLINICAL NOTES

THROMBOLYSIS FOR ST-ELEVATION MYOCARDIAL INFARCTION TREATMENT

In the past, ST elevation myocardial infarction was treated with thrombolytic drugs that converted plasminogen to plasmin relying on its action to break clots. These drugs (alteplase, streptokinase and tenecteplase) have been superseded by emergency percutaneous coronary intervention. Alteplase is still the drug of choice in patients with life threatening pulmonary embolism.

of a clot. Conversion of plasminogen to plasmin is achieved by tissue plasminogen activator (tPA) or by urokinase.

Tissue plasminogen activator

tPA is released from activated endothelial cells and is the most important activator of fibrinolysis. It binds to plasminogen, cleaving it to form plasmin, but will only interact with plasminogen bound to fibrin, i.e., will only release plasmin in the area of a thrombus.

Antifibrinolytic factors

Thrombin-activated fibrinolysis inhibitor, plasminogen activator inhibitor and α_2-antiplasmin, act to oppose fibrinolysis. The extent of fibrinolysis thus depends on the balance between fibrinolytic promotors (such as tPA) and these antifibrinolytic factors.

OVERVIEW OF HAEMOSTASIS

The role of platelets, the clotting cascade and fibrinolysis in haemostasis are outlined in Fig. 6.6.

COAGULATION ASSAYS

PT, APTT and thrombin time (TT) are tests used to assay various aspects of the coagulation cascade. A summary of their normal range and some common causes of abnormal results are shown in Table 6.3.

Specific factor assays can be used to identify deficiencies of single coagulation factors. This is of relevance in haemophilia, where a factor assay indicates the level of factor in the blood which correlates to the severity of disease.

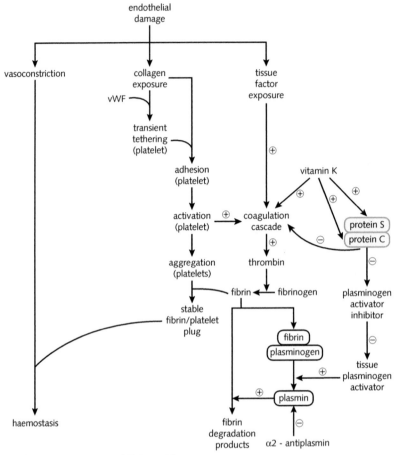

Fig. 6.6 Overview of haemostasis. *vWF,* von Willebrand factor.

Table 6.3 Coagulation assays

Test	Normal range	Possible causes
PT: prolonged (with APTT normal)	12–14 seconds	Factor VII deficiency Warfarin treatment Mild vitamin K deficiency Early liver disease
APTT: prolonged (with PT normal)	30–36 seconds	Factor VIII deficiency Factor IX deficiency Factor XI deficiency Factor XII deficiency Von Willebrand disease heparin treatment Lupus anticoagulant
PT and APTT: both prolonged	As previous	DIC Direct FXa inhibitor treatment (e.g., rivaroxaban) Direct thrombin inhibitor treatment (e.g., dabigatran) Warfarin overdose Severe vitamin K deficiency Combined factor deficiencies in advanced liver disease

Table 6.3 Coagulation assays—cont'd

Test	Normal range	Possible causes
TT prolonged	10–12 seconds	DIC Heparin and LMWH treatment Direct thrombin inhibitor treatment (e.g., dabigatran) Inherited disorder of fibrinogen Low fibrinogen (see causes later)
Fibrinogen low	2–4.5 g/L	DIC Massive transfusion Severe liver disease Postthrombolysis
Fibrinogen high	2–4.5 g/L	Acute or chronic inflammation scenarios Pregnancy Trauma Specific cancers e.g., Hodgkin lymphoma

APTT, Activated partial thromboplastin time; DIC, disseminated intravascular coagulation; LMWH, low-molecular-weight heparin; PT, prothrombin time; TT, thrombin time.

CLINICAL NOTES

PROTHROMBIN TIME (PT)

The PT correlates with the activity of the extrinsic pathway. A normal PT is 10–14 seconds, but the normal range varies slightly with the laboratory.

CLINICAL NOTES

ACTIVATED PARTIAL THROMBOPLASTIN TIME (APTT)

This correlates with intrinsic pathway activity. Normal range is 30–40 seconds but the normal range varies slightly with the laboratory.

D-dimers

Small fibrin fragments, termed 'D' fragments, are produced by high levels of thrombin and FXIIIa, i.e., when the coagulation cascade is active. They are thus present in large quantities in conditions such as DIC or large thrombus formation. D-dimers are detectable in plasma; their absence is indicated by a negative D-dimer assay, which confidently excludes significant thrombosis, such as deep vein thrombosis (DVT) or pulmonary embolism (PE). However; D-dimer presence does not automatically verify thrombosis—high levels are also seen in infection, inflammation, after surgery or trauma.

CLOTTING FACTOR DISORDERS

Acquired factor deficiencies

Vitamin K deficiency

Vitamin K deficiency is most commonly secondary to diseases causing fat malabsorption, as vitamin K is a fat-soluble vitamin. Gastrointestinal disease and biliary obstruction are common causes of fat malabsorption and thus vitamin K deficiency.

A high proportion of dietary vitamin K is liberated from ingested food by commensal bacteria in the gastrointestinal (GI) tract. Patients on long-term broad-spectrum antibiotics which indiscriminately kill these bacteria are also at risk of vitamin K deficiency. Thus patients who have a prolonged stay in intensive care units, often on antibiotics and poor nutrition, typically develop vitamin K deficiency.

Levels of the vitamin K-dependent factors (II, VII, IX and X) are reduced, prolonging the PT. In severe cases, the APTT may also be prolonged. Treatment is with oral or parenteral supplementation.

Liver disease

All clotting factors are synthesized hepatically (except vWF). Liver disease advanced enough to impair hepatic synthetic function is therefore typically hallmarked by clotting factor deficiency. Likewise, fibrinogen levels are low and fibrinogen dysfunctional in severe liver disease. In addition, advanced cirrhosis may cause portal hypertension with secondary splenomegaly, increasing splenic platelet sequestration and lowering their numbers. Reduced hepatic thrombopoietin synthesis impairs platelet production. All these factors together make for an increased bleeding tendency in advanced liver disease.

Disseminated intravascular coagulation

DIC is an immensely dangerous condition resulting from a pathologic and widespread systemic activation of coagulation cascades. This results in formation of platelet microthrombi, and generalized widespread fibrin deposition. Fibrin deposition then activates fibrinolytic pathways, generating fibrin degradation products (FDPs). FDPs inhibit further fibrin polymerisation, further impairing coagulation. Two serious consequences of these processes are:

- Small vessel occlusion by microthrombi causes distal ischaemia and organ dysfunction
- Consumption of fibrinogen, clotting factors and platelets leads to bleeding and haemorrhage

The PT, APTT and TT are all prolonged, and fibrinogen and platelet count are significantly lowered. The small vessel microthrombi lead to shearing of red blood cells, leading to formation of 'fragments' or schistocytes. This scenario is MAHA. DIC is provoked by large-scale exposure of the circulation to procoagulants, including tissue factor, from which the circulation is usually protected. Underlying mechanisms may include:

- Widespread damage to vascular endothelium
- Severe intravascular haemolysis
- Bacterial lipopolysaccharides in severe infection

Sepsis, trauma, burns, malignancy and massive blood loss are typically severe physiologic derangements predisposing to DIC.

Management of disseminated intravascular coagulation

As patients with DIC are critically ill, acute treatment involves resuscitation via an airway, breathing, circulation (ABC) approach. Supportive care, often in high-dependency or intensive care where ventilatory or haemodynamic support is available in case of organ failure, is almost always warranted. The mainstay of management of DIC is treatment of the underlying disorder that provoked the DIC. Haematologic management is essentially supportive and centres around appropriate transfusion with platelets and fresh-frozen plasma (to replace clotting factors). Cryoprecipitate (to restore fibrinogen) is also used, but only if the patient is bleeding or an invasive procedure is required. Aggressively correcting hypothermia and acidosis will facilitate regaining functional haemostasis.

HEREDITARY FACTOR DEFICIENCIES

Von Willebrand disease

Von Willebrand disease is the most common hereditary bleeding disorder. It affects up to 1% of the population,

though the majority are asymptomatic. Plasma vWF is a carrier protein for FVIII, prolonging its survival in the circulation. Bleeding symptoms thus occur when plasma levels are sufficiently decreased or the vWF is defective. Since vWF is also vital for transient tethering of platelets in primary haemostasis, the usual clinical manifestations resemble those of platelet disorders, i.e., easy bruising, prolonged mucocutaneous bleeding following dental extractions, menorrhagia or epistaxis. See Table 6.4 for clinical differentiation between the three most common hereditary clotting factor deficiencies.

Type 1 is the most common form of the disease. Endothelial synthesis of vWF is normal, but release into the circulation is impaired, resulting in low plasma vWF levels. This inadequate exocytosis can be managed in an acute bleeding scenario by treatment with desmopressin.

Types 2 and 3 cause more severe disease and are managed in specialist centres. The first line treatment for types 2 and 3 is FVIII (vWF is bound to FVIII) or vWF concentrate.

Haemophilia A: factor VIII (8) deficiency

Haemophilia A is caused by a deficiency of FVIII. As an X-linked recessive condition, it overwhelmingly affects males. Male prevalence of haemophilia A is 1 in 5000; this is unaffected by geography, ethnicity or social class. Thirty-three percent of cases arise in absence of family history, which likely represents spontaneous or 'de novo' mutations of the FVIII gene. Bleeding frequency and severity correlates with the plasma level of FVIII. Seventy percent of haemophilia A patients are classified as having severe haemophilia (Table 6.5).

Table 6.4 Differentiation between the three most common hereditary clotting factor deficiencies

Feature	Haemophilia A and B	Von Willebrand disease
Deficient factor	Factor VIII (haemophilia A) Factor IX (haemophilia B)	vWF
Inheritance pattern (excluding de novo cases)	X-linked	Variable, usually autosomal dominant
Most likely sites of bleeding	Joints, muscles	Mucocutaneous
Platelet count	Normal	Normal
Platelet function	Normal	Impaired
PT	Normal	Normal
APTT	Prolonged	Normal/prolonged
Bleeding time	Normal	Prolonged

APTT, Activated partial thromboplastin time; PT, prothrombin time; vWF, von Willebrand factor.

Table 6.5 Quantifying the severity of haemophilias A and B

Concentration of coagulation factor (% of normal)[a]	Clinical implications
50%–100%	None
25%–50%	Increased bleeding occurs only following severe extensive trauma
5%–25% (Mild)	Severe bleeding occurs postsurgery, or mild bleeding episodes following minor trauma
1%–5% (Moderate)	Severe bleeding episodes following minor trauma
<1% (Severe)	Spontaneous bleeding, predominantly into joints or muscle tissue

[a] *The deficient factor is factor VIII in haemophilia A, whereas in haemophilia B it is factor IX that is deficient.*

Treatment is with factor replacement therapy and supportive transfusions as needed. In addition, desmopressin and tranexamic acid may be used to enhance existing FVIII activity. Prophylactic treatment with FVIII is currently recommended in children with severe haemophilia A.

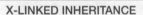

CLINICAL NOTES

X-LINKED INHERITANCE

As for all X-linked diseases, daughter of an affected male is an obligate carrier, and sons are unaffected. Daughters of carrier women have 50% chance of being carriers themselves, but the sons will be always affected.

CLINICAL NOTES

RECURRENT TRANSFUSIONS

As with all patients that habitually receive transfusions, there is a significant risk of the patient developing antibodies, making future transfusions much more challenging.

ETHICS

Before donor screening programmes and development of recombinant factors, iatrogenic blood-borne infections such as hepatitis B and C and human immunodeficiency virus were a significant cause of comorbidity in haemophilia patients. With haemophilia causing an average of 31 bleeding episodes per person annually, these patients typically undergo enormously frequent transfusions. As always, it is important not to demonstrate any prejudice towards patients positive for such diseases.

Haemophilia B: factor IX (9) deficiency

Haemophilia B (also known as 'Christmas disease') is caused by a deficiency of FIX. Like haemophilia A, it is X-linked, thus patients are almost always men. The two diseases are clinically indistinguishable, laboratory coagulation factor assays being required to differentiate them. Haemophilia B is however five times less common. Treatment is similar to haemophilia A management, but with FIX replacement (rather than FVIII). FIX has a longer half-life than FVIII, thus fewer factor replacements are required.

Clinical presentation of haemophilias (A and B)

Haemarthrosis (bleeding into joints) is the most common feature of haemophilia, followed by muscular haematomas; together representing 95% of presentations. Nose bleeds, GI bleeds, haematuria and prolonged bleeding following surgery or dental extraction may also be the presenting complaint in haemophilia. A normal PT with an abnormal APTT is strongly suggestive of haemophilia (A or B) in a patient presenting with bleeding.

Complications of haemophilias (A and B)

Acute complications include compartment syndrome, haematoma compression of the respiratory tract, massive loss of circulating volume and intracranial haemorrhage. Chronic complications include chronic joint pain and joint destruction from repeated haemarthroses as well as other bleeding sequelae such as brain damage from haemorrhagic stroke.

Factor replacement therapy in haemophilia A or B

In haemophilia A, factor VIII is replaced with recombinant FVIII, whilst in haemophilia B, Factor IX is replaced with recombinant FIX. In an emergency, if recombinant factors are unavailable, then prothrombin complex concentrates or 'NovoSeven' may be used. Most transfusion laboratories do keep at least one emergency dose of factor concentrates. Plasma-derived factor concentrates are no longer recommended in the United Kingdom.

During acute bleeding episodes, patients should administer their own supply of recombinant factor, and attend hospital if necessary. Replacement should be aimed to correct to 100% of normal levels for 'severe' or life-threatening bleeds. All other 'minor' bleeds (e.g., haemarthroses, muscle haematomas or oral mucosal and muscular bleeds) should be corrected to 30% to 50% of normal levels.

Other clotting factor deficiencies

Hereditary deficiencies of the other coagulation factors are rare. However, in specific areas, the prevalence of a certain hereditary deficiency may be high. Examples include:

- High prevalence of FXI deficiency among Ashkenazi Jews
- High prevalence of FVII deficiency in Northern Italy

THROMBOSIS

A pathologic thrombus can develop in both the arterial or venous circulation. Arterial thromboembolism is the underlying pathology in MI and ischaemic cerebrovascular accident (and thus the leading cause of death in the developed world). Venous thrombi can form anywhere but are most common in the deep veins (DVT) of the legs. Embolisation of such a venous clot to the pulmonary vasculature (PE) can be fatal.

HINTS AND TIPS

DEFINITIONS: THROMBOSIS VERSUS THROMBUS

Formation of a clot is termed 'thrombosis.' A clot remaining at the site of formation is a 'thrombus.' However; if dislodged, the thrombus is referred to as a thromboembolism, which is always pathologic.

Virchow triad describes three factors which predispose to thrombus formation:

- Haemodynamic disruption (turbulence or stasis)
- Endothelial injury/dysfunction
- Hypercoagulability

Haemodynamic disruption

Normally blood flow is nonturbulent (laminar). Any factors causing nonlaminar (turbulent) flow or stasis can potentially activate the coagulation system, leading to thrombosis.

A ubiquitous clinical scenario predisposing to venous thrombosis is immobility. Calf muscle activity pumps venous blood in the lower limbs back towards the heart (the 'calf-muscle pump'). In immobility, this pumping action is absent and stasis of the venous blood predisposes to thrombosis.

Another common clinical scenario (this time predisposing to arterial thrombosis) is atrial fibrillation (AF). Ineffectual atrial emptying caused by absent atrial systole causes relative stasis and thrombi formation within the atria. When these thrombi ultimately leave the heart, they lodge in the cerebral circulation, causing ischaemic stroke. Patients with AF are thus often anticoagulated (if drugs cannot reimpose rhythm control) to reduce the risk of this occurring.

Conversely, mechanical heart valves cause significant turbulence to blood flow through the heart, and likewise present a profound risk factor for arterial thromboembolism. These patients are therefore always anticoagulated.

Endothelial injury/dysfunction

Endothelial injury/dysfunction may occur in context of a myriad of scenarios, including shear stress, atherosclerosis, infection, inflammation and immune-mediated damage. This results in activation of primary haemostasis and consequently thrombosis.

Hypercoagulability

Alteration to the usual constituents of blood can abnormally increase the tendency to thrombosis. The thrombophilias are haemostatic disorders that increase the tendency of blood to clot. These may be inherited or acquired (more common).

SECONDARY (ACQUIRED) THROMBOPHILIAS

Specific conditions associated with an increased incidence of thrombosis are outlined in Table 6.6.

Antiphospholipid antibody syndrome

Also known as lupus anticoagulant syndrome, antiphospholipid (APL) antibody syndrome. This disorder is diagnosed when serum antiphospholipid antibodies are identified following a typical clinical event. The main complications of this syndrome are arterial and/or venous thromboses and pregnancy-related complications such as recurrent miscarriage. The disease can be idiopathic or secondary to other autoimmune disorders, e.g., systemic lupus erythematosus (SLE).

Table 6.6 Factors associated with increased thrombosis

Factor	Mechanism
Immobilisation	Venous stasis
Obesity	Chronic inflammation Impaired fibrinolysis
Pregnancy	Lower limb venous stasis (IVC compression) Increased levels of coagulation factors I, II, VII, VIII, IX and X Reduced levels of protein S
Oestrogen therapy	Increased plasma levels of factors II, VII, IX and X Reduced levels of antithrombin and tPA
Cigarette smoking	Abnormal endothelial and platelet function
Certain cancers	Secretion of tumour factors with FX activating properties
Nephrotic syndrome	Renal loss of clotting factor proteins
Myeloproliferative disorders	Increased viscosity caused by hypercellularity and secondary disrupted flow dynamics
Sickle-cell anaemia	Abnormal platelet activation Abnormal activation of coagulation cascades Vasoocclusion (by sickled cells) and impaired blood flow
Lupus anticoagulant syndrome	See Clinical notes box later:

IVC, inferior vena cava; *tPA*, tissue plasminogen activator.

APL antibody syndrome is diagnosed by either demonstration of APL antibodies or the presence of lupus anticoagulant. The latter test interferes with the APTT test (artefactually prolonging the result), however unlike other causes of prolonged APTT that increased the risk of bleeding, this is a prothrombotic condition.

PRIMARY (HEREDITARY) THROMBOPHILIAS

Factor V (FV) Leiden

FV Leiden is a mutant form of FV. A point mutation of the FV gene (resulting in an arginine → glutamine substitution) renders mutated FV relatively resistant to inactivation by activated protein C. This mutation thus predisposes to venous thrombosis in the following hypercoagulable states:

- Use of the oral contraceptive pill
- Pregnancy
- Surgery and immobility
- Other thrombophilias

This disorder has a UK incidence in Caucasians of 5% and likely accounts for the majority of cases of inherited thrombophilia responsible for VTE. However, most people carrying FV Leiden will never suffer a thromboembolic event.

Antithrombin deficiency

AT deficiency is an autosomal dominant condition affecting 1 in 2000 people. Deficiency is either caused by a reduction in AT quantity (type 1) or functionality (type 2). Homozygosity is lethal. Heterozygotes have 50% of normal plasma AT levels, a reduction which typically results in a thrombotic event below the age of 50 years. AT-deficiency thrombosis is often severe and recurrent. Both subtypes require lifelong warfarin anticoagulation.

Deficiencies of proteins C and S

Protein S deficiency and protein C deficiency are clinically indistinguishable. Deficiency is either caused by a reduction in quantity (type 1) or functionality (type 2). Heterozygotes have 50% of normal levels of protein C or S. Clinical features are similar to AT deficiency, but the thrombotic risk is lower.

Defective fibrinolysis

Abnormal variants of both plasminogen and fibrinogen are associated with reduced fibrinolysis and increased thrombotic tendency.

Prothrombin allele G20210A

Between 2% and 3% of the population have this prothrombin variant, which increases prothrombin levels and thus thrombotic risk. It is the second most common thrombophilia, after FV Leiden.

Hyperhomocysteinaemia

Elevated plasma homocysteine increases the risk of both venous and arterial thrombosis.

VENOUS THROMBOEMBOLISM

DVT occurs most commonly in deep veins of the lower limbs. Unilateral swelling, tenderness and erythema (redness) of the overlying skin are suggestive of a DVT. The Well's score may be used to determine if exclusion of a DVT with a negative D-dimer test or a Doppler ultrasound scan is warranted which must be excluded with a negative D-dimer test or a Doppler ultrasound scan.

WELL'S SCORE

This is a validated risk stratification tool used to estimate the probability of a deep vein thrombosis (DVT), before implementing more discriminating tests such as D-dimers and ultrasound scanning. It scores 1 point for presence of each of the risk factors (active cancer, paralysis/lower limb immobility, previous confirmed DVT or major surgery in the last 12 weeks) and examination findings (unilateral pitting oedema on suspect limb, collateral superficial venous dilation, calf circumference ≥3 cm than asymptomatic calf, unilateral swelling of entire leg, tenderness localized to deep venous regions). Where an alternative diagnosis is at least as likely as a DVT to account for the symptoms and signs, -2 points are scored. Scores range from -2 to +9, and a score of 1, 0, -1 or -2 suggest a DVT is unlikely.

The main danger of DVT is embolisation to the pulmonary vasculature. However, postthrombotic syndrome (chronic changes to skin and tissue overlying the zone of the DVT) is an important chronic complication. DVTs are common, particularly in hospital patients with risk factors. Treatment is necessary to reduce the likelihood of PE.

Clinical presentation of pulmonary embolism

Whilst massive PE present with cardiovascular collapse and loss of consciousness or cardiac arrest, small PE may be subtle and nonspecific in their presentation. A high index of suspicion is essential, particularly in patients with risk factors. The following symptoms may suggest a PE: breathlessness, cough (+/- blood), chest pain and sweating.

Marked tachypnoea (respiratory rate > 25 breath per minure), tachycardia (≥120 beats per minute), hypotension (systolic blood pressure ≤ 90 mmHg) and peripheral capillary oxygen saturation measured by pulse oximetry (SpO2) ≤ 92% or arterial partial pressure of oxygen (pO2) < 13 kPa are particularly worrisome and warrant exclusion of PE with a negative D-dimer scan, especially if associated with a normal chest X-ray.

Diagnosis is with computed tomography pulmonary angiogram (CT-PA) or a ventilation perfusion (VQ) scan. Treatment is immediate parenteral anticoagulation, or in case of haemodynamic instability thrombolysis may be offered.

ANTICOAGULATION

The main use of anticoagulants is to prevent inappropriate thrombus formation or extension of an existing thrombus.

Anticoagulants do not affect platelet plug formation (primary haemostasis), nor do they destabilise existing thrombi. They act at specific stages in the coagulation cascade to ultimately prevent fibrin formation. The type of anticoagulant and duration of use depends on the indication for treatment. Important indications for anticoagulation therapy include:

- Prophylaxis against thrombosis, e.g., postoperatively, prolonged immobilisation, atrial fibrillation, mechanical heart valves
- Treatment postthromboembolic event (DVT, PE, arterial thrombosis or MI)
- During certain invasive procedures, e.g., cardiopulmonary bypass or haemofiltration

People given anticoagulants must have appropriate monitoring (e.g., APTT in intravenous heparin, INR with warfarin) to safely titrate the dose they receive. The main complication of anticoagulant use is haemorrhage. Patients at high-risk of bleeding are relatively or absolutely contraindicated for anticoagulation. Examples of high-risk factors for bleeding include:

- Ongoing active internal bleeding
- History of haemorrhagic stroke
- Recent eye, brain or spinal cord surgery
- Severe liver disease
- Severe thrombocytopenia
- Peptic ulcers
- Oesophageal varices
- Frequent mechanical falls

Important variables for the commonly used anticoagulants are summarized in Table 6.7.

Warfarin

Warfarin is a functional vitamin K antagonist and thus impairs levels of the vitamin-K-dependent factors (VII, IX, X and II (affected most → least). Proteins C and S are also inactivated by warfarin. The PT (presented as INR) is used

INTERNATIONAL NORMALIZED RATIO (INR)

This is the measured prothrombin time (PT) divided by an agreed 'normal' PT, and corrected for reagent and instrument interlaboratory variability. A high INR equates to a more prolonged PT, i.e., increased tendency to bleed, or alternatively less tendency to clot. A raised INR indicates underactivity of the extrinsic pathway, such as is seen in warfarinized patients. Although the INR is a test specifically designed to assess the anticoagulation with warfarin, it is often used interchangeably with PT.

Table 6.7 Comparison of unfractionated heparin (UFH), low-molecular-weight heparins (LMWH), warfarin, dabigatran and the anti-Xa inhibitors (rivaroxaban, apixaban and edoxaban)

Drug	Warfarin	UFH	LMWH	Dabigatran	Rivaroxaban, Apixaban and Edoxaban
Mechanism of anticoagulant action	Vitamin K epoxide reductase inhibition (reduced levels of II, VII, IX, X)	Antithrombin potentiation	Antithrombin potentiation and anti Xa	Direct thrombin inhibition	Direct Factor Xa inhibition
Administration route	Oral	IV or SC	SC	Oral	Oral
PT	Prolonged	Normal/mildly prolonged	Normal	Normal	Normal/mildly prolonged
APTT	Prolonged (especially at higher levels)	Prolonged	Normal/mildly prolonged	Normal/mildly prolonged	Normal
TT	Normal	Prolonged	Normal/mildly prolonged	Normal/mildly prolonged	Normal
Test used to Monitor	INR	APTT	Anti-Xa (only certain circumstances)	None approved for routine use	None approved for routine use
Reversal	Vitamin K Prothrombin complex concentrate (PCC)	Protamine	Protamine	Idarucizumab, ('Praxbind')	Under development

APTT, Activated partial thromboplastin time; INR, international normalized ratio; IV, intravenous; PT, prothrombin time; SC, subcutaneous; TT, thrombin time.

to monitor warfarin's anticoagulatory effect, since the factors affected by warfarin impair the extrinsic pathway more than the intrinsic pathway.

Target INR ranges vary with treatment indication and are shown in Table 6.8. As warfarin has a half-life of 40 hours, a dose change usually takes 4–5 days to influence the INR.

Since warfarin crosses the placenta and is teratogenic, it is contraindicated in early pregnancy whilst foetal organogenesis is occurring. Heparin does not cross the placenta and is therefore safer in early pregnancy when anticoagulation is necessary.

Warfarin treatment interferes with numerous other drug actions, and its own action is affected by multiple drugs. Common examples are given in Table 6.9.

Table 6.8 Target ranges: INR for specific indications

Indication	Target INR range
Atrial fibrillation	2–3
Mechanical heart valve (aortic)	2.5–3.5
Mechanical heart valve (mitral)	3–4
DVT prophylaxis	2–3
DVT/PE treatment dose	2–3

DVT, Deep vein thrombosis; INR, international normalized ratio; PE, pulmonary embolism.

Table 6.9 Drugs interacting with warfarin

Potentiate action (increase INR)	Attenuate action (decrease INR)
Alcohol	Certain antiepileptics (carbamazepine, phenytoin)
SSRIs	Azathioprine
Certain antibiotics (cephalosporins, macrolides, fluoroquinolones, metronidazole)	Rifampicin
Tricyclic antidepressants	
Thyroxine	

INR, International normalized ratio; SSRIs, selective serotonin reuptake inhibitors.

Warfarin overdose

Treatment hinges on stopping further administration and administering oral/parenteral vitamin K or prothrombin complex concentrate (PCC) depending on how excessively raised the INR is and the presence/severity of any bleeding complications (see Chapter 7: Combined clotting factor concentrates). Local guidelines will be available to direct management and haematology input is advisable. PCC contains factors II, VII, IX and X, i.e., the vitamin K-dependent factors which are depleted by warfarin. Its use can result in thrombotic complications.

Unfractionated heparin

Heparin is a glycosaminoglycan that binds to and potentiates antithrombin. Standard (unfractionated) heparin contains molecules ranging in weight from 5000 to 30,000 kDa. The different chain lengths affect both activity and clearance; larger molecules are more rapidly cleared from the circulation. The APTT is used to monitor and titrate unfractionated heparin therapy.

Low-molecular-weight heparins

LMWHs have a mean molecular weight of 5000 kDa. LMWHs are very commonly used as prophylaxis against DVT and at higher doses in the acute management of DVT and PE. Their anticoagulant activity is monitored only in renal failure, extremes of weight and pregnancy, by anti-Xa assay. The risk of complications is less for LMWH than for unfractionated heparin. In addition, LMWH differ from unfractionated heparin because:

- It has greater activity against FXa relative to its antithrombin activity
- It has reduced protein binding and clearance
- Interactions with platelets are reduced

Fondaparinux

Fondaparinux is a synthetic indirect FXa inhibitor, related to LMWH. It mediates its effect by potentiating antithrombin. It exhibits no thrombin inhibition and carries almost no risk of heparin-induced thrombocytopenia (HIT), so is often used where patients have a history of suspected HIT.

Direct oral anticoagulants

These are anticoagulants with novel alternative mechanisms of action to conventional heparin and warfarin. Importantly, with the exception of dabigatran, reversal agents have not yet been developed. This is relevant in an acute haemorrhage scenario, where no mechanism is available to reverse the drug-mediated anticoagulation. Vitamin K, PCC and protamine are ineffective at reversing these drugs. Various mechanisms underpin the activity of these anticoagulants, which are discussed as follows.

> **RED FLAG**
>
> **REVERSAL OF DABIGATRAN**
>
> A reversal agent, idarucizumab, ('Praxbind') is available for use in acute haemorrhage scenarios.

Direct thrombin inhibition

Inhibition of thrombin and thus prevention of the fibrinogen→fibrin conversion underpins the anticoagulant action of oral dabigatran (trade named 'Pradaxa'). It is appropriate in most anticoagulation scenarios, and in particular is widely used for postoperative VTE prophylaxis, in elective hip or knee replacements. It offers two major advantages over warfarin:

- A highly predictable dose response: no regular monitoring (i.e., blood tests) is required
- Drug-drug interactions are few, since it does not inhibit/induce cytochrome P450 enzymes

Other drugs that also exert their anticoagulant action by thrombin inhibition, but are administered parenterally, include bivalirudin and argotraban.

Direct FXa inhibition

Inhibition of FXa prevents formation of the prothrombinase complex (X-FVa-Ca^{++}) and thus thrombin cannot be cleaved from prothrombin, ultimately preventing the final fibrinogen → fibrin step of coagulation. Oral drugs exploiting this mechanism include rivaroxaban, apixaban and edoxaban.

THROMBOPROPHYLAXIS

All hospital inpatients, particularly those undergoing surgery, are at high risk of VTE. All inpatients must therefore have their individual VTE risk assessed and documented. Typical assessment tools allow balancing of individual thrombosis risk factors against protective factors, allowing the best method of prophylaxis for each patient to be determined and implemented.

Mechanical thromboprophylaxis approaches include regular mobilisation, compression stockings and pneumatic intermittent compression devices. Pharmacologic thromboprophylaxis may include any of the anticoagulants, but subcutaneous LMWH are the most commonly used drugs.

THERAPEUTIC FIBRINOLYSIS

Whilst anticoagulants prevent extension of existing clots and new clot formation; they cannot destroy existing clots. To destroy clots, intravenous fibrinolytic 'clot-busting' drugs are needed. Since they do not discriminate between physiologic and pathologic thrombi, degrading both equally, they carry a high risk of bleeding complications and have numerous side effects. Their use is therefore restricted to:

- Life-threatening PE or MI where alternative treatments are not feasible or have failed
- Ischaemic cerebrovascular strokes within 3 hours of first symptom appearance

Thrombolysis in ischaemic stroke

Fibrinolytic drugs are given intravenously if <3 hours has elapsed from the first appearance of symptoms and CT imaging has excluded haemorrhage as the cause of the stroke. Treatment aims to restore cerebral blood supply to brain tissue distal to the clot. There are two drugs currently in use:

- Recombinant human tPA (first-line preferred treatment where available). Alteplase, reteplase and tenecteplase are all recombinants
- Streptokinase, derived from group A β-haemolytic streptococci. It binds to plasminogen, forming a complex that activates other plasminogen molecules. Allergic reactions are common

Absolute contraindications to fibrinolytic ('thrombolysis') treatment for ischaemic stroke include:

- Intracranial haemorrhage (historic or current)
- Neurosurgery, head trauma or stroke in last 3 months
- Active internal bleeding
- Arteriovenous malformation, aneurysm or neoplasm
- Platelet count <100
- Anticoagulant use

● Chapter Summary

- Haemostasis consists of the sequence of vasoconstriction, primary haemostasis and finally secondary haemostasis
- Primary haemostasis consists of specific changes to platelets (adhesion, activation and aggregation) which results in formation of a platelet plug at the site of the developing clot
- Secondary haemostasis consists of activation of the coagulation cascades, ultimately converting soluble fibrinogen to insoluble fibrin and stabilising the clot
- Antiplatelet drugs reduce the probability of thrombus formation by inhibiting key stages in platelet activation and are used where inappropriate thrombus formation is likely, e.g., cardiovascular disease
- Thrombocytopenia may result from shortened lifespan or reduced production. Platelets may also be functionally impaired, which may lead to the same set of symptoms as a reduced platelet count, i.e., increased tendency to bleed including spontaneously
- The coagulation pathways are cascades of clotting factor activation, which convert a platelet plug to a mature clot (secondary haemostasis). The traditional models were subdivided into extrinsic, intrinsic and common pathways, whilst the currently accepted model consists of an initiation phase followed by an amplification phase
- Coagulation disorders may be hereditary, e.g., the haemophilias, or acquired (more common), e.g., disseminated intravascular coagulation. They may arise from either platelet (thrombophilias) or coagulation cascade dysfunction
- The important diagnostic parameters for initial assessment of blood clotting capacity are the prothrombin time (PT), the activated partial thromboplastin time (APTT) and the fibrinogen concentration
- Thromboprophylaxis (treatment to prevent inappropriate thrombus formation e.g., deep vein thrombosis or pulmonary embolism) is very important, particularly in hospitalized patients. The most common thromboprophylactic drugs are heparins (including low-molecular-weight heparins) and warfarin
- Fibrinolytic drugs degrade fibrin and therefore disintegrate stable clots. They are used to limit serious/life-threatening complications secondary to acute pathologic thrombus formation e.g., myocardial infarctions (MIs) are likely, and superior treatment (such as angioplasty in the case of an MI) is unavailable

Transfusion products

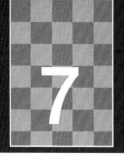

7

INTRODUCTION

The term 'blood transfusion' refers to the therapeutic use of any of the particular components or 'blood products' obtained from donation of whole blood, e.g., red cells, platelets, fresh frozen plasma (FFP) and its derivatives. Nowadays, whole blood transfusion has become extremely uncommon and is only rarely used. Storage temperatures and 'shelf-lives' of the various blood products are given in Table 7.1.

Donation process

In the United Kingdom (UK), donated blood comes from healthy, unpaid volunteers. Volunteers must be aged 17–65 years at their first donation and must weigh >50 kg to donate. Regular donors cannot donate more frequently than every 16 weeks (women) or 12 weeks (men). A fingerprick (haemoglobin) [Hb]) is performed to avoid donation in patients with undiagnosed anaemia. Donors may donate whole blood or a single component, e.g., platelets (where the technique of apheresis is used).

Table 7.1 Storage temperatures and shelf-lives of donated blood components

Blood Component	Storage features	Maximum shelf life	Storage solution	Approximate volume per unit/bag/pool/pack	Usage instructions at room (i.e., ward) temperature	Usual duration of intravenous administration
Red cells	4°C (±2°C)	35 days	Saline, adenine, glucose, mannitol (SAGM)	~220–340 mL per unit	Use within 4 hours of removal from blood fridge. May be returned to blood bank within 30 minutes, but no longer	1.5–3 hours per unit
Platelets	Agitated, 22°C (±2°C)	5–7 days	citrate-phosphate-dextrose (CPD) and plasma	~340 mL (pool) ~150 mL (apheresis unit)	Use within 2 hours of removal from the agitator. May be returned to blood bank within 30 minutes, but no longer	20–30 min per pool/unit
Granulocytes (BUFFY COAT)	22°C (±2°C), but must *not* be agitated	24 hours	White cell additive solution	~60 mL per pack (10 packs represent a typical adult dose)	Must be infused as soon as possible after collection from donor	The entire dose should be infused over 1–2 hours
Fresh frozen plasma (FFP)	<−25°C	36 months	None	~270 mL per bag	Must use within 4 hours of thawing. Must be thawed at 37°C. Once thawed, FFP cannot be returned to blood bank	20–30 mins per bag

Continued

Table 7.1 Storage temperatures and shelf-lives of donated blood components—cont'd

Blood Component	Storage features	Maximum shelf life	Storage solution	Approximate volume per unit/bag/pool/ pack	Usage instructions at room (i.e., ward) temperature	Usual duration of intravenous administration
Cryoprecipitate	<−25°C	36 months	None	190 mL per pool (2 pools represent a typical adult dose)	Must use within 4 hours of thawing. Must be thawed at 4°C. Once thawed, cryoprecipitate cannot be returned to blood bank.	~10 min per pool
Fractionated plasma products						
Immunoglobulins	22°C	Up to 3 years	Saline Glycine	Use immediately after opening		
Clotting factors	<30°C	Up to 3 years	Typically powder for reconstitution	Use immediately after reconstitution		
Albumin	<25 °C	Up to 3 years	Saline	Use immediately after opening		

Infection screening questionnaire

A screening questionnaire is completed before every donation to identify and exclude (or defer) donation from individuals at high risk of having an undiagnosed transmittable 'blood-borne' infection. It also screens for general health, to avoid potential detriment of donation to the donor or recipient.

Donor exclusion or deferral is based on criteria that evolve with scientific consensus opinions. Current examples of permanent exclusion criteria include:

- Current or past infection with hepatitis B, C, human immunodeficiency virus (HIV), human T-lymphotropic virus (HTLV) or syphilis
- Intravenous (IV) drug use, even historic. This includes bodybuilding drugs and injectable tanning agents, as well as habit-forming drugs of abuse
- Sex workers (those receiving/have ever received money or drugs for sex)

12-month deferral criteria include:

- Sexual contact in the last 12 months (even barrier protected) with anyone meeting the permanent exclusion criteria
- Sexual contact in the last 12 months (even barrier protected) with anyone who has been sexually active in a geographic area with high prevalence of HIV infection

- Sexual contact in the last 12 months (even barrier protected) with a man that has sex with other men

For up to date eligibility, exclusion and deferral criteria for potential blood donors, please visit (http://www.transfusionguidelines.org.uk/).

Whole blood donation: sample collection

If a patient passes the screening questionnaire and is fit to donate, whole blood is drawn from a large vein in the antecubital fossa of the arm. The whole process usually takes <30 minutes. Collection volume is determined by the height and weight of the donor, since it is important not to remove >15% of the donor's circulating blood volume (this could potentially cause hypovolaemic complications).

After collection, donations are ABO and RhD typed as well as being screened for the presence of antibodies that can potentially cause problems for a recipient. Mandatory infection screening tests are also performed on every sample.

Apheresis: sample collection

Apheresis allows collection of a single component of blood such as platelets from the donor. The component of choice is extracted from the blood and the remainder of the blood returned to the donor. Since most of the collected blood is returned, a much larger amount of the select component can be taken. In the case of platelets, a single donor may provide one unit. Otherwise, platelets derived from four donors are combined ('pooled') to make up an adult therapeutic dose (ATD) or 'pool.' Apheresis allows the platelet recipient to be exposed to products derived from a single rather than multiple donors. This reduces the chance of adverse reactions and infection transmission. Apheresis also facilitates provision of human leukocyte antigen (HLA)–matched platelets.

Infection screening tests performed on all collected samples

The minimum mandatory infection screen on donated samples includes hepatitis B, C, HIV, HTLV, hepatitis E virus and syphilis (Table 7.2), although note that additional screening for cytomegalovirus (CMV), trypanosoma cruzi, West Nile virus and malarial antibodies can be used if a specific infection risk is identified. Importantly, there is as yet no test capable of detecting prion diseases.

Note that these tests are screening rather than diagnostic. The HIV test will not, for example, reveal infection in an individual that has recently acquired the virus and not yet seroconverted (i.e., generated antibodies against the virus) with absent or low viraemia (virus present in the blood that is tested for with the HIV nucleic acid test). This highlights the importance of the screening questionnaire as this minimizes the chances of an individual with a recently acquired asymptomatic infection donating blood.

Whole blood donation processing

Collected samples are anticoagulated with citrate phosphate dextrose. The sugar allows the red cells to sustain their glycolytic metabolism, whilst the citrate sequesters coagulation factors which would otherwise cause clotting. The phosphate acts as a buffer. Samples are removed at this stage for blood grouping and infection screening. The remaining sample is then leucodepleted. The leucodepleted sample is then separated into plasma, platelets and red cells.

Leucodepletion

Leucodepletion is the process of removing white cells from a blood product to reduce risk of white-cell borne infection including variant Creutzfeldt–Jakob disease (vCJD) transmission and immune reactions in the recipient, including the dreaded transfusion-associated graft–versus-host disease (GVHD).

RED CELL ANTIGENS

Transfused red cells must be ABO compatible (Box 7.1.). To understand this concept, it is important to have an appreciation of red cell antigens.

> **RED FLAG**
>
> **ABO INCOMPATIBLE TRANSFUSION**
>
> IgM antibodies in the recipient's plasma bind to antigens on the donor red cells. This activates the complement pathway leading to intravascular destruction (haemolysis) of red cells and a huge release of inflammatory cytokines. These cause shock, renal impairment and disseminated intravascular coagulopathy. This scenario is often fatal and most commonly arises because of human error leading to accidental transfusion of an ABO incompatible blood type.

Red cell antigens are molecules capable of provoking an immune response. The surface membrane of the red cell is studded with numerous different molecules, and these can all potentially act as antigens. They do not provoke an immune response in the individual that has synthesized them, because they are 'self' antigens in their native physiologic host. However, if transfused into an individual that does not possess the same array of antigens on their native red cells, an immune response occurs. This can be fatal.

As one would expect, there are different red cell antigens; the most clinically important are the ABO system and the Rhesus antigens.

THE ABO ANTIGEN SYSTEM

The ABO system refers to various forms of the 'H' antigen. This is an oligosaccharide molecule expressed at the surface of red cells. Its physiologic function is unknown.

Table 7.2 Mandatory infection screening tests performed on all collected samples

Infection	Parameter used for testing
Hepatitis B	Hepatitis B surface antigen (HBsAg) HBV DNA
Hepatitis C	Anti-HCV antibodies HCV RNA testing
HIV 1+2	Anti-HIV 1 antibodies Anti-HIV 2 antibodies HIV RNA testing
HTLV	Anti-HTLV I antibodies Anti-HTLV II antibodies
Syphilis	Syphilis antibodies (antitreponemal Ab)
HEV	HEV RNA

Ab, Antibody; DNA, deoxyribonucleic acid; HBV, hepatitis B virus; HCV, hepatitis C virus; HEV, hepatitis E virus; HIV, human immunodeficiency virus; HTLV, human T-lymphotropic virus; RNA, ribonucleic acid.

'O' antigen

If the H antigen is unmodified, the antigen is known as the 'O' antigen.

'A' antigen

If the H antigen has an N-acetylgalactosamine moiety added, it becomes the 'A' antigen. If the person possesses the gene for the relevant galatosaminyltransferase enzyme (the A antigen gene), the native H antigen is modified in this way, forming the A antigen. Red cells therefore express A antigens at their surface.

'B' antigen

If the H antigen has an added galactose moiety, the resulting antigen is the 'B' antigen. If the person possesses the gene for the relevant galatosyltransferase enzyme (the B antigen gene), the native H antigen is modified in this way, forming the B antigen. The red cells therefore express B antigens at their surface.

ABO blood group

The blood group is determined by the antigens expressed on the red cells. Presence of exclusively O antigens correlates to blood group O. Presence of exclusively A antigens, or A antigens accompanied by O antigens corresponds to blood group A. Presence of exclusively B antigens, or B antigens accompanied by O antigens corresponds to blood group B. Presence of A and B (but no 'O') antigens corresponds to blood group AB (Table 7.3). In this way, the ABO genes are codominant.

Genetics of the A, B and O antigens

There are three alleles: A, B and O. Each allele corresponds to the antigen expressed at the red cell surface. Since there are two copies of each allele in a person's genome, there are six possible combinations (genotypes): O/O, A/O, A/A, B/O, B/B and A/B.

There are only four phenotypes, however: both A/O and A/A correspond to a blood group A, and B/O and B/B correspond to blood group B. Regardless of whether there are one or two copies of an 'A' antigen gene, the blood group is 'A,' except where a single 'A' allele coexists with a 'B' allele, when the blood group is 'AB.' Alleles for A and B antigens are considered codominant to each other. As the 'O' antigen is simply an unmodified 'H' carbohydrate, heterozygous A/O or B/O individuals, (see Table 7.3) will express both O and A or O and B antigens respectively.

Anti-A and anti-B antibodies

Unlike antibodies formed by exposure to foreign antigens, immunoglobulin (Ig) M antibodies arise against A or B antigens (even in the absence of direct exposure by a transfusion of foreign type A or B red cells). This phenomenon arises in response to structurally similar antigens present on intestinal bacteria and/or ingested food molecules. For example, people with blood group A (genotype A/A or A/O) possess anti-B antigens even without ever having been exposed to the 'B' antigen. Anti-A and/or anti-B antigens are typically present by 6 months of age. These anti-A, anti-B IgM antibodies are considered 'natural antibodies' since no sensitizing event is necessary for their generation.

Significantly, since the 'O' antigen is an unmodified 'H' carbohydrate, and the 'A' and the 'B' antigens are simply

Table 7.3 Blood group, corresponding red cell antigens, genotype, antibodies and ABO compatibilities

Blood group	Genotype	Red cell antigens on native red cells	Antibodies	ABO compatibility: i.e., can receive red cells from donors with blood group(s):	ABO incompatibility: must NOT be transfused with red cells from donors with blood group(s):
O[a]	O/O	O only	Anti-A Anti-B	O	A, B or AB
A	A/A	A only	Anti-B	O and A	B or AB
	A/O	A and O			
B	B/B	B only	Anti-A	O and B	A or AB
	B/O	B and O			
AB	A/B	A and B	None; immune tolerant to A, B and O antigens	A, B, O, AB	Can safely receive transfusion from all ABO types [b]

[a] Group O blood type patients (O/O genotype) are termed 'universal donors,' since their red cells do not exhibit A or B antigens and thus can be safely transfused to any blood type without causing an ABO incompatibility reaction.
[b] Group AB blood type patients (A/B genotype) are termed 'universal recipients,' since they can safely accept any ABO type. This is because they have immune tolerance to both A and B antigens as these are normally expressed on their own red cells.

modified 'H' carbohydrates, the 'O' antigen does not provoke an immune response in A/A, A/O, B/B, B/O or A/B genotype individuals. This principle has very important clinical implications.

Clinical significance

The clinical significance of blood groups arises from the necessity of ensuring ABO compatibility between the blood product donor(s) and the recipient. Incompatibility will provoke an immediate and severe immune response in the transfusion recipient, because of exposure to A and/or B nonself antigens. Essentially, this means that the blood group type of the donation blood must not contain the antigens that the recipient's own red cells do not express.

Mechanism of immune intolerance

In an individual who does not normally express an antigen on their own red cells, IgM antibodies to the nonnative antigens will be present. If nonnative (foreign) antigens are introduced to a transfusion recipient by an ABO-incompatible red cell transfusion, the recipient's immune system will recognize the antigen as foreign and commence complement-mediated destruction.

In a group O patient (O/O), antibodies to A and B antigens are present. Group O patients must not receive red cells expressing these antigens, i.e., red cells from A/O, A/A, B/O, B/B or A/B genotyped individuals.

In a group A patient (A/O or A/A), anti-B antigens are present. Group A patients must not receive red cells expressing the B antigen, i.e., those from B/O, B/B or A/B genotyped individuals. They can, however, safely receive blood from group O individuals (O/O) as these red cells do not express a 'foreign' antigen (remember the H representing group O is also present in group A and B albeit in a modified form).

In a group B patient (B/O or B/B), anti-A antigens are present. Group B patients **must not** receive red cells expressing the A antigen, i.e., those from A/O, A/A or A/B genotyped individuals. They can safely receive blood from group O individuals (O/O) for the same reasons as stated earlier (see Table 7.3).

THE Rh ANTIGEN (PREVIOUSLY TERMED 'RHESUS ANTIGEN') SYSTEM

Please note that many texts still refer to the Rh antigen as the 'rhesus' antigen, but it is now more correctly described as the Rh antigen. There are five Rh antigens that may be expressed on an individual's red cells: C, c, D, E, and e. D is the most clinically significant. Presence of a single 'D' allele confers Rh positive status (it is dominant). Rh positive individuals are therefore DD or Dd, and Rh-negative individuals dd. Predominance of Rh negativity is strongly determined by race. Less than 1% of Africans and Asians are Rh negative, whilst up to 15% of Caucasians are Rh negative.

Antibodies against Rh D are usually IgG, as opposed to the IgM antibodies commonly targeted against A and B antigens. Clinical implications of the IgG nature of anti-D antigens include that RhD incompatible transfusion reactions are usually inconsequential. However, IgG are able to cross the placenta (unlike the larger IgM). The clinical significance of this is that Rh disparity between mother and fetus (specifically between a Rh −ve mother and a Rh +ve fetus) can lead to placental transfer of anti-Rh D maternal antibodies. This is in contrast to the large, bulky IgM anti-A and anti-B antibodies, accounting for why ABO mother-fetus incompatibility is of no consequence.

Also in contrast to the ABO system, antibodies to Rh D ('anti-D') are only present in Rh D −ve individuals that have experienced a sensitizing event. A 'sensitizing event,' refers to an event which leads to development of anti-D antibodies. Transfusion with Rh D +ve cells to a Rh −ve recipient is a sensitizing event.

Sensitizing events in pregnancy

Most clinically relevant sensitizing events occur in pregnancy if the Rh −ve woman is carrying a Rh +ve fetus. These include:

- Normal pregnancy (small amounts of fetal blood enter the maternal circulation)
- Maternal trauma during pregnancy
- Ectopic pregnancy
- Abortion
- Amniocentesis/chorionic villous sampling

Prevention of maternal development of anti-D (Rh −ve mothers only)

If a female of childbearing age develops anti-D antibodies, during any subsequent pregnancy, the anti-D IgG will cross the placenta. This may result in haemolytic disease of the fetus or haemolytic disease of the newborn (see later). It is therefore important to prevent the development of anti-D antibodies in Rh −ve females of childbearing age.

Management of Rh −ve females in this age bracket therefore involves:

- Avoiding transfusion of Rh +ve red cells
- Prophylactic anti-D at particular stages prenatally and postnatally
- Treating any sensitizing events in pregnancy with anti-D as soon as possible

Anti-D immunoglobulin

Anti-D Ig is derived from donated plasma of Rh −ve individuals that possess a high level of the anti-Rh D antibody. Since it is derived from blood donation, it is considered a blood product. Intramuscular anti-D Ig administered to a

Rh −ve mother will coat any fetal red cell D antigens that have entered the maternal circulation, before maternal anti-D antibodies can be generated. This may protect any Rh +ve fetuses that the mother may carry in future pregnancies from immune haemolysis, hydrops and Rh haemolytic disease of the newborn.

Haemolytic disease of the fetus
If the fetus is Rh +ve fetus and the mother has developed IgG anti-D antibodies from a previous sensitizing event, they will cross the placenta and may lead to 'haemolytic disease of the fetus' (HDF). HDF manifests with immune haemolysis and hydrops fetalis (prenatal heart failure in utero).

Haemolytic disease of the newborn
Haemolytic disease of the newborn (HDN) is the postnatal manifestation of transplacental maternal transfer of anti-D IgG antibodies. Haemolytic anaemia may cause pallor in the newborn, or even jaundiced at or soon after the birth (within 36-hours postdelivery). Splenomegaly may be present. If in utero heart failure (hydrops) was present because of HDF, the baby will also have severe oedema, pallor and respiratory distress. Treatment following delivery may include red cell transfusion, noninvasive or mechanical ventilatory support, IV Ig and exchange transfusion.

OTHER RED CELL ANTIGENS

Other red cell antigens which may be encountered include: Kell, Duffy, Kidd, Lewis, 'P', 'I' and 'MN'. Maternofetal incompatibility of some of these antigens may also cause non-Rh haemolytic disease the newborn, with anaemia and jaundice. These antigens are also significant in patients with diseases warranting regular or frequent transfusions, e.g., patients with thalassaemia, sickle cell disease or myelodysplastic syndrome.

RED CELL TRANSFUSIONS

Red cell transfusions are indicated for restoring oxygen carrying capacity in patients with low [Hb] or blood loss, when alternative treatment strategies are ineffective or inappropriate. Acute indications include acute significant blood loss in a context of trauma, surgery or obstetrics, or any other cause of haemorrhagic shock. Severe haemolytic anaemia causes a drop in [Hb] that may warrant transfusion. It is important to be guided by the rate of red cell loss (rather than merely the magnitude of loss), as illustrated by the trend in serial [Hb] across consecutive samples.

Nonurgent indications include symptomatic anaemia of any cause (see Chapter 3: Anaemia). Certain diseases (e.g., beta thalassaemia major) render individuals permanently transfusion-dependent.

Selection of appropriate donated red cells for transfusion
Cross-matching
Transfused red cells issued to a particular individual must have been fully cross-matched by the issuing laboratory. This consists of three components: grouping, antibody screening and testing the patient's sample against the intended transfusion product. A request (including the number of units required) for blood 'cross-match' should only be made when a red cell transfusion is definitely and appropriately clinically indicated.

Grouping
A blood sample is tested by the laboratory to identify the ABO and Rh status of the patient before any transfusion.

Antibody screening
The patient's plasma is then exposed to a panel of red cells which possess specific blood group antigens other than ABO and Rh. This screens for presence of common anti-red cell antigen antibodies that may be present in the patient's plasma. If present, these would cause a transfusion reaction if donor cells bearing the particular antigen were transfused. If identified, the blood bank will only issue red cells lacking such antigens.

Serologic cross-matching
'Cross-matching' describes incubation of a small sample of the intended donor blood unit (group compatible and common antibody-screened) with the intended recipient's plasma. This will identify any atypical antibodies present in the intended recipient's blood that would result in a transfusion reaction if transfused with particular unit of blood. Evidence of incompatibility can thus be safely identified, avoiding a potentially catastrophic transfusion reaction.

Group and Save (or Group and Screen)—'G&S'
A request for blood 'G&S' is done when red cells might be required for transfusion. The request does not need to indicate the number of units that could potentially be required. This commonly requested process (e.g., before surgery with anticipated significant blood loss), refers to grouping and common antibody screening of a patient's blood sample. The sample is then stored ('saved') in the laboratory for seven days. In the event of a cross-matched sample request being made, the laboratory can immediately test the patient's plasma against the planned unit of red cells intended for donation. As it has already been grouped and antibody screened, this allows more rapid issuing of fully cross-matched blood.

Emergency cross-matching

The full cross-matching process takes time. In emergencies, where ABO group is unknown, red cells that are known to be group O and Rh D negative can be transfused immediately. Once blood group status is known, 'group specific' blood can then be issued (taking ~25 minutes), whilst full serologic cross-matching is performed (taking ~45 minutes, assuming no antibodies in the planned recipient).

Other features important for selecting appropriate donation products

Irradiated red cells

Gamma irradiation of red cells (also platelets and granulocytes) is performed within 14 days of collection. After this, shelf-life is only 14 days. All granulocyte concentrates are irradiated. Irradiated red cells (and platelets) are reserved for patients at risk of GVHD (see transfusion-associated graft versus host disease). This includes recipients

- With severely impaired cell-mediated immunity, e.g., severe combined immunodeficiency
- With haematologic diseases such as Hodgkin lymphoma
- Following particular chemotherapeutic drug exposure, e.g., fludarabine or bendamustine

An updated list of at-risk diseases and settings is available at www.bcshguidelines.com.

Cytomegalovirus negativity

Red cells or platelets should be CMV negative (i.e., derived from donors confirmed as CMV −ve) in certain situations. Although previously the list included recipients of allogeneic transplants, it is now accepted that universal leucodepletion of blood products effectively eliminates the CMV transmission risk. The current indications are now therefore limited to scenarios where the recipient is:

- A baby <12-months-old,
- Pregnant and CMV −ve
- Person with HIV and CMV −ve
- Intrauterine (fetal transfusions)

Granulocytes must be CMV negative when intended for transfusion to patients known to be seronegative for CMV infection.

Washed red cells

Sequential washing of the cells removes most traces of residual donor plasma. Washing is performed for red cells destined for recipients with a history of recurrent severe allergic or febrile reactions to previous red cell transfusions.

Administration of red cells

Consent

Whenever possible, the patient should provide informed consent for transfusion.

Confirming correct blood and correct recipient

Around 1 in 13,000 transfusions are administered to the wrong patient. It is vital for rigorous measures to be taken to minimize potential error.

CLINICAL NOTES

ERROR REDUCTION IN TRANSFUSION

Appropriate measures to take to reduce errors include:

- Repeated identity and document checking, ideally with two people *and* the patient at all stages from pretransfusion sample collection to commencement of transfusion
- A final pretransfusion check should be performed at the bedside including the patient
- If available electronic transfusion management technology with barcode recognition should be used as an additional level of positive patient identification
- Avoidance of unnecessary transfusions
- Avoidance of out-of-hours transfusions
- Adherence to local transfusion guidelines

Filtering and warming

Any indwelling cannula may be used for blood transfusion, but the larger the diameter the better. Standard blood-giving sets contain a mesh filter. Gravity or active pumping may be used. Active warming of the sample to 37°C with a dedicated blood-warmer is optimal, particularly for rapid transfusions. Red cells in a nonemergency situation are usually infused over 90–120 minutes. Drugs must never be added to the blood bag.

Monitoring

Patients receiving a red cell transfusion should at a minimum have their pulse rate, respiratory rate, blood pressure (BP), temperature measured before starting the transfusion and then 15 minutes after the start of the transfusion and up to 60 minutes after the transfusion has ended.

ALTERNATIVES TO RED CELL TRANSFUSIONS

Some individuals are averse to receiving blood products. This may be because of concern about the associated risks, or religious beliefs.

For such individuals, alternatives to blood transfusion are necessary. Unfortunately, most of these alternatives are only practical when the scenario of potential blood loss, e.g., surgery, is known about well in advance. They are not therefore useful in cases of emergency haemorrhage.

Clinically, these measures are inferior, but these alternative options need to be available in the context of valid, informed refusal of transfusion by an adult with capacity. With children under 16 years of age, the law differs.

Emergency alternatives to red cell transfusion

The only practical alternative to transfusion in an emergency haemorrhage scenario is an attempt to restore the depleted circulation volume with crystalloid or colloid. Whilst this approach may temporarily restore organ perfusion pressure in haemorrhage, it will not compensate for the impairment of oxygen delivery to organs and tissues, since this is a function of the reduced oxygen carrying capacity imposed by the red cell loss. It will also cause haemodilution of remaining red cells, clotting factors and platelets. If a cell-saver (see later) is present, this may be lifesaving, but they are not universally available and even cell-savers are unacceptable to those with some particular beliefs.

Nonemergency alternatives to red cell transfusion

- Intraoperative cell salvage: this refers to red cells lost in the surgical field being aspirated, washed and returned to the patient. This technique relies on the availability of the automated cell-saver equipment and staff trained and competent in its use. It can be particularly beneficial in certain 'clean' surgeries e.g., knee and hip replacements but is not applicable in cancer resections or where any infective material may be present.
- Prior autologous donation: an individual can donate their own blood in advance of the situation where a need for red cell transfusion is anticipated. This can then be transfused as needed if and when the need arises. However, this strategy is not appropriate if the patient's predonation Hb is low.

- Erythropoiesis-stimulation: this strategy administers erythropoietin to increase the patient's red cell counts in advance of planned surgery. The rationale is that the impact of exsanguination will be minimized by the increased haematocrit.
- Normovolaemic haemodilution: immediately before surgery, blood is collected from the patient. The volume collected is replaced by crystalloid or colloid, restoring intravascular volume. The intravascular blood is however now haemodiluted. For a given volume of surgical blood loss, a smaller number of red cells are lost, reducing the impact on [Hb] levels. Immediately postoperatively, the collected blood is 'returned' to the patient.

OTHER TRANSFUSION PRODUCTS

Platelets

One unit of platelets is known as a 'pool' (as it represents the platelets of four pooled whole blood donations) or an adult therapeutic dose (ATD). Platelets must be stored at room temperature (22–24°C) on agitators to avoid aggregation. Their shelf-life is 5 days.

One ATD typically raises the platelet count by 20–40 $\times 10^9$. A single ATD should be infused over a period of 15–30 minutes. Platelets should only be transfused to recipients with the same blood group as the donors. The cause of thrombocytopenia should ideally be identified before platelets transfusion, as it is contraindicated in thrombotic thrombocytopenic purpura (see Chapter 6: Thrombotic thrombocytopenic purpura) and heparin-induced thrombocytopenia (see Chapter 6: Heparin-induced thrombocytopenia). Indications for platelet transfusion include:

- Haemorrhage:
  o When platelet count is $<100 \times 10^9$ (intracranial or intraocular haemorrhage)
  o When platelet count is $<50 \times 10^9$ (all other haemorrhages)
  o As part of a massive transfusion protocol in the context of major haemorrhage
  o In patients known to be on antiplatelet drugs (e.g., aspirin, clopidogrel, etc.)
- Prophylactic
  o Extremely low platelet count ($<10 \times 10^9$)
  o Very low platelet count ($<20 \times 10^9$) in presence of risk factors for bleeding, e.g., sepsis
  o Low platelet count ($<50 \times 10^9$) before major surgery with potential significant blood loss, e.g., laparotomy

Certain complications (transfusion-related lung injury [TRALI], bacterial contamination, allergic and febrile reactions) are more common with platelet transfusions than with red cell transfusions.

Granulocyte concentrates

Granulocytes (neutrophils) are occasionally prescribed as daily transfusions to neutropenic patients with life-threatening bacterial or fungal infection. They must ABO and Rh D compatible and fully cross-matched because of persistence of red cells and platelets (typically two ATD's worth of platelets per unit). They are irradiated to reduce the chance of transfusion-associated GVHD.

Plasma derivatives

Because of concern about potential transmission of vCJD via transfusion products, British donor-derived plasma has not been used for FFP, human albumin solution, clotting factor concentrates (single or combined) or Ig for the last 20 years.

Fresh frozen plasma

FFP is obtained by apheresis or whole blood donations. Following leucodepletion, rapid freezing preserves the activity of the highly labile coagulation factors. FFP contains the normal array of clotting factors, albumin and Igs, in physiologic proportions. The minimum dose is 12–15 mL/kg. Indications for FFP transfusion include:

- Acquired coagulation defect caused by deficits of multiple clotting factors, for example:
  o DIC
  o Decompensated liver disease.
  o As part of massive transfusion in major haemorrhage
  o Where prothrombin complex concentrate (PCC) or single clotting factor concentrates are unavailable, FFP may be substituted for provision of the requisite clotting factor(s).
- Plasma exchange e.g., for thrombotic thrombocytopenic purpura

Compatibility of FFP is different to that with red cells. A patient should ideally receive FFP donated by a patient with the same blood group as them (Table 7.4). The universal donor/recipient label is swapped for FFP: blood group O can receive FFP from any group but can only donate FFP to other blood group O patients. This is because group O plasma contains anti-A and anti-B antibodies, thus should only be given to group O patients. Group AB plasma, conversely, contains neither anti-A nor anti-B antibodies, so is acceptable to all groups.

Immunoglobulins

Normal immunoglobulins

The Igs extracted from several thousand blood donations are pooled and used as replacement therapy for patients with severe Ig deficiency. They can be administered intravenously (IV Ig) or subcutaneously (SC Ig). As IV Ig at high doses is immunosuppressive, it can also be used for treatment of some autoimmune diseases, e.g., immune thrombocytopenic purpura
(see Chapter 6: 'Immune thrombocytopenic purpura').

Table 7.4 Fresh frozen plasma compatibility

Blood group	Native red cell antigens	Plasma antibodies	Can receive FFP safely from blood groups	Can donate FFP safely to blood groups
O	O	Anti-A Anti-B	O, A, B or AB	O only
A	A and O	Anti-B	A, AB	A, O
B	B and O	Anti-A	B, AB	B, O
AB	A and B	None	AB	AB, A, B, O

FFP, Fresh frozen plasma.

Specific immunoglobulins

If a patient that has not previously developed immunity towards a particular pathogen by previous infection or vaccination, they will not possess antibodies against that pathogen. If then exposed to that pathogen and it has the potential to cause serious illness, specific Igs can be used if available.

Specific Igs are obtained from screened and vaccinated donors that identified to have a very high antibody levels against the relevant pathogen. Most commonly used in the UK are:

- Tetanus Ig, which is given to patients that have *not* recently completed a tetanus toxoid vaccination course if they are injured by a mechanism likely to involve clostridium tetanus exposure (e.g., soil-contaminated cuts, foreign body penetrations, human/animal bites)
- Hepatitis B Ig, which is given to unvaccinated individuals that sustain a high-risk injury such as a needlestick injury
- Rabies virus Ig and varicella zoster virus Ig are used, but have only a narrow range of specific indications

The most commonly used specific Ig is anti-D (see Anti-D immunoglobulin), which is derived from Rh −ve donors with particularly high levels of anti-D antibodies.

Human albumin solution (HAS)

Albumin solution contains albumin purified from plasma. It contains no antibodies or clotting factors and can be given without regard to the recipient's blood group. It is available in various concentrations. Indications are largely for treatment of complications of liver failure or nephrotic syndrome. Severe hypersensitivity reactions can occur.

Cryoprecipitate

Cryoprecipitate is the insoluble precipitate formed by thawing FFP at 4°C. It contains factors VIII and XIII, vWF and fibrinogen. An adult dose represents two 'pools' (each pool representing 5 donations). Adult indications for cryoprecipitate include:

- As part of a massive transfusion protocol in the context of a major haemorrhage
- Hypofibrinogenaemia (i.e., [fibrinogen] <1.5 g/dL) and haemorrhage
- Disseminated intravascular coagulation (DIC)
- Severe liver failure
- Bleeding postthrombolysis
- Factor VIII concentrate is unavailable for a haemophilia A patient with bleeding (this is very, very rare as most transfusion laboratories keep emergency doses of recombinant factor VIII)

Single clotting factor concentrates

With the exception of factors V, X and II, all other factors are available as single-factor concentrates. They are used for treatment of coagulation deficiency diseases, e.g., haemophilias A and B. Recombinant factors are now widely used in bleeding disorders. This eliminates the risk of viral or prion transmission associated with regular/frequent exposure to donor FFP (as the source of the required factor(s).

Combined clotting factor concentrates: prothrombin complex concentrate

Prothrombin complex concentrate (PCC) contains factors II, VII, IX and X. These are the vitamin K-dependent factors. PCC thus rapidly reverses the effect of warfarin when someone is bleeding. PCC has completely replaced the traditional use of FFP in this particular context; it has greater efficacy and less risk of serious allergic reaction and transfusion-associated circulatory overload (TACO). PCC is also sometimes used in the coagulopathy associated with fulminant liver disease. It replaces the four specific factors most deficient in this condition (i.e., the vitamin K-dependent factors). Also the fluid balance of these critically-ill patients is extremely challenging; in this context, the volume of FFP required to restore factor levels could potentially be highly detrimental. PCC is also used in hereditary deficiencies of II and X. Never confuse Octaplex (a PCC brand) with Octaplas.

OCTAPLEX VERSUS OCTAPLAS

Octaplex is a brand of prothrombin complex concentrate, most commonly used in warfarin overdose. Octaplas, on the other hand, is a brand of solvent detergent treated fresh frozen plasma (FFP). The detergent inactivates bacteria and most encapsulated viruses, including hepatitis B and C and human immunodeficiency virus. FFP donations destined for the Octaplas product are sourced from countries with a low risk of variant Creutzfeldt–Jakob disease.

TRANSFUSION COMPLICATIONS

There are several different types of reactions that may occur in response to a transfusion. All may occur with any transfused product, but some are more likely with certain components. The consequences can range from mild to catastrophic. Clinical classification is by time elapsed following the start of transfusion, i.e., acute (within 24 hours) or delayed (>24 hours). For ease of understanding, the important reactions are classified here by underlying mechanism (Fig. 7.1).

Management in suspected acute transfusion reaction

Whenever an acute transfusion reaction is suspected, the transfusion should be paused. The patient should be assessed

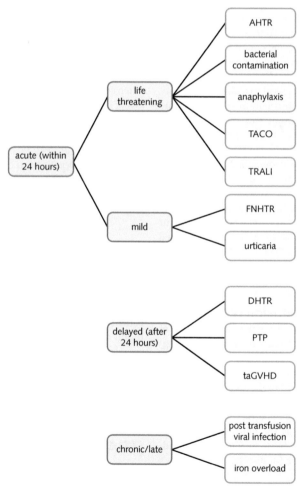

Fig. 7.1 Classification of transfusion reactions according to time of onset following the transfusion. *AHTR*, Acute haemolytic transfusion reaction; *DHTR*, delayed haemolytic transfusion record; *FNHTR*, febrile nonhaemolytic transfusion reaction; *PTP*, posttransfusion purpura; *TACO*, transfusion-associated circulatory overload; *TA-GVHD*, transfusion-associated graft-versus-host disease; *TRALI*, transfusion-associated lung injury.

by a clinician and vital signs measured. If the patient is well and vital signs normal, a nonsevere transfusion reaction is likely, and the transfusion may be resumed. Appropriate medication may be prescribed, e.g., paracetamol for febrile nonhaemolytic transfusion reaction, for symptomatic relief. However, if the patient is unwell, the giving set should be disconnected, and the cannula flushed with saline. Resuscitation using an airway, breathing, circulation approach should be commenced, with critical care input and senior supervision. Specific immediate management relevant to the suspected diagnosis, (e.g., intramuscular adrenaline and IV fluid boluses in suspected anaphylaxis) should be urgently undertaken. The culprit unit should be retained and returned urgently to the blood bank for further testing and to allow recall of associated donations if appropriate.

Haemolytic transfusion reactions

ABO incompatible transfusion
The most severe and feared acute haemolytic transfusion reactions are caused by ABO incompatibility. This occurs in 1/180,000 red cell transfusions. Anti-A or anti-B IgM antibodies in the recipient bind to the donor A or B antigens. Complement binding is initiated and intravascular destruction (haemolysis) of donor red cells takes place. C3a and C5a cause vasodilation and increased vascular permeability, causing intravascular fluid redistribution into tissues and profound distributive hypotension and shock. This may be compounded by acute renal failure. Release of tissue thromboplastin from lysed red cells can lead to DIC. Death occurs in 15% of cases of ABO incompatibility and may result from as little as 30 mL of transfused ABO incompatible blood. Patients are anxious (often experiencing a sensation of impending doom), flushed, feel extremely unwell, and may complain of abdominal or loin pain. Symptoms occur soon after the start of the transfusion. Dark urine caused by haemoglobinuria (indicating the release filtration of free Hb from the lysed red blood cells [RBCs]) is a classical sign pointing to intravascular haemolysis.

Other haemolytic transfusion reactions
Less severe haemolytic transfusion reactions arise because of IgG antibodies which react with other red cell antigens, e.g., Rh, Kell, etc. The haemolysis is extravascular (i.e., reticuloendothelial and splenic removal of antibody-coated donor cells, rather than destruction within the vascular system). It typically occurs more gradually (i.e., a 'delayed' complication) and is less catastrophic. Haemoglobinuria is not a feature of extravascular haemolysis and as the bilirubin is unconjugated, it binds to albumin is unable to be filtered by the kidneys. It thus cannot be present in (or discolour) the urine.

Febrile nonhaemolytic reactions

An isolated pyrexia (≥38°C or ≥1.5°C above baseline, if baseline <37°C) not associated with any other derangement

in blood oxygen saturation (SpO$_2$), respiratory rate (RR), heart rate (HR) or BP may be managed by temporarily pausing the transfusion and/or administering an antipyretic such as paracetamol. Increased frequency of observations should be implemented. Shivering, myalgia and nausea may accompany the fever. Febrile nonhaemolytic reactions occur in 1% to 2% of red cell transfusions and represent the most common transfusion reaction.

However, a rise in temperature >2°C above baseline, or any derangement of other observations or symptoms suggestive of a haemolytic or bacterial contamination reaction should warrant immediate cessation of transfusion and be managed as for all suspected acute transfusion reactions.

Hypersensitivity reactions

Anaphylaxis
Anaphylaxis may occur because of red cells, but is more common with FFP and plasma-rich transfusion products such as platelets. This is a potentially fatal acute complication of transfusion. Pallor, tachycardia, desaturation and hypotension may be accompanied by an urticarial rash. Oedema causes an expiratory wheeze (bronchospasm), inspiratory stridor (laryngospasm) and swelling of the lips and tongue. Increased vascular permeability causes the hypotension which may progress to severe distributive shock, loss of consciousness and death.

CLINICAL NOTES

The clinical significance of 70 mL/kg body weight is that this volume represents the entire circulating volume. For a 75-kg adult, this is 5.25 L.

Mild allergic reaction
Itching ('pruritus') or an urticarial rash unaccompanied by a change in vital signs or any more worrisome symptoms most likely represents a mild allergic reaction. However, the patient should be fully assessed, and the more serious transfusion reactions clinically excluded. Mild allergic reactions are relatively common acute transfusion reactions, most often seen during platelet or FFP transfusions, but can also occur with other blood product transfusions. Antihistamines (e.g., chlorphenamine) may reduce the symptoms.

Transfusion-related lung injury (TRALI)

Severe breathlessness and a productive cough with frothy pink sputum occurring within less than 6 hours (more typically within 2 hours) of transfusion may suggest TRALI, an important acute complication of transfusion. Hypotension caused by abnormal redistribution of intravascular fluid into the lung parenchyma is not uncommon. A fever may be present. TRALI results from donor antibodies reacting with the recipient's leucocytes. Inflammatory sequestration in the lungs leads to noncardiogenic pulmonary oedema (with an acute respiratory distress syndrome-type picture on the chest X-ray). Treatment is supportive; supplementary oxygen with ventilation in a critical care setting if required.

Transfusion-related circulatory overload

TACO describes new onset (or exacerbation of existing) pulmonary oedema within less than 6 hours of a transfusion. This manifests as acute respiratory distress (breathlessness, ↑RR and desaturation) and is associated with signs of intravascular hypervolaemia, e.g., elevated jugular venous pressure, hypertension and tachycardia. Patients with low body weight that receive a large volume transfusion, e.g., in massive haemorrhage, are at particularly risk. Similarly, patients with preexisting cardiac or renal insufficiency, hypoalbuminaemia and iatrogenic fluid overload are at high risk. TACO and TRALI are occasionally difficult to distinguish; Table 7.5 provides useful distinguishing features.

Infection

Bacterially contaminated transfusion product

This most often occurs with platelets (as they are stored at 22°C), but rarely occurs with red cells. An acute, severe

Table 7.5 Differentiating between TACO and TRALI

Clinical features	TRALI	TACO
Onset after transfusion	Usually <2 hours	Within 6 hours
Tachycardia	Yes	Yes
BP	Hypotensive or normotensive	Hypertensive or normotensive
Respiratory distress (↑RR, ↓SpO2, dyspnoeic)	Yes	Yes
Pyrexia	Likely	Unlikely
Fluid challenge	Improves, or no change	Worsens
Diuresis	Worsens	Improves
Underlying mechanism	Intravascular hypovolaemia caused by abnormal fluid redistribution	Intravascular hypervolaemia

BP, Blood pressure; RR, respiratory rate; SpO2, blood oxygen saturation; TACO, transfusion-associated circulatory overload; TRALI, transfusion-related lung injury.

response is seen very soon after the transfusion starts. Symptoms and signs may be very similar to an acute haemolytic or hypersensitivity reaction, with hypotension, shock and reduction in consciousness. Rigors and elevation of temperature >2°C above baseline may distinguish bacterial contamination from these other serious acute transfusion reactions.

Viral infection from infectious donation

Chronic viral infection secondary to transfusion with blood products derived from a virally infected donor represents a rare but important delayed complication of transfusion. The risks are <1 in 1.2 million for hepatitis B, <1 in 7 million for HIV and <1 in 28 million for hepatitis C.

Transfusion-associated graft-versus-host disease

This delayed complication of transfusion is fortunately very rare, as it is usually fatal. It arises because of lymphocyte contamination of a transfusion product. Routine leucodepletion minimizes the chance of this occurring. When it does occur, the lymphocytes may establish themselves in recipient tissues and generate an immune response against the recipient's cells. Symptoms typically develop within 30 days posttransfusion, and include rash, pyrexia, diarrhoea, deranged liver function tests and bone marrow aplasia.

Patients with impaired cell-mediated immunity are at particular risk for transfusion-associated GVHD, hence their requirement for irradiated red cell, platelet and granulocyte transfusions.

Iron overload

This is a delayed complication associated with multiple or recurrent transfusions (see Chapter 2: Iron overload).

Posttransfusion purpura

This delayed transfusion reaction typically manifests between 5 and 12 days following a transfusion (see Chapter 6: Posttransfusion purpura).

MASSIVE HAEMORRHAGE

Definitions vary as to what constitutes a 'massive' haemorrhage, but the following are reasonable:

- >150 mL blood loss/minute
- >70 mL blood loss per kg body weight (Box 7.8) in a 24-hour period
- >35 mL blood loss per kg body weight in a 3-hour period

- uncontrolled bleeding leading to reduction in the systolic blood pressure to <90 mmHg and a tachycardia >100 beats per minute

In all scenarios, the primary priority is obtaining haemostasis. Transfusion of appropriate blood products should aim to:

- maintain a sufficient intravascular volume to maintain end-organ perfusion pressure
- prevent an excessive fall in Hb impairing the oxygen delivery to perfused tissues

In practice, massive haemorrhage requires massive transfusion; i.e., transfusion of red cells in large amounts accompanied by appropriate platelet transfusions, FFP and cryoprecipitate. All UK hospitals have algorithms (major haemorrhage protocols) which should be activated as soon as a major haemorrhage is recognized. These guidelines will dictate the initial ratio of RBC:FFP:platelets:cryoprecipitate that should be administered whilst awaiting laboratory results for more tailored guidance. One of the commonly used ratio 4:4:1 (RBC:FFP:platelets) for the first major haemorrhage pack (MHP) and followed by the second MHP which has all the aforementioned in same ratio but added two pools of cryoprecipitate.

Complications associated with massive transfusions

All the usual complications associated with transfusion are possible, but the necessary large-volume transfusions required in massive haemorrhage scenarios are particularly likely to cause TACO. There is also significant risk of the following complications:

- Hypothermia
- Hypocalcaemia
- Hyperkalaemia
- Dilutional coagulopathy
- Metabolic acidosis

Chapter Summary

- Blood donation is a standardized process nationwide. A questionnaire attempts to exclude donations from people that have a high risk of having transmissible blood-borne infections, e.g., hepatitis or HIV.
- Donated whole blood is usually separated into components, which may contribute to pooled donation units, e.g., platelets, or represent a single transfusion unit, e.g., red cells. Plasma (fresh frozen plasma) and protein components such as immunoglobulins are also used, as are all cellular blood components.
- Different blood products have specific requirements in terms of processing, storage solution and temperature and lifespan.
- Donated products may undergo various procedures following their separation from whole blood, e.g., irradiation or washing in the case of red cells; such activities may be required where the product is destined for a particular subgroup of recipients.
- Careful consideration as to whether transfusion of any blood product is indicated, is important and should be done on a person-specific and context-specific basis as blood products represent a scarce and valuable resource.
- A person's blood group (the phenotype) is determined by the array of antigens expressed at the surface of their red cells (determined by genotype). A, B and O antigens can be present, and their combination(s) determines the blood group.
- An individual's blood group determines the blood type of the donor individual that they can safely receive blood products from (ABO compatibility). Transfusion of incompatible blood products, e.g., type AB blood to a type O individual can be fatal.

- Most wrong blood type (group-incompatible) transfusions are caused by human error, despite multiple checkpoints in the system from requesting to administering blood products.
- Rh –ve women of childbearing age that require a blood transfusion must receive Rh –ve red cells. Since exposure of the Rh antigen to a Rh –ve woman is likely to cause complications with any future babies she may carry.
- The 'group and save' of a blood sample identifies the patient's blood group and retains the serum for any necessary cross-matching of group compatible units in the event of a red cell transfusion becoming necessary. Full cross-matching of a serum sample with a unit of group-compatible blood that is provisionally intended for a particular patient is necessary before every transfusion.
- In scenarios of massive haemorrhage, adherence to specific transfusion protocols is necessary to minimize complications.
- Complications of transfusion can be divided into immediate (e.g., ABO incompatibility), early (e.g., transfusion associated lung injury) or late (e.g., infection).

Principles of immunology

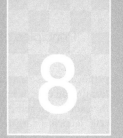

8

AN INTRODUCTION TO IMMUNOLOGY

The immune system is represented throughout the body and plays a role in most pathological processes. It works as a network with many different components; to get your head around immune function and malfunction, it helps to have an idea of the overall picture before diving into the details.

This chapter aims to introduce the bigger picture of immunology whilst avoiding the detail, which will be covered later. Try to understand the concepts and links that are covered here and revisit them as you progress through the later chapters.

The need for an immune system

The threat of many different types of infection is present for all living things. Methods to defend against these threats are required and have evolved as the nature of pathogens has also evolved. Humans face encounters with a multitude of pathogens, from aerosols of virus particles to multicellular parasites. These threats are diverse in their mechanisms of entry into the body (e.g., broken skin, airway mucosa, contaminated food), as well as their strategies of attack within the body and methods of reproduction. For example, pathogens can replicate within cells or populate the lumen of the gastrointestinal tract. Many of these pathogens can rapidly mutate, meaning that a threat that the body has encountered before may not appear in the same way if encountered again. Therefore, an immune system must be broad in its recognition of pathogens and in its mechanisms of response, yet swift enough to destroy a rapidly reproducing population.

The body also regularly encounters a plethora of harmless organisms that share characteristics with pathogens. In addition, the environment we live in and the tissues of the body itself contain many molecules that are a similar structure to molecules found on the surfaces of pathogens. For this reason, the immune system must be regulated to attack the harmful and tolerate the harmless.

Problems that arise in the immune system can lead to a breakdown in this balance:

- A fault in system function could lead to severe and repeated infection
- A loss of immune regulation could lead to unnecessary tissue damage

These immunologic problems are explored in Chapter 12.

Innate immunity

The first response of the immune system that is commonly seen is inflammation. This is an orchestration of cellular and molecular components, aimed at preventing pathogen entry and spread. It is nonspecific and can be activated by stimuli such as trauma, as well as directly by pathogens. No previous exposure is needed to form an inflammatory response—it meets the need for a broad recognition of pathogens, with a swift response to them. The initial inflammatory response is part of a larger division of the immune system termed the *innate* immune system. The innate immune system is made up of cellular, humoral and physical defences, all tasked with the initial prevention of infection.

The innate immune system involves families of cells and proteins which:

- Recognize and kill pathogens
- Process their remains
- Alert other components of the immune system to the presence of pathogens

The full detail of the innate immune system is covered in Chapter 9.

HINTS AND TIPS

Pathogens are detected by the innate immune system in many ways, including pattern recognition molecules, opsonization (when immune molecules mark a pathogen for destruction) and antibody binding.

Adaptive immunity

The innate immune system's nonspecific nature means that it is inefficient at clearing infections, this can result in tissue damage. A response targeted to each pathogen is required, but the diversity of pathogens makes this difficult. The immune system tackles this by creating large populations of cells, each with subtly different recognition molecules. This makes up the *adaptive* immune system. These cells can recognise a great range of molecular motifs, some of which may originate on pathogens, but some molecules that they recognise could be found on the tissues of the body itself. Signals from the innate immune system activate the adaptive immune system when an infection is taking place—this way, adaptive immune cells are only activated if a pathogen is present and they recognise that pathogen. These activated adaptive immune cells divide, forming an effective population in the immune system. If the same pathogen infects the body again, these selected cells launch a targeted response against that pathogen, eradicating it more effectively than with the innate immune response alone. As a result, a population of adaptive immune cells evolves according to the body's exposure to pathogens.

There are many branches to the adaptive immune system, these are covered in Chapter 10. Some adaptive immune cells can kill pathogens or infected body cells directly, some produce molecules (antibody) directed against pathogens and some are involved in the overall coordination of the immune response. This coordination is an important concept in immunology—it is the ability of the immune system to respond appropriately to infection, depending on the type of pathogen that is encountered. The innate and adaptive immune systems are compared in Table 8.1, components of each system are summarized in Table 8.2.

Table 8.1 Essential differences between the innate and adaptive immune systems

	Innate immune system	Adaptive immune system
Response to pathogens	Rapid—response does not change with repeated exposure	Slower—requires repeated exposure to develop
Specificity	Each component can defend against various types of pathogen (it is not antigen specific)	Each component can only defend against one type of pathogen (it is antigen specific)
Mechanisms of defence	Broad and are effective against many pathogens (e.g., phagocytosis, complement)	Specific to each pathogen (e.g., antibody)

Table 8.2 Components of the innate and adaptive immune systems

	Innate system	Adaptive system
Cellular components	Monocytes/macrophages Neutrophils Eosinophils Basophils Mast cells Natural killer cells	B cells/plasma cells T cells
Molecular components	Complement Cytokines Acute phase proteins Interferons	Antibody Cytokines

HINTS AND TIPS

T cells coordinate the adaptive immune response, as well as eradicating certain pathogens. B cells secrete antibody, which neutralizes pathogen directly and aids the innate immune system in pathogen recognition.

The link: presentation of antigen

Adaptive immunity is driven by the recognition of small molecular units found on pathogens, these units are called antigen. In infection, innate immune cells kill pathogens and process their remains to produce antigen. This is then presented to adaptive immune cells by professional antigen presenting cells, linking the innate and adaptive immune systems. The adaptive immune system then coordinates the response, as described earlier. This process of antigen presentation is also used by the majority of body cells to flag up any intracellular infection to the immune system. Antigen presentation and recognition is covered in more detail in Chapter 10.

Chapter Summary

- Pathogens vary greatly in nature
- A broad and efficient immune system is required to prevent infection whilst avoiding tissue damage
- The innate immune system is broad in its recognition of pathogens and can activate the adaptive immune system
- The adaptive immune system is more targeted, it develops with pathogen exposure and is driven by antigen presentation from the innate immune system
- An ineffective immune system can result in severe infection, an unregulated immune system can result in tissue damage

The innate immune system

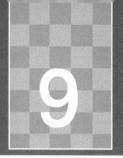

9

Innate defences can be classified into three main groups:
1. Barriers to infection
2. Cells
3. Serum proteins and the complement system

BARRIERS TO INFECTION

Physical and mechanical

Skin and mucosal membranes act as physical barriers to the entry of pathogens. Tight junctions between cells prevent the majority of pathogens from entering the body. The flushing actions of tears, saliva and urine protect epithelial surfaces from colonization. High oxygen tension in the lungs, and body temperature, can also inhibit microbial growth.

In the respiratory tract, mucus is secreted to trap microorganisms. They are then mechanically expelled by:

- Beating cilia (mucociliary escalator)
- Coughing
- Sneezing

Chemical

The growth of microorganisms is inhibited at acidic pH (e.g., in the stomach and vagina). Lactic acid and fatty acids in sebum (produced by sebaceous glands) maintain the skin pH between 3 and 5. Enzymes such as lysozyme (found in saliva, sweat and tears) and pepsin (present in the gut) destroy microorganisms.

Biological (normal flora)

A person's normal flora is formed when nonpathogenic bacteria colonize epithelial surfaces. Normal flora protects the host by:

- Competing with pathogenic bacteria for nutrients and attachment sites
- Producing antibacterial substances

The use of antibiotics can disrupt the normal flora, making pathogenic organisms more likely to cause disease.

CLINICAL NOTES

CLOSTRIDIUM DIFFICILE

Hospitalized patients that are being treated with certain antibiotics are at greater risk of developing a *Clostridium difficile* (*C. diff*) infection because of the disruption of the patient's normal gut flora. *C. diff* infection causes watery diarrhoea, nausea and abdominal pain; possible complications include toxic megacolon and sepsis. The infection can rapidly spread between patients on a ward so adequate hand washing and isolation of infected patients is essential.

CELLS OF INNATE IMMUNITY

The cells of the innate immune system consist of:

- Phagocytes
- Natural killer cells
- Degranulating cells

Phagocytes

Phagocytes (macrophages and neutrophils) engulf and then destroy pathogens. Macrophages are long-lived sentinel cells stationed at likely sites of infection; upon infection, they release cytokines that recruit the shorter-lived but more actively phagocytic neutrophils.

Neutrophils (for structure and production, see Chapter 1: Neutrophils)

Neutrophils comprise 50% to 70% of circulating white cells. Neutrophils arrive quickly at the site of inflammation and in the act of killing pathogens they die; in fact, dead neutrophils are the major constituent of pus. Neutrophils migrate from the bloodstream in response to tissue damage, complement proteins and chemicals released by macrophages (see Chapter 11). They are phagocytes so have an important role in engulfing and killing extracellular pathogens.

The process of phagocytosis and the mechanisms of killing are shown in Fig. 9.1. During inflammation, neutrophil production is stimulated by the cytokine granulocyte colony-stimulating factor. A high neutrophil count is part of the acute phase response (see later). Neutrophils can be activated and recruited either by interleukin (IL)-8 and tumour necrosis factor (TNF) secreted by macrophages, or by IL-17 secreted by T cells of the adaptive immune system.

CLINICAL NOTES

NEUTROPENIC SEPSIS

Neutropenic individuals are at an increased risk of serious bacterial infections and sepsis. Neutropenic sepsis is often difficult to detect because of the decreased immune response to pathogens; any suspicion of infection should be investigated, and the patient treated accordingly.

Monocytes and macrophages

Monocytes and macrophages comprise the other major group of phagocytic cells. Monocytes account for 5% to 10% of the circulating white cell count and circulate in the blood for approximately 8 hours before migrating into the tissues, where they differentiate into macrophages; these macrophages can live for decades. Some macrophages become adapted for specific functions in particular tissues, e.g., Kupffer cells in the liver, glial cells in the brain and osteoclasts in bone.

In comparison to monocytes, macrophages:

- Are larger and longer-lived
- Have greater phagocytic ability
- Have a larger repertoire of lytic enzymes and secretory products

Macrophages phagocytose and destroy their targets using similar mechanisms to neutrophils. The rate of phagocytosis can be greatly increased by opsonins, such as immunoglobulin (Ig) G and the complement protein C3b. Neutrophils and macrophages have receptors for these opsonins, which may be bound to the antigenic surface. Intracellular pathogens, e.g., *Mycobacterium,* can prove difficult for macrophages to kill. They are either resistant to destruction inside the phagosome or can evade by entering the macrophage cytoplasm. For the immune system to act against these pathogens, T cell help is required.

In addition to phagocytosis, macrophages can secrete a number of compounds into the extracellular space, including cytokines (TNF, IL-8 and IL-1) and hydrolytic enzymes. Macrophages are also able to process and present antigen in association with class II major histocompatibility complex (MHC) molecules.

Macrophages express a wide array of surface molecules including:

- Receptors for complement and the Fc portion of IgG
- Pattern recognition molecules (PRMs)
- Cytokine receptors, e.g., TNF-α and interferon-γ (IFN-γ)
- MHC and B7 molecules (to activate the adaptive immune response)

Macrophages can be activated by:

- Cytokines such as IFN-γ
- Contact with complement or products of blood coagulation
- Direct contact with the target through PRM stimulation

Following activation, macrophages become more efficient phagocytes and have increased secretory and microbicidal activity. They also stimulate the adaptive immune system by expressing higher levels of MHC class II molecules and secreting cytokines.

In comparison to neutrophils, macrophages:

- Are longer-lived (they do not die after dealing with pathogens)
- Are larger (diameter 25–50 μm), enabling phagocytosis of larger targets
- Move and phagocytose more slowly
- Retain Golgi apparatus and rough endoplasmic reticulum and can therefore synthesize new proteins, including lysosomal enzymes and secretory products
- Can act as antigen-presenting cells

Killing by phagocytes

The process of phagocytosis allows cells to engulf matter that needs to be destroyed. The cell can then digest the material in a controlled fashion before releasing the contents. The process of phagocytosis is shown in Fig. 9.1.

Natural killer cells

Natural killer (NK) cells develop from lymphoid progenitor cells, but unlike the other types of lymphocytes (T cells and B cells, see Chapter 10) their function mainly lies in the innate immune response. NK cells use cell-surface receptors to identify virally modified or cancerous cells. Similar to macrophages, NK cells do not require T cell help to kill pathogens but function more effectively when T helper cells secrete IFN-γ. One set of receptors activates NK cells, initiating killing; others inhibit the cells:

- Activating receptors include calcium-binding C-type lectins, which recognize certain cell-surface carbohydrates.
- Inhibitory receptors include killer-cell immunoglobulin-like receptors (KIRs). KIRs are members of the immunoglobulin gene superfamily (see Chapter 10) and recognize class I MHC molecules on other cells.

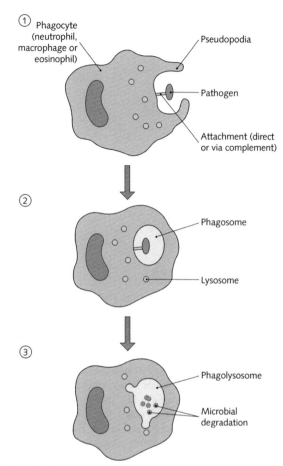

① Phagocyte (neutrophil, macrophage or eosinophil)

Pseudopodia

Pathogen

Attachment (direct or via complement)

②

Phagosome

Lysosome

③

Phagolysosome

Microbial degradation

Fig. 9.1 Phagocytosis. Pseudopodia surround the pathogen (1). They fuse around the organism, producing a vesicle known as a phagosome (2). Lysosomes fuse with the phagosome to form phagolysosomes (3). Proteins within the lysosome, and other granules that fuse with the phagolysosome, lead to degradation of the organism. The microbial products are then released.

Because the C-type lectin receptors are activated by carbohydrates on normal host cells, the KIR system acts to prevent NK cells from attacking the host. Conversely, a cell that is not expressing class I MHC molecules will not activate the KIR system so would be attacked by NK cells. This is useful in eliminating body cells that have downregulated class I MHC because of viral infection (e.g., herpes) or mutation; the lack of MHC I in these infected or mutated cells evades attack from T cells but this same MHC I deficiency causes NK cells to attack.

NK cells can also destroy antibody-coated target cells irrespective of the presence of MHC molecules, a process known as antibody-dependent cell-mediated cytotoxicity. This occurs because killing is initiated by cross-linking of receptors for the Fc portion of IgG1 and IgG3. NK cells are not clonally restricted, have no memory and are not very specific in their action. They induce apoptosis in target cells (Fig. 9.2) by:

- Ligation of Fas or TNF receptors on the target cells; NK cells produce TNF and exhibit Fas ligand (FasL).

This initiates a sequence of caspase recruitment and activation, resulting in apoptosis.

- Degranulation by NK cells, which releases perforins and granzymes. Perforin molecules insert into and polymerize within the target cell membrane. This forms a pore through which granzymes can pass. Granzyme B then initiates apoptosis from within the target cell cytoplasm.

The induction of apoptosis is a crucial tool for the immune system. It can be used for targeted killing of infected or mutated cells and is also a key part of the development of the adaptive immune system (see Chapter 10).

HINTS AND TIPS

Fas receptors are found on human cells. Once they bind to the Fas ligand, they stimulate apoptosis.

Degranulating cells

Mast cells and basophils (Chapter 1: Basophils)

Mast cells and basophils have similar functions but are found in different locations; basophils comprise <1% of circulating white cells, whereas mast cells are resident in the tissues.

High concentrations of mast cells are found close to blood vessels in connective tissue, skin and mucosal membranes. The two types of mast cell—mucosal and connective tissue—differ in their tissue distribution, protease content and secretory profiles.

Mast cells function by discharging their granule contents. Degranulation is triggered by cross-linking of high-affinity receptors for the Fc portion of IgE (Fig. 9.3). Cross-linkage results in an influx of calcium ions into the cell, which induces release of pharmacologically active mediators from granules (Table 9.1). This mechanism allows mast cells to attack larger organisms living in lumens, such as tapeworms, which otherwise would evade immune attack. Mast cell activation releases leukotrienes, which attract eosinophils to the site of parasitic infection. This plays an important role in the development of an episode of a type I hypersensitivity, with the mast cells and basophils providing the early phase response and the eosinophils mediating the late phase response. This underlies the allergic response (see Chapter 12).

HINTS AND TIPS

During severe allergy (anaphylaxis, see Chapter 12: Anaphylaxis) mast cell tryptase levels increase for a few hours. This is a useful diagnostic test for anaphylaxis.

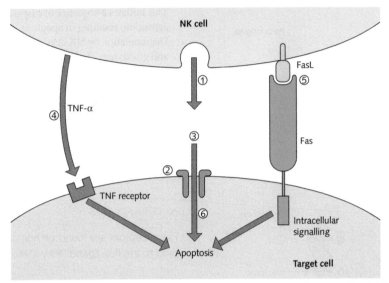

Fig. 9.2 Mechanism of killing by natural killer (NK) cells. Activation of NK cells in the absence of an inhibitory signal results in degranulation (1). Perforins form a pore in the target cell, allowing entry of granzymes (2) (3). Tumour necrosis factor (TNF) produced by NK cells acts on the target cell's receptors (4). Fas ligand (FasL) interacts with target cell Fas (5). Intracellular signalling from Fas TNF receptors and granzymes results in apoptosis (6).

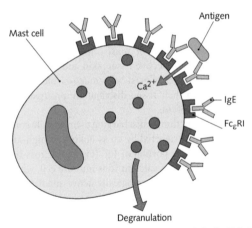

Fig. 9.3 Activation of mast cells by immunoglobulin E (IgE). IgE, produced by plasma cells, binds via its Fc domain to receptors on the mast cell surface. Cross-linking of these receptors by an antigen causes an influx of calcium ions (Ca^{2+}) into the cell. Calcium ions cause a rapid degranulation of inflammatory mediators from the mast cell. *FcεRI*, High-affinity IgE receptor.

Eosinophils Chapter 1: Eosinophils

Eosinophils comprise 1% to 3% of circulating white cells and are found principally in tissues. They are derived from the colony-forming unit for granulocytes, erythrocytes, monocytes and megakaryocytes (CFU-GEMM) and their maturation is similar to that of the neutrophil (see Chapter 1). They are important in the defence against parasites and cause damage by extracellular degranulation. Their granules contain major basic protein, cationic protein, peroxidase and perforin-like molecules. Peroxidase generates hypochlorous acid, major basic protein damages the parasite's outer surface (as well as host tissues) and cationic protein acts as a neurotoxin, damaging the parasite's nervous tissue.

SOLUBLE PROTEINS

The soluble proteins that contribute to innate immunity (Table 9.2) can be divided into antimicrobial serum agents and proteins produced by cells of the immune system.

Acute phase proteins

The acute phase response is a systemic reaction to infection or tissue injury, where macrophages release cytokines IL-1, IL-6 and TNF; these cytokines reach the liver through the circulation. The liver responds by increasing its production of certain plasma proteins. These so-named acute phase proteins (APPs) are:

- C-reactive protein (CRP)
- Complement components
- Fibrinogen
- α_1-Antitrypsin
- Haptoglobulin

The change in plasma concentration is accompanied by fever, leucocytosis, thrombocytosis, catabolism of muscle proteins and fat deposits. Symptomatically, this

Table 9.1 Mast cell mediators and their actions

Mediator[a]		Action
Primary	Histamine	Increased capillary permeability, vasodilatation, smooth muscle contraction
	Serotonin	Increased capillary permeability, vasodilatation, smooth muscle contraction, platelet aggregation
	Heparin	Anticoagulation
	Proteases	Activates complement (C3)
	Platelet-activating factor	Increased mucus secretion
		Platelet aggregation and activation, increased capillary permeability, vasodilatation, chemotactic for leucocytes, neutrophil activation
Secondary	Leucotrienes (C4, D4, B4)	Vasodilatation, smooth muscle contraction, mucus secretion, chemotactic for neutrophils
	Prostaglandins (D2)	Vasodilatation, smooth muscle contraction, chemotactic for neutrophils, potentiation of other mediators
	Bradykinin	Increased capillary permeability, vasodilatation, smooth muscle contraction, stimulation of pain nerve endings
	Cytokines	Various

[a] Mast cells contain many preformed (primary) mediators that are stored in granules. They can also synthesize new (secondary) mediators when they are activated

Table 9.2 The soluble proteins of innate immunity

	Protein	Notes
Secreted agents	Lysozyme	Bactericidal enzyme in mucus, saliva, tears, sweat and breast milk Cleaves peptidoglycan in the cell wall
Innate antimicrobial serum agents	Lactoferrin	Iron-binding protein that competes with microorganisms for iron, an essential metabolite
	Complement	Group of 20 proenzymes activation leads to an enzyme cascade, the products of which enhance phagocytosis and mediate cell lysis Alternative pathway can be activated by nonspecific mechanism
	Mannan-binding lectin	Activates the complement system
	C-reactive protein	Acute phase protein, produced by the liver Binds C-polysaccharide cell wall component of bacteria and fungi Activates complement via classical pathway Opsonizes for phagocytosis
Proteins produced by cells of the innate system	Interferon-α	Produced by virally infected cells
	Interferon-β	Induces a state of viral resistance in neighbouring cells by: Inducing genes that will destroy viral DNA Inducing MHC class I expression
	Interferon-γ	Mainly produced by activated NK cells Activates NK cells and macrophages

MHC, Major histocompatibility complex; NK, natural killer.

change contributes to what is described as severe fatigue—'malaise'. Synthesis of APPs is enhanced by cytokines secreted by macrophages and endothelial cells. The main APP is CRP.

The extent of the rise in the plasma concentration of different APPs varies:

- Increased several folds above normal levels: α_1-glycoprotein, α_1-proteinase inhibitor, haptoglobulin, fibrinogen
- 100–1000-fold increase: CRP.

The concentration of other plasma proteins, most notably albumin and transferrin, falls.

C-reactive protein

Levels of CRP rise within hours of tissue injury or infection. The actions of CRP are outlined in Table 9.2. CRP elevation can be slight (e.g., cerebrovascular accident), moderate (e.g., myocardial infarction) or marked (e.g., bacterial infections).

> **HINTS AND TIPS**
>
> Tumour necrosis factor-α, interleukin (IL)-1 and IL-6 released by macrophages stimulate the liver to produce the acute phase proteins.

Erythrocyte sedimentation rate

The erythrocyte sedimentation rate (ESR) is an index of the acute phase response. It is especially representative of the concentration of fibrinogen and α-globulins. Elevated fibrinogen levels cause red cells to form stacks (rouleaux), which sediment more rapidly than individual blood cells.

> **HINTS AND TIPS**
>
> In chronic inflammation, high C-reactive protein and erythrocyte sedimentation rate persist. The resulting catabolism of muscle and fat may lead to severe weight loss.

> **CLINICAL NOTES**
>
> **THE ACUTE PHASE RESPONSE**
>
> The acute phase response provides us with chemical markers of inflammation that can be measured. In a child presenting with abdominal pain, a C-reactive protein (CRP) level can aid the clinician in their diagnosis. A normal CRP can allow more conservative management whereas a raised CRP would indicate an inflammatory response and necessitate urgent treatment, such as surgery in differentiating the abdominal pain in constipation from that of appendicitis. The erythrocyte sedimentation rate (ESR) takes more time than CRP to become elevated—CRP rises within 2 hours of the insult and falls within a day after the insult resolves, making it a more sensitive and

therefore preferable test (Fig. 9.4). The neutrophil count is often used to monitor inflammation; both neutrophil count and CRP level are simple, cheap and fast to measure.

For these reasons the neutrophil count and CRP are often used, in conjunction with clinical signs, to see if inflammation is taking place and when it has recovered. The white cell count and ESR are useful markers measured in chronic inflammatory diseases. Some hospitals now measure plasma viscosity instead of ESR. However, ESR levels are still crucial for the diagnosis and monitoring of rheumatologic conditions such as giant cell (temporal) arteritis and systemic lupus erythematosus.

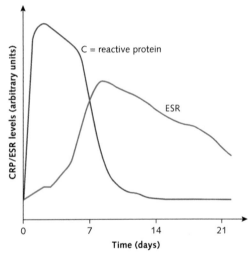

Fig. 9.4 Comparison of the change in C-reactive protein (CRP) levels and erythrocyte sedimentation rate (ESR) following an inflammatory stimulus.

The complement system

The complement system (so-called because its actions are complementary to the function of antibody) is, in fact, much older in evolutionary terms than antibody and is equally as important.

Complement is a collection of over 20 serum proteins that are always at high levels in the blood of the healthy individual. The complement system may seem complex with all the alphanumerical naming and active and inactive components. Thinking about it simply, it is a system that has three methods of activating a common pathway, which in turn has three results or effectors. The reason for the large number of proteins is to allow amplification; many of the components of complement are proenzymes that, when cleaved, activate more complement. This is similar to the amplification of clotting factors in the coagulation cascade seen in Chapter 6.

The three pathways that activate the complement system are the classical, the alternative and the lectin. All pathways result in the activation of the complement component C3 to C3 convertase. An overview of the complement system is given in Fig. 9.5.

The classical pathway

The classical pathway was discovered first and involves the activation of complement by the Fc portion of antibody. IgM is particularly good at activating complement as it is a pentamer (has five Fc portions):

- Fc activates C1
- C1 activates C2 and C4
- C2 and C4 activate C3 (C3 convertase)

The alternative pathway

C3 is an unstable molecule and without inhibition, spontaneously breaks down to the very reactive C3b; C3b reacts with two common chemical functional groups, the amino and hydroxyl groups. C3b is therefore neutralized quickly by water. However, with many pathogens made up of proteins and carbohydrates that contain these functional groups, C3b attaches to the pathogen and is not broken down by water. C3b then reacts with more complement components to form C3bBb; this is C3 convertase. This reaction does not occur on body cells because of the expression of endogenous complement inhibitors (see later).

The lectin pathway

Mannan-binding lectin (MBL), which is a normal component of serum, binds to carbohydrates found on the cell wall of certain bacteria and fungi (e.g., *Salmonella, Neisseria, Candida albicans*). MBL also binds to MBL-associated

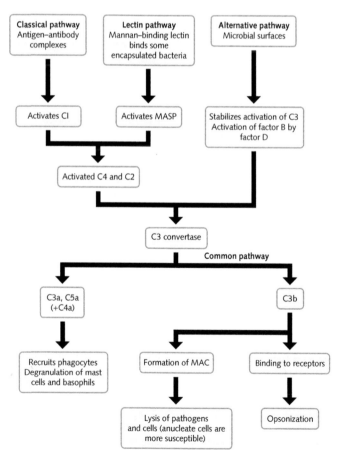

Fig. 9.5 Overview of the complement system. Cell lysis by complement is caused by formation of the membrane attack complex (MAC). This is formed when C5b, C6, C7, C8 and C9 bind together to form a 10-nm pore in the cell surface. *MASP*, Mannan-binding lectin associated serine protease.

serine proteases (MASP). This complex bears structural homology to the C1 complex. MASP then acts on C4 and C2 to generate the C3 convertase of the classical pathway.

C3 convertase

With the production of C3 convertase, all three pathways converge. C3 convertase has enzymatic effects against C3 and enables the production of large quantities of C3b, thus producing a major amplification step in the complement pathway.

Effectors of complement

C5 is now cleaved into C5a and C5b. C5b then triggers the activation of C6–C9. These form the membrane attack complex (MAC). The MAC attacks pathogens by inserting a hole in their cell membrane; the pathogen then dies via osmotic lysis. The MAC appears to be the only way the immune system has of killing one family of bacteria, the *Neisseria* (a family that includes meningococcus and gonococcus).

The cleaved fragments C3a and C5a are anaphylotoxins which are chemoattractant for other immune cells which follow the concentration gradient to the infection. Complement also opsonizes bacteria as macrophages have receptors for C3b.

These functions are summarized in Table 9.3.

Inhibitors of complement

As we have seen, complement can activate spontaneously through the alternative pathway. Complement is regulated by inhibitory molecules which are necessary to prevent complement-mediated damage of healthy cells. There are nine complement inhibitors which act at various levels throughout the pathway:

- Membrane cofactor protein, complement receptor type 1, C4b-binding protein and factor H: these prevent assembly of C3 convertase
- Decay accelerating factor: this accelerates decay of C3 convertase
- C1 inhibitor: inhibits C1
- Factor I and membrane cofactor protein: cleave C3b and C4b
- CD59 (protectin): prevents the formation of the MAC

Deficiency in any one of these inhibitory components can result in disease:

- Hereditary angioedema: deficiency of C1 inhibitor leads to unbalanced, spontaneous activation of the early complement pathway, causing life-threatening swellings
- Atypical haemolytic-uraemic syndrome: genetic deficiency in a complement inhibitor called Factor I leads to activation of the late complement cascade, leading to red cell destruction

INNATE IMMUNE SYSTEM PATTERN RECOGNITION MOLECULES

Pattern recognition molecules are required for the detection and elimination of pathogens. We have already come across the recognition molecules MBL and C1b in the complement system and seen how they function to defend the body. These are found in solution in the serum and are classified as collectins, being composed of collagen-like and lectin portions. Lectins are any protein that binds sugar molecules, usually on the surface of bacteria, e.g., MBL binds to the sugar mannose.

Nucleotide-binding and oligomerization domain (NOD) is a pattern recognition molecule found across the body, including in epithelial cells in the gut. It recognizes certain bacterial cell wall components and stimulates an immune response. The *NOD* gene is mutated in some individuals with Crohn disease.

Toll-like receptors (TLRs) are a family of about a dozen pattern recognition molecules. When they bind their ligand, they send a signal to innate immune system cells which then secrete cytokines. They have a few important clinical roles. In sepsis, TLR-4 is stimulated by vast amounts of lipopolysaccharide found on bacterial cell walls. This causes release of large amounts of TNF from macrophages, which in turn activates nitrous oxide synthase causing a fall in blood pressure and organ perfusion.

Drugs designed to bind and stimulate TLRs are being used in situations where it is helpful to stimulate a more powerful immune response, for example in some vaccines and cancer treatments.

Table 9.3 Functions of complement

Function	Notes
Cell lysis	Insertion of MAC causes lysis of gram-negative bacteria Nucleated cells are more resistant to lysis because they endocytose MAC
Inflammation	C3a, C4a, C5a cause degranulation of mast cells and basophils C3a and C5a are chemotactic for neutrophils
Opsonization	Phagocytes have C3b receptors, which means phagocytosis is enhanced when pathogens are coated in C3b
Solubilization and clearance of immune complexes	Complement prevents immune complex precipitation and solubilizes complexes that have already been precipitated Complexes coated in C3b bind to CR1 on red blood cells. The complexes are then removed in the spleen

MAC, Membrane attack complex.

CLINICAL NOTES

SEPSIS

Sepsis is when the body's immune response to infection becomes dysregulated, putting the body at risk of organ failure and death. This can be caused by infection, most commonly bacterial but also viral. The role of over activation of the innate immune system in sepsis has been detailed earlier, with the example of Toll-like receptor–4 receptor activation leading to a fall in blood pressure. It is important to identify and treat sepsis as fast as possible; Fig. 9.6 shows a typical scenario in which a patient develops sepsis. Sepsis should be suspected in any patient that develops signs of systemic infection (tachycardia, tachypnoea, pyrexia, hypotension, decrease in blood oxygen saturation, decreased level of consciousness) and has a likely source of infection (urinary tract infection, respiratory tract infection, septic arthritis, meningitis, etc.). The 'Sepsis 6' describes the package of management that should be started immediately and aims to prevent organ failure and death:

1. Give high-flow oxygen
2. Take blood cultures and consider other source cultures
3. Give intravenous antibiotics
4. Give a fluid challenge (e.g., 500 mL 0.9% NaCl)
5. Measure serum lactate and other blood tests (full blood count, C-reactive protein, urea and electrolytes, blood gases)
6. Monitor urine output

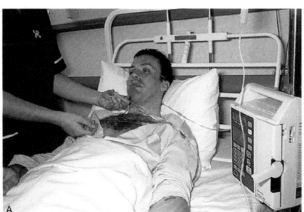
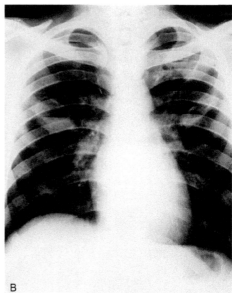

Fig. 9.6 (A and B) A 30-year-old patient is admitted with cerebral oedema following a road traffic collision. He is treated with high dose corticosteroids, intubated, has a urinary catheter inserted and has multiple venous cannulas inserted. While recovering he develops a productive cough with a respiratory rate of 23 breaths per minute, has a temperature of 38.2°C, a systolic blood pressure of 96 mmHg and a pulse of 124 beats per minute. This patient has sepsis. Many factors in his initial treatment predispose him to this. A chest radiograph shows abscesses typical of Staphylococcal pneumonia, suggestive of a source of infection. The 'Sepsis 6' should be started immediately and a senior review sought. (Reprinted with permission from Helbert M. Immunology for Medical Students 3rd edn. Philadelphia: Elsevier, 2016.)

Chapter Summary

- The innate immune system provides a broad defence against pathogens. It is made up of barriers to infection, cellular defences and soluble proteins.
- Barriers to infection can be physical, e.g., skin, chemical, e.g., stomach acidity, or biological, e.g., gut flora.
- Cells of the innate immune system are phagocytes (e.g., macrophages, neutrophils), natural killer cells and degranulating cells (e.g., mast cells, eosinophils). Phagocytes generally target extracellular pathogens, natural killer cells kill virally infected or cancerous host cells and degranulating cells generally target multicellular pathogens (e.g., worms).
- Acute phase proteins and the complement system make up the soluble protein fraction of the innate immune system.
  - Acute phase proteins are produced in response to infection and contribute to the innate immune defence in many ways. They are often measured to aid in diagnosing infection (e.g., C-reactive protein).
  - Complement proteins directly attack pathogens and alert the immune system to their presence. The complement system is activated via multiple pathways, either by bacterial cell wall components or antibody bound to pathogens.
- Pattern recognition molecules enable the innate immune system to detect pathogens. Overstimulation of pattern recognition molecules by large amounts of pathogen contributes to the symptoms of sepsis.

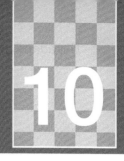

The adaptive immune system 10

The adaptive immune system provides lasting immunity, specific to each pathogen that it encounters. It is made up of various cells and secreted molecules that contribute to its two main branches: humoral and cell-mediated immunity. Humoral immunity involves the production of antibody; cell-mediated immunity is the development of a cellular response against infected or cancerous body cells. A key component of both of these branches is the immunoglobulin domain.

THE IMMUNOGLOBULIN DOMAIN

Pathogen recognition is central to the functioning of the adaptive immune system. It is largely mediated by a family of proteins that all contain very similar amino acid sequences—the immunoglobulin domain. This domain is approximately 110 amino acids in length; the polypeptide chain in each domain is folded into seven or eight antiparallel beta strands. These strands are arranged to form two opposing sheets, linked by a disulphide bond and hydrophobic interactions.

The group of molecules that contain the immunoglobulin domain are referred to as the immunoglobulin superfamily. All molecules in the immunoglobulin superfamily extend from the surface of cells or are secreted from cells.

Members of the immunoglobulin superfamily include:

- B cell receptors (Fig. 10.1)
- T cell receptors (TCR; Fig. 10.2)

- Major histocompatibility complex (MHC) molecules (Fig. 10.3)
- T cell accessory molecules such as CD4 (Fig. 10.5)
  - Immunoglobulin (Fig. 10.8).
  - Certain adhesion molecules, e.g., ICAM-1, ICAM-2 and VCAM-1.

Structure of B and T cell surface antigen receptors

Structure of B cell receptors

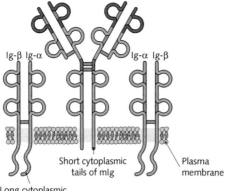

Ig-β Ig-α   Ig-α Ig-β

Short cytoplasmic tails of mIg

Plasma membrane

Long cytoplasmic tails are involved in signal transduction

▬▬ Interchain disulphide bond

Fig. 10.1 Structure of the B cell surface receptor. Membrane-bound immunoglobulin is nonsignalling. It associates with two Ig-α/Ig-β heterodimers (members of the immunoglobulin gene superfamily), which have long cytoplasmic domains capable of transducing a signal.

The B cell surface receptor consists of a membrane-bound immunoglobulin (mIg) molecule associated with two Ig-α/Ig-β heterodimers (also members of the immunoglobulin superfamily). mIg recognizes the conformational structure

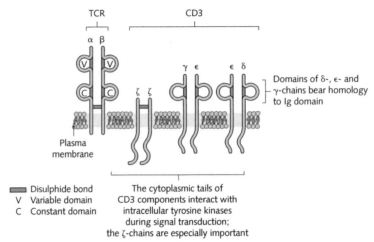

Fig. 10.2 Structure of the T cell surface antigen receptor. Negative charges on the transmembrane portion of CD3 components interact with positive charges on the T cell receptor (TCR). This maintains the complex. Antigen is detected by the TCR, but the signal is transduced by CD3.

(shape) of antigenic epitopes while the Ig-α/Ig-β heterodimers are thought to mediate signal transduction (Fig. 10.1). The role of B cells in adaptive immunity is covered in the section on humoral immunity later in this chapter.

Structure of T cell surface receptors

Antigen recognition by T cells differs from antigen recognition by B cells. T cells require the antigen to have been processed and presented to them as opposed to B cells, which simply recognize free-floating antigenic epitopes. This processing and presentation of antigen is carried out by antigen presenting cells (APCs), e.g., macrophages, and involves the MHC, which will be described later.

The T cell surface antigen receptor is made up of two parts: the TCR and CD3. Both the TCR and CD3 are members of the immunoglobulin superfamily. The TCR recognizes and binds antigen, while CD3 is involved in signal transduction. Therefore CD3 is functionally analogous to the Ig-α/Ig-β heterodimer in B cells.

The TCR is a heterodimer, comprising α- and β-chains. It is structurally similar to the immunoglobulin Fab region (see the section on humoral immunity). Each of the α- and β-chains is made up of two immunoglobulin domains, one variable and one constant, linked by a disulphide bond. As in the variable domains of immunoglobulin, three variable regions on each chain combine to form the antigen-binding site.

CD3 is made up of three polypeptide dimers, consisting of four or five different peptide chains. The dimers are γε, δε and ζζ (found in 90% of CD3 molecules) or ζη (Fig. 10.2).

The major histocompatibility complex (MHC)

MHC is a generic term for a group of molecules produced by higher vertebrate species. The MHC molecule functions as a 'window' to the inside of cells; it is the platform on which antigens are presented to the immune system. Human leucocyte antigen (HLA) is the term used to describe human MHC.

COMMON PITFALLS

All nucleated cells express some form of major histocompatibility complex. This enables any infected cell to present antigens from intracellular pathogens to the immune system.

The MHC genes

MHC genes exhibit considerable diversity; there are more than 100 identified alleles for human leucocyte antigen B (HLA-B). This means that most individuals will be heterozygous at most MHC gene loci. Therefore any two randomly selected individuals are very unlikely to have identical HLA alleles. Diversity of the MHC increases the chance that a person will be able to mount an adaptive response against a pathogen. The MHC genetic loci are tightly linked, so that one set is inherited from each parent. A complete set of major histocompatibility complex (MHC) alleles inherited from one parent is referred to as a haplotype and is found on the short arm of chromosome 6. The MHC genes are divided into three regions, each region encoding one of the three classes of the MHC: class I, class II and class III. The MHC alleles exhibit codominance, which means that both alleles are expressed. The HLA haplotype is the main identified genetic factor in autoimmune disease (for more detail see Chapter 12: Role of human leucocyte antigen).

individual. The polymorphism of the MHC is largely concentrated in the peptide-binding cleft.

MHC restriction

T cells are only able to recognize antigen in the context of self-MHC molecules (self-MHC restriction), as opposed to B cells, which recognize free antigen. CD8$^+$ T cells recognize antigen only in association with MHC class I molecules (MHC class I restricted). CD4$^+$ cells recognize antigen only in association with MHC class II molecules (MHC class II restricted).

Structure of the MHC

MHC class I and class II molecules are glycoproteins expressed on the cell surface and consist of cytoplasmic, transmembrane and extracellular portions (Fig. 10.3). MHC class I and class II are both members of the immunoglobulin superfamily. MHC class III molecules have other roles unrelated to immune function and are not covered here.

Both class I and class II molecules bind specific peptides. Class I molecules from one individual are not likely to bind the same peptides as class I molecules from an unrelated

MHC function: antigen processing and presentation

MHC molecules do not present whole antigen, the antigen being degraded into peptide fragments before binding can occur. There are different pathways of antigen processing for MHC class I and class II (summarized in Fig. 10.4). Class I molecules are found on nearly all nucleated cells. MHC class I molecules present endogenous antigens, such as those found in cells infected by viruses or intracellular bacteria. Thus CD8$^+$ T cells recognize virally altered cells and destroy them (see Chapter 11).

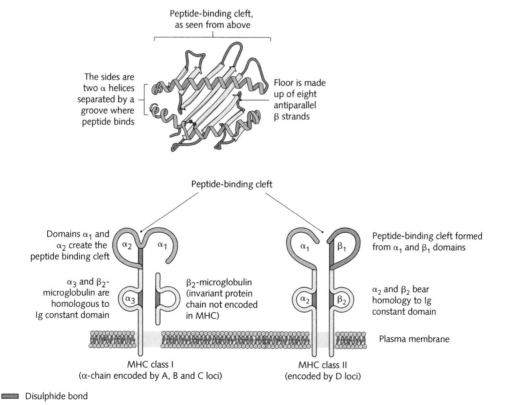

Fig. 10.3 Structure of major histocompatibility complex (MHC) class I and class II molecules. The peptide-binding cleft of a class I molecule is also shown as seen from above.

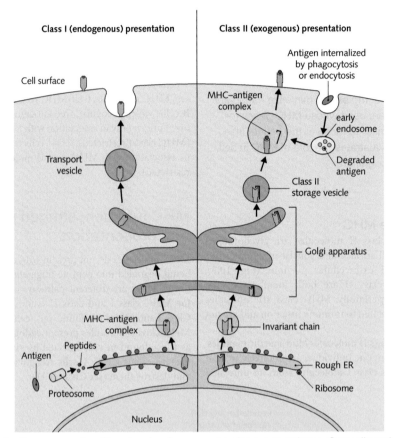

Fig. 10.4 Routes of antigen processing. Class I molecules present endogenous antigens. Cytosolic antigen is degraded by proteosomes and transported into the rough endoplasmic reticulum (ER), where peptides are loaded onto major histocompatibility complex (MHC) class I molecules. The MHC–peptide complex is transported via the Golgi apparatus to the cell surface. Class II molecules present exogenous antigens that have been phago- or endocytosed into intracellular vesicles. The MHC molecule is transported from the rough ER to the vesicle by the invariant chain (Ii). It is displaced from the MHC molecule by processed antigen, which is then presented at the cell surface.

MHC class II molecules present exogenous antigen that may have been phagocytosed or endocytosed into intracellular vesicles. Professional APCs process and present antigen to CD4$^+$ T cells in association with MHC class II molecules. These cells express high levels of MHC class II molecules. Professional APCs include:

- Dendritic cells, including Langerhans' cells
- Macrophages
- B cells

The differences between MHC class I and class II molecules are summarized in Table 10.1.

Function of CD4 and CD8

CD4 and CD8 are 'accessory' molecules that play an important role in the T cell–antigen interaction. CD4 and CD8 have two important functions:

- They bind MHC class II and class I molecules, respectively, thereby strengthening the T cell–antigen interaction.

Table 10.1 Differences between major histocompatibility complex class I and class II molecules

	Class I	Class II
Size of bound peptide	8–9 amino acids	13–18 amino acids (binding cleft more open)
Peptide from	Cytosolic antigen	Intravesicular or extracellular antigen
Expressed by	All nucleated cells, especially T cells, B cells, macrophages, other APCs, neutrophils	B cells, macrophages, other APCs, epithelial cells of the thymus, activated T cells
Recognized by	CD8+ T cells	CD4+ T cells

APC, Antigen-presenting cells

- Signal transduction.

The role of CD4 and CD8 in antigen–receptor binding is shown in Fig. 10.5.

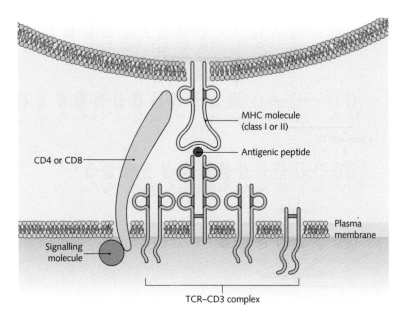

Fig. 10.5 The role of CD4 and CD8 in T cell receptor–major histocompatibility complex (TCR–MHC) antigen interaction. CD4 or CD8 is closely associated with the TCR complex. They bind MHC in a restricted fashion (CD8 to class I only, CD4 to class II only). Binding is antigen-independent and strengthens the bond between TCR and a complementary peptide–MHC complex. Molecules associated with CD4 or CD8 are then able to transduce a signal.

GENERATION OF ANTIGEN RECEPTOR DIVERSITY

The immune system may encounter approximately 20^8 possible antigens, each requiring a corresponding receptor if host defence is to be effective. The human genome contains only 30,000 genes and so a 'one gene per antigen receptor' code is simply not possible. Instead, this diversity is achieved by genetic recombination, a process in which segments of information are cut and pasted from genes. This enables each gene to produce many different receptors.

TCR and immunoglobulin (i.e., antibodies and mIg) are the only genes to undergo genetic recombination.

Genetic rearrangements

Before genetic recombination occurs, the gene segments are in 'germline configuration'. Rearrangement only occurs in the variable domain, which codes for the antigen-binding site of the receptor; the remaining structure must remain constant for the receptor to function. Each variable domain is encoded by a random combination of one of each of the V, D and J exons (nucleic acid sequences). The C exons encode the constant regions.

Following rearrangement, the clonal progeny of each B cell will produce immunoglobulin of a single specificity. Rearrangement is completed and functional immunoglobulin chains are produced before the B cell encounters antigen (Fig. 10.6).

The presence of multiple V, D and J gene segments (and the apparently random selection of these segments) generates considerable diversity, which can be calculated (Table 10.2).

A similar process occurs in T cells: α- and γ-chain variable domains have V and J segments; β- and δ-chains have V, D and J segments.

Junctional diversity

The formation of junctions between the various gene segments produces an opportunity for increased diversity, where nucleotides are added or subtracted at random to form the joining segments.

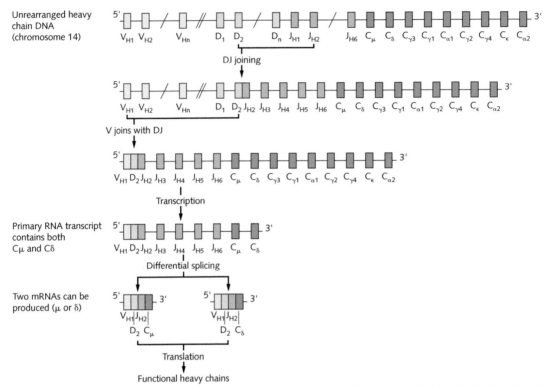

Fig. 10.6 Genetic rearrangement of immunoglobulin genes. Rearrangement of the heavy chain is similar to that of the light chain, although the join between D and J segments occurs first. In an unstimulated B cell, the heavy-chain mRNA that is transcribed contains both the Cμ and Cδ segments. The mRNA can be differentially spliced such that both IgM and IgD will be produced. They will both exhibit the same antigen-binding specificity.

Table 10.2 Calculation of antibody diversity

Mechanism of diversity		Number of combinations	
	Light chain	Light chain	Heavy chain
Random joining of gene segments	100 × 5 = 500	100 × 6 = 600	75 × 30 × 6 = 13,500
Random chain associations	(500 + 600) × 13,500 = 1.5 × 10⁷		

Given that a light chain can associate with any heavy chain and considering the number of gene segments present in germline DNA, it is possible to calculate the number of different molecules that can be produced. The extent of the contribution of junctional flexibility, N-nucleotide addition and somatic hypermutation is not known but will be significant.

Junctional flexibility and N-nucleotide addition

When exons are spliced, there are slight variations in the position of segmental joining. In addition, up to 15 nucleotides can be added to the D–J and the V–DJ joints. This occurs only in heavy chains and is catalysed by terminal deoxynucleotidyl transferase (TdT).

Both junctional flexibility and N-nucleotide addition can disrupt the reading frame, leading to non-functional rearrangements. However, formation of productive rearrangements increases antibody diversity. The V–J, V–DJ and VD–J joints fall within the antigen-binding region of the variable domain. Therefore diversity generated at these joints will impact on the antigen specificity of the Ig molecule.

Somatic hypermutation

Somatic hypermutation is a process that increases the affinity of an antibody for its antigen and is also called affinity maturation. This occurs after the immune system is exposed to an antigen. B cells that are dividing by mitosis to increase in number in order to combat infection are allowed to undergo mutation in their variable domain (the only cells in the body permitted to do so). Some mutations decrease the antibody's specificity for the antigen and apoptosis is stimulated in these cells. Other mutations result in antibodies with increased specificity, these B cells are allowed to survive (the mutation is positively selected for). Antibodies produced later in the primary and secondary immune response will therefore have an increased affinity for antigen.

The TCR does not exhibit somatic hypermutation. Diversity is generated only in developing T cells, which undergo apoptosis if they are either self-reactive or nonfunctional.

Class switching

This is the process whereby a single B cell can produce different classes of immunoglobulin that have the same specificity. The mechanism is not well understood but involves 'switch sites', i.e., DNA sequences located upstream from each heavy chain C gene segment. Possible mechanisms include:

- Differential splicing of the primary transcript (Fig. 10.6)
- A looping out and deletion of intervening heavy chain C gene segments (and introns)
- Exchange of C gene segments between chromosomes

This process underlies the class switch from IgM in the primary response to IgG, IgA or IgE in the secondary response. Cytokines are important in controlling the switch.

Recognition molecules and their diversity are crucial for the generation of a specific, adaptive immune response. The adaptive immune response can be humoral or cell-mediated.

HUMORAL IMMUNITY

B cells and antibody production

The humoral immune response is brought about by antibodies, which are particularly efficient at eliminating extracellular pathogens. Antigen and therefore pathogens can be cleared from the host by a variety of effector mechanisms, which are dependent on antibody class or isotype (see Tables 10.3 and 10.4):

- Activation of complement, leading to lysis or opsonization of the microorganism
- Antibody-dependent cell-mediated cytotoxicity (ADCC)
- Neutralization of bacterial toxins and viruses
- Mucosal immunity (IgA-mediated)
- Degranulation of mast cells (IgE and IgG mediated)

COMMON PITFALLS

Activated and differentiated B cells are known as plasma cells. It is these plasma cells that produce antibodies.

B cells are activated by antigen in a T-cell-independent or dependent fashion. T helper (Th) cells are primed by APCs, which present antigen to Th cells in conjunction with MHC class II molecules. B cells are stimulated by antigen interacting with B cell receptors. Primed Th cells interact with B cells that also express antigen–MHC complexes. This interaction induces a sequence of surface receptor binding and cytokine production that results in B-cell activation, proliferation and differentiation. An overview of B-cell activation is given in Fig. 10.7.

HINTS AND TIPS

Primary lymphoid organs (the thymus and bone marrow) are where lymphocytes are created and undergo early development. Secondary lymphoid organs (the spleen and lymph nodes) maintain lymphocytes and are involved in initiating an immune response.

B cells are activated within follicles found in secondary lymphoid structures only if they encounter specific antigen, namely foreign antigen. During proliferation, variable regions of the immunoglobulin genes within B cells undergo somatic hypermutation. Follicular dendritic cells present antigen, to which the B cells with the highest affinity will bind. This causes the expression of bcl-2, which prevents B cells undergoing apoptosis. Therefore the highest-affinity B cell clones are positively selected. B cells require help from T cells to produce antibodies. Activated Th cells provide the help needed by producing cytokines (IL-2, IL-4, IL-5, and IL-6). This acts as a further method of regulation within the immune system, as both B cells and T cells need exposure to the offending antigen in order for a response to be evoked.

The clonal selection of B cells that respond only to foreign antigen is an example of tolerance. This means that B cells that react to autoantigen (and therefore would attack body tissues) are destroyed by apoptosis, i.e., B cells 'tolerate' autoantigen. This is explored more in the section on tolerance later in this chapter.

Structure and function of antibody

The structure of immunoglobulin G (IgG) is shown in Fig. 10.8.

Immunoglobulin molecules (using IgG as an example) are composed of two identical heavy and two identical light chains, linked by disulphide bridges. The light chains consist of one variable and one constant domain, while the heavy chain contains one variable and three constant domains. Digestion of IgG with papain (papaya proteinase 1, an enzyme derived from papayas) produces two types of fragment:

1. Two Fab fragments consisting of the light chain and two domains of the heavy chain (denoted VH and CH1). These fragments bind antigen.

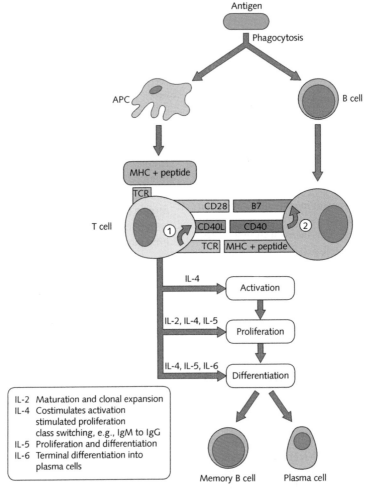

Fig. 10.7 Overview of the humoral immune response. Activated and differentiated B cells, known as plasma cells, produce antibody. B cells are activated by antigen in a T-cell-independent or dependent fashion, as described in the text. (1) Binding of the T cell receptor (TCR) to major histocompatibility complex (MHC) induces the T cell to produce CD40L, which binds to CD40 on the B cell, producing a major stimulatory signal. (2) CD28 on the T cell then interacts with B7 on the B cell (costimulatory signal). Cytokines are also involved; their actions are shown in the diagram. *APC*, antigen presenting cells.

2. One Fc fragment consisting of the remainder of the heavy chain (CH2 and CH3). This fragment binds complement.

The light chain

The light chain is comprised of a variable domain at the amino (N) terminal and a constant domain at the carboxy (C) terminal.

The constant region can be κ or λ, but both light chains within an immunoglobulin molecule will be the same; ≈ 60% of human light chains are κ.

The heavy chain

The heavy chain has a variable domain attached to several constant domains. There are five classes of immunoglobulin in humans: IgG, IgA, IgM, IgE and IgD. The heavy chain determines the class. The heavy chain can be γ (IgG), α (IgA),

μ (IgM), ε (IgE) or δ (IgD). IgG, IgA and IgD have three constant domains with a hinge region; IgM and IgE have four constant domains but no hinge region. There is little known about IgD that is relevant and it will not be considered.

The variable domain

Each variable domain exhibits three regions that are hypervariable. The hypervariable regions on both light and heavy chains are closely aligned in the immunoglobulin molecule. Together, they form the antigen-binding site and therefore determine the molecule's specificity.

The hinge region

The hinge allows movement and therefore greater interaction with epitopes. The hinge region is also the site of the interchain disulphide bonds.

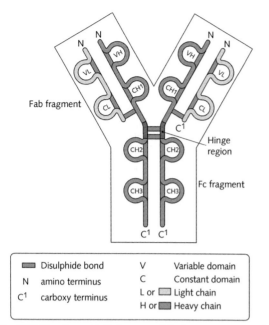

	Disulphide bond	V	Variable domain
N	amino terminus	C	Constant domain
C^1	carboxy terminus	L or	Light chain
		H or	Heavy chain

Fig. 10.8 Structure of IgG. Immunoglobulins are composed from two identical light chains and two identical heavy chains. The chains are divided into domains, each of which is an immunoglobulin fold. The variable domains form the antigen-binding site. Digestion of the immunoglobulin molecule with papain produces an Fc portion (which binds complement) and two Fab portions (which bind antigen).

Classes of antibody

The different properties of the immunoglobulin classes are shown in Table 10.3. Different immunoglobulin classes and subclasses are specific to each species. IgG and IgE are monomeric, while secreted IgA (sIgA) is usually present as a dimer and secreted IgM as a pentamer. The sIgA molecule is made up of two IgA monomers: a J chain and a secretory piece. The IgA dimer (J chain) is produced by submucosal plasma cells and enters the mucosal epithelial cell via receptor-mediated endocytosis, binding to the poly-Ig receptor. Having passed from the basal to the luminal surface of the epithelial cell, the IgA dimer is secreted across the mucosa, with part of the poly-Ig receptor (the secretory piece) still attached.

The functions of antibodies

The functions of immunoglobulins are shown in Table 10.4.

Lymphatic drainage and lymph nodes

Lymph nodes provide a site for lymphocytes to interact with antigen and other cells of the immune system.

At the arterial end of capillaries, water and low-molecular-weight solutes are forced into tissue spaces as a result of high hydrostatic pressure, creating interstitial fluid. Most interstitial fluid returns to the venous circulation at the venous end of capillaries (due to osmotic pressure gradients). The remainder leaves the interstitial space via the lymphatic system as lymph. Lymphatic vessels are present in almost all tissues and organs of the body.

Lymphatic circulation

The lymphatic system acts as a passive drainage system to return interstitial fluid to the systemic circulation; lymph is not pumped around the body. Lymph vessels therefore contain

Table 10.3 Properties of the immunoglobulin classes

	IgG	IgA	IgM	IgE
Physical properties				
Molecular weight (kDa)	150	300	900	190
Serum concentration (mg/mL)	13.5	3.5	1.5	0.0003
Number of subunits	1	2	5	1
Heavy chain	γ	α	μ	ε
Biological activities				
Present in secretions	✗	✓	✓	✗
Crosses placenta	✓	✗	✗	✗
Complement fixation	✓	✓	✓✓✓	✗
Binds phagocytic receptors	✓	✗	✓	✗
Binds mast cell receptors	✓	✗	✗	✓
Other features				
Main role	Main circulatory Ig for secondary immune response	Major Ig in secretions	Main Ig in primary immune response	Allergy and antiparasitic response

Ig, Immunoglobulin

Table 10.4 Summary of the functions of immunoglobulins

Function	Notes
Opsonization	Phagocytic cells have antibody (Fc) receptors, thus antibodies can facilitate phagocytosis of antigens
Agglutination	Antigens and antibodies (IgG or IgM) clump together because immunoglobulin can bind more than one epitope simultaneously. IgM is more efficient because it has a high valency (10 antigen-binding sites)
Neutralization	Binding to pathogens or their toxins prevents their attachment to cells
Antibody-dependent cell-mediated cytotoxicity (ADCC)	The antibody–antigen complex can bind to cytotoxic cells (e.g., cytotoxic T cells, NK cells) via the Fc component of the antibody, thus targeting the antigen for destruction
Complement activation	IgG and IgM can activate the classical pathway; IgA can activate the alternative pathway
Mast cell degranulation	Cross-linkage of IgE bound to mast cells and basophils results in degranulation
Protection of the neonate	Transplacental passage of IgG and the secretion of sIgA in breast milk protect the newborn

sIgA, Secretory immunoglobulin A; *NK,* natural killer.

numerous valves to prevent backflow of lymph. Afferent lymph vessels carry lymph into lymph nodes. They empty into the subcapsular sinus and lymph percolates through the node. Each node is drained by only one efferent vessel.

Lymph returns to the circulation at lymphovenous junctions. These are located at the junction of the right subclavian vein and right internal jugular vein (which empties the right lymphatic duct) and at the junction of the left subclavian vein and left internal jugular vein (which empties the thoracic duct). Lymphatic drainage of the body is not a symmetrical left-right split; the right lymphatic duct drains the right arm and thorax, the rest of the body drains to the left lymphatic duct.

Lymph nodes

Lymph nodes act as filters, 'sampling' lymphatic fluid (and therefore plasma) for bacteria, viruses and foreign particles. APCs, loaded with antigen, also migrate through lymph nodes. They are present throughout the lymphatic system, often occurring at junctions of the lymphatic vessels. Lymph nodes frequently form chains and may drain a specific organ or area of the body.

Lymph nodes act as sites for initiation of the adaptive immune response. Antigen is sampled, processed and presented by several professional APCs (macrophages and dendritic cells). It is in the lymph nodes that B and T cells first encounter antigen and hence where they are activated and initiate the adaptive immune response.

Lymphocyte recirculation

Lymphocytes move continuously between blood and lymph. Efferent lymph contains more lymphocytes than afferent lymph because:

- Antigenic challenge results in stimulation and proliferation of lymphocytes
- Lymphocytes enter the lymph node directly from blood

Lymphocyte recirculation is essential for a normal immune response (Fig. 10.9). Approximately 1%–2% of the lymphocytic pool recirculates each hour. This increases the chances of an antigenically committed lymphocyte encountering complementary antigen.

Lymphocytes tend to recirculate to similar tissues. For example, an activated lymphocyte that has migrated from the skin to a local lymph node is most likely to migrate back to the skin following transport in the blood. Similarly, lymphocytes activated in mucosal-associated lymphoid tissue (MALT) will return to MALT. This recirculation is governed by the expression of molecules on both the lymphocyte and surface endothelium. These molecules, called integrins, confer specificity to lymphocyte recirculation. This fine tuning of lymphocyte recirculation is known as lymphocyte homing. Areas of endothelium through which lymphocytes migrate are known as high endothelial venules (HEVs).

Lymphadenopathy

Lymph nodes can become enlarged (lymphadenopathy) for several reasons, including infection. Causes of lymphadenopathy are outlined in Chapter 1.

Mucosal-associated lymphoid tissue

MALT consists of unencapsulated subepithelial lymphoid tissue found in the gastrointestinal, respiratory and urogenital tracts (Fig. 10.10).

It can be subdivided into:

- Organized lymphoid tissue, e.g., tonsils, appendix, Peyer patches
- Diffuse lymphoid tissue located in the lamina propria of intestinal villi and lungs

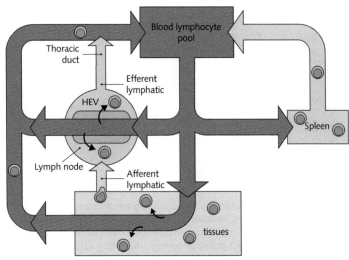

Fig. 10.9 Lymphocyte recirculation. Lymphocytes can enter lymph nodes via specialized high endothelial venules or in lymph. They leave the node in lymph that is returned to the systemic circulation via the right lymphatic duct or thoracic duct. *HEV*, high endothelial venule.

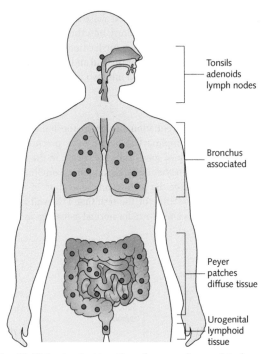

Fig. 10.10 Anatomical location of mucosal-associated lymphoid tissue (MALT). MALT is found in the nasal cavity, throat, respiratory tract, gastrointestinal tract and urogenital tract. Immune cells activated in MALT will return only to other mucosal sites.

Organized lymphoid tissue

Respiratory tract

MALT in the nose and bronchi includes the:

- Lingual, palatine and nasopharyngeal tonsils
- Adenoids
- Bronchial nodules

The respiratory system is exposed to a large number of organisms every day, most of which are cleared by the mucociliary escalator. Microorganisms that are not removed are presented by dendritic cells in the bronchi and stimulate germinal centres.

Gastrointestinal tract

Peyer patches are organized submucosal lymphoid follicles present throughout the large and small intestine, particularly prominent in the terminal ileum. The structure of a Peyer patch is shown in Fig. 10.11.

Food and harmless bacteria living in the gut contain many potentially antigenic substances. The immune system generally does not react to these. This is referred to as oral tolerance and is at least in part mediated by epithelial cells in gastrointestinal MALT, which secrete transforming growth factor β (TGF-β). This has a suppressive effect on local T cells, which is thought to prevent an immune response to peptides in food.

CELL-MEDIATED IMMUNITY

Cell-mediated immunity is mediated by T lymphocytes, macrophages and natural killer (NK) cells. The cell-mediated immune system is involved in the elimination of:

- Intracellular pathogens and infected cells (mainly viruses, mycobacteria and fungi)
- Tumour cells
- Foreign grafts

The thymus plays an important role in cell-mediated immunity because it is the site of T cell maturation (hence they are called 'T' cells!).

Gut lumen

Fig. 10.11 Structure of a Peyer patch. Peyer patches are found in the gastrointestinal tract. Microbes are transported across specialized epithelial M cells in pinocytotic vesicles into a dome-shaped area. Antigen-presenting cells then process and present antigen to T cells. T helper cells can then activate B cells within the follicle. Some of the B cells do not differentiate into plasma cells, but migrate into germinal centres where they undergo high affinity and class switching maturation. Peyer patches also play a key role in the development of oral tolerance.

T cell development and the thymus

The aim of T cell development and maturation is to select for T cells with receptors that can recognize foreign antigen in conjunction with self-MHC, while also destroying any that do not bind to self-MHC or any that bind to proteins in the body (autoantigens). This process occurs in the thymus.

The thymus is a gland with two lobes, located in the anterior part of the superior mediastinum, posterior to the sternum and anterior to the great vessels and upper part of the heart. It can extend superiorly into the root of the neck and inferiorly into the anterior mediastinum. It receives its blood supply from the inferior thyroid and internal thoracic arteries. Each lobule is divided into two regions (Fig. 10.12):

- An outer cortex
- An inner medulla

T lymphocyte differentiation begins in the bone marrow (see Chapter 1: Lymphocytes) before early precursor cells migrate to the thymus, specifically the cortex. In the thymus, immature T lymphocytes undergo random recombination of their TCR genes (see the section on Generation of antigen receptor diversity). Some of the resulting TCR will be specific for pathogens and others for normal autoantigens. These

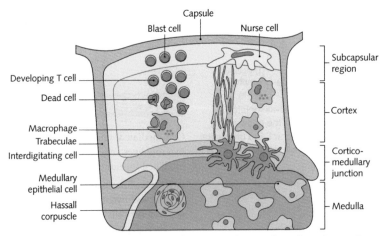

Fig. 10.12 Structure of a thymic lobule. Developing T cells (thymocytes) move from the subcapsular region to the medulla of the thymus during maturation. Several different types of stromal cell support them. Many thymocytes undergo apoptosis (particularly in the cortex) and are phagocytosed by macrophages.

developing T cells then migrate towards the medulla where they encounter specialized epithelial cells. These epithelial cells express MHC class I and class II molecules. Developing T cells that are able to bind self-MHC to some extent (as required for their function) will proliferate, resulting in positive selection. Furthermore, T cells that interact with MHC class I lose their CD4 (they are now CD8 T cells) and T cells that interact with MHC class II lose their CD8 (becoming CD4 T cells); this is MHC restriction. T cells that do not interact with the MHC molecules undergo apoptosis, as they do not receive a protective signal as a result of the TCR–MHC interaction. The thymic epithelial cells also have a unique mechanism for expressing many of the body's proteins (e.g., insulin) and peptides from these proteins are displayed on MHC class I and class II molecules. T cells that recognize this autoantigen can be forced to undergo apoptosis—this is central tolerance (see section on tolerance later in this chapter).

A much smaller and more mature group of thymocytes survives to enter the medulla. Thymocytes continue to mature in the medulla and eventually leave the thymus, via postcapillary venules, as mature, antigen-specific, immunocompetent T cells. In total, only 1%–5% of thymocytes in the thymus reach maturity, the remainder undergoing programmed cell death (apoptosis). The T cells that leave the thymus have been selected because they can recognize self-MHC, but those that recognize self-MHC plus autoantigen have been deleted. This process is summarized in Fig. 10.13.

T lymphocytes

Functions of different T cell phenotypes

The different types of T cell can be differentiated by cell-surface molecules and function. There are two different types of TCR, which have different functions. T cells expressing αβ-TCRs account for at least 95% of circulatory T cells. They become cytotoxic, helper or suppressor cells and, unless specified otherwise, account for all the T cells mentioned in this book. T cells expressing a γδ-TCR are present at mucosal surfaces and their specificity is biased towards certain bacterial and viral antigens.

T helper cells

T helper (Th) cells play a key role in the development of the immune response. They determine the epitopes to be targeted by the immune system. This is achieved through their interactions with processed antigen, as presented by APCs in conjunction with MHC class II molecules. They also determine the nature of the immune response directed against target antigens, e.g., cytotoxic TCR or antibody response. Finally, they are required for normal B cell function (see "B cells and antibody production" earlier in this chapter). Overall, they orchestrate the immune response according to the nature of the threat faced.

Most Th cells are CD4$^+$ and can be divided into five subsets on the basis of the cytokines they secrete and hence the actions they have:

1. Th0
2. Th1
3. Th2
4. Th17
5. Regulatory T cells (Treg)

Th0 cells arise as a result of initial short-term stimulation of naïve T cells and are capable of secreting a broad spectrum of cytokines. Prolonged stimulation of Th0 cells results in the emergence of Th1 and Th2 subsets. The cytokines released by the Th1 and Th2 subsets modulate one another's secretion. The different cytokine profiles of the Th1, Th2 and Th17 subsets reflect their different immunological functions (Table 10.5).

Most immune responses involve more than one subset of T cells. For example, staphylococcus (an extracellular bacterium) stimulates both Th2 and Th17 responses. On the other hand, some responses become very polarized. For example, the immune system relies almost exclusively on Th1 cells to respond to mycobacterium tuberculosis, an intracellular pathogen.

The fifth type of Th cell, Treg, has two main regulatory roles. The first is to dampen the immune response once an infection has been brought under control. The second is to regulate self-reactive T cells that have not developed central tolerance in the thymus. Their action is via cytokines, including transforming growth factor-β (TGF-β) and IL-10. Tregs also have a role in oral tolerance (described in the section on tolerance later in this chapter).

Cytotoxic T cells

Most cytotoxic T (Tc) lymphocytes are CD8$^+$ and recognize antigen in conjunction with MHC class I molecules (endogenous antigen). Therefore they are involved in defending against intracellular pathogens, i.e., viruses and some bacteria. They lyse target cells via the same mechanisms as NK cells (see Chapter 9: Natural killer (NK) cells).

T cell activation

T cells are activated by interactions between the TCR and peptide bound to MHC. Activation also requires a 'second message' from the antigen-presenting cell. This process, termed costimulation, is shown in Fig. 10.14.

Superantigens

T cells can be activated in a non-specific fashion by superantigens. Superantigens cross-link between the V-β domain of the TCR and an MHC class II molecule on an APC. Cross-linking is independent of the peptide-binding cleft but depends on the framework region of the V-β domain. This means that one superantigen is able to activate about 5% of T cells, far more than a normal antigen. Staphylococcal enterotoxin is an example of a T cell superantigen, causing Toxic Shock Syndrome (see 'Clinical notes').

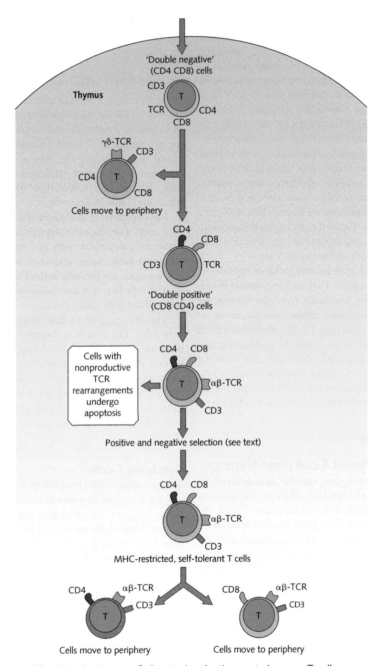

Fig. 10.13 Development of T cells in the thymus. Cells entering the thymus to become T cells are negative for CD4, CD8, CD3 and the T cell receptor (TCR). Rearrangement of the genes encoding the TCR will produce three cell lines: (1) CD4⁺ αβ-TCR; (2) CD8⁺ αβ-TCR; and (3) CD4⁻CD8⁻ γδ-TCR. The β- or γ-chain genes rearrange first. If a functional β-chain is formed, both CD4 and CD8 are upregulated and the α-chain gene rearranges. The resultant T cells are positively selected if their TCR is functional, but negatively selected if they react too strongly. The majority of thymocytes will undergo apoptosis due to positive or negative selection. *MHC*, major histocompatibility complex.

Table 10.5 Differences between the T helper 1, T helper 2 and T helper 17 cell subsets

Cytokines secreted	Th1 cells IL-2, IFN-γ, TNF-β	Th2 cells IL-4, IL-10	Th17 cells IL-17
Functions	• Responsible for classical cell-mediated immunity reactions such as delayed-type hypersensitivity and cytotoxic T cell activation • Involved in responses to intracellular pathogens; for example, viruses, some protozoa and fungi, and some bacteria • Activate macrophages	• Promote B cell activation • Involved in allergic diseases and responses to helminthic infections	• Promote neutrophil activation and migration • Involved in responses to extracellular bacteria and fungi

Th1, T helper 1; *Th2*, T helper 2; *Th17*, T helper 17.

CLINICAL NOTES

TOXIC SHOCK SYNDROME

Toxins produced by staphylococci and streptococci can act as superantigens, producing the clinical picture of toxic shock syndrome (TSS), where a seemingly innocuous stimulus such as a graze can lead to fever, a diffuse macular rash and sepsis. There is an association between tampon use and *Staphylococcus aureus* TSS with many known deaths as a result. Management of TSS is the same as that of sepsis (see Chapter 9). Antibiotic therapy should cover *S. aureus* and *Streptococcus pyogenes*.

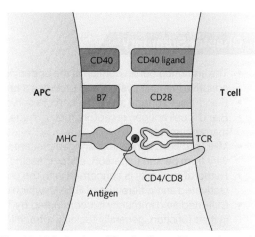

Fig. 10.14 Activation of T cells. Several interactions with antigen-presenting cells (APCs) are required to activate T cells. The T cell receptor (TCR) and CD4 or CD8 bind to major histocompatibility complex (MHC) and antigens. CD28 on the T cell binds to B7 on the APC, providing a co-stimulatory signal. *MHC*, major histocompatibility complex.

TOLERANCE

Tolerance is the ability of the immune system to ignore certain peptides that have the potential to trigger an immune response. The need for 'self-tolerance' is logical; immune activation by endogenous peptides would be damaging to tissues. Tolerance also includes harmless environmental antigens such as food or pollen. A breakdown in tolerance to either endogenous or environmental antigens can result in autoimmune disease or allergies (covered extensively in Chapter 12).

Central tolerance

Central tolerance is achieved through negative selection. As previously described, T cells (in the thymus) and B cells (in the bone marrow) are eliminated if they are self-reactive. Central tolerance is not complete: only the most self-reactive lymphocytes are deleted, ensuring that a wide lymphocyte repertoire is maintained. Additionally, some self-reactive T cells develop into regulatory T cells (Tregs) instead of being eliminated.

Peripheral tolerance

In the periphery, self-antigens do not generally elicit an immune response. Several mechanisms prevent autoantigen reactive T cells from causing autoimmune disease. These include:

- Lack of the costimulation required for T cell activation: costimulatory molecules such as CD40 or CD28 are found on APCs but not on other body tissues.
- Tregs secrete IL-10 and TGF-β in the presence of autoantigen reactive T cells. These cytokines suppress surrounding T cells.

Oral tolerance

A degree of tolerance is required because the gastrointestinal tract is full of antigens that have the potential to trigger an immune response. Epithelial cells in the gastrointestinal tract secrete TGF-β, causing any T cell that recognizes an antigen found in food or on harmless gut bacteria to become a Treg specific to that antigen. These Tregs also play a role in the peripheral tolerance to the harmless gastrointestinal antigens.

CLINICAL NOTES

Oral tolerance is emerging as a way to treat allergies and autoimmune disease. Grass pollen allergy (hay fever) can be managed by long-term sublingual administration of grass pollen. The Th2 cells that mediate the allergy are effectively switched off by Tregs created during the oral administration of grass pollen antigen.

Chapter Summary

- The immunoglobulin domain is the underlying basic structure of many components of the adaptive immune system and provides a basis for antigen recognition.
- B and T cell surface antigen receptors serve this antigen recognition function.
- B and T cell antigen receptors require huge diversity, which is achieved through genetic rearrangement.
- MHC provides a means of antigen presentation to the adaptive immune system. Its genes vary from person to person, encompassing the spectrum of possible antigen.
- Humoral immunity is concerned with the production of antibody from plasma cells (activated and differentiated B cells, which develop in bone marrow).
- Cell-mediated immunity is coordinated by T cells. These develop in the thymus and vary in their function, generally tackling intracellular infections and tumour cells.
- Self-reactive B and T cells are eliminated in development. This is central tolerance.

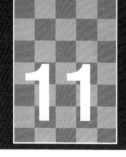
RESPONSE TO TISSUE DAMAGE

Inflammation is a nonspecific response evoked by tissue injury. The aims of the process are:

- Removal of the causative agent, e.g., microbes or toxins
- Removal of dead tissue
- Replacement of dead tissue with normal tissue or scar formation

CLINICAL NOTES

Inflammation is defined clinically by four cardinal signs: rubor, dolor, calor and tumor (redness, pain, heat and swelling). These are key observations in almost every clinical examination and are often best found by comparing one side with the other, for example feeling the temperature of both legs simultaneously when looking for cellulitis.

Acute inflammation

Acute inflammation is the immediate response to cell injury. It is of short duration (a few hours to a few days) and is triggered by a range of insults, including physical trauma, chemical or thermal damage and infection. Both innate and adaptive immune cells initiate the acute inflammatory response. Infection is sensed by resident macrophages through Toll-like receptors, which then release cytokines, attracting neutrophils to the site of infection. In other instances (such as parasitic worm infection), inflammation is initiated by resident mast cells, which tend to attract eosinophils. CD4$^+$ T lymphocytes play a central role in acute inflammation: they are activated by macrophages and produce many of the chemical mediators of acute inflammation (Table 11.1). Once inflammation has been initiated, several changes occur in vascular endothelium to allow attachment and extravasation of leucocytes—primarily neutrophils but also monocytes and lymphocytes. Attachment and extravasation require the presence of surface molecules on both the endothelium and leucocytes.

Vascular changes

Tissue injury and the ensuing immune response result in the release of chemical mediators (cytokines, chemokines and histamine) that act on local blood vessels. The main changes that occur are:

- Vasodilatation: causing increased blood flow and therefore redness and heat
- Slowing of the circulation and increased vascular permeability: formation of an inflammatory exudate results in swelling
- Entry of inflammatory cells, especially neutrophils, into the tissues

Leucocyte extravasation

The majority of cells that respond in acute inflammation are neutrophils, required for their phagocytic behaviour. Neutrophils adhere to the vessel wall and then pass between the endothelial cells into the tissues, where they follow the increasing chemokine concentration gradient to the site of inflammation (chemotaxis). This is a multistep process involving:

- Margination: adherence of neutrophils to the vessel wall. There are two phases to margination. The first is 'tethering and rolling' and the second is 'activation and strengthening'. Neutrophils adhere to vessel walls via cell adhesion molecules (CAMs).
- Diapedesis (extravasation): neutrophils move between endothelial cells into the tissue.
- Chemotaxis: due to the release of several chemotactic agents (Table 11.1).

CAMs are either members of the immunoglobulin superfamily, the selectin family or the integrin family. Integrin molecules allow immune cells to target specific sites, a process known as homing (as seen in Chapter 10). To interact

Table 11.1 Overview of the mediators of acute inflammation

Action	Mediators
Increased vascular permeability	Histamine, bradykinin, C3a, C5a, leukotrienes C$_4$, D$_4$, E$_4$, PAF
Vasodilatation	Histamine, prostaglandins, PAF
Pain	Bradykinin, prostaglandins
Leucocyte adhesion	LTB$_4$, IL-1, TNF-α, C5a
Leucocyte chemotaxis	C5a, C3a, IL-8, PAF, LTB$_4$, fibrin and collagen fragments
Acute phase response	IL-1, TNF-α, IL-6
Tissue damage	Proteases and free radicals

IL, Interleukin; LT, leukotriene; PAF, platelet-activating factor; TNF, tumour necrosis factor.

successfully with the extracellular matrix, neutrophils must express β_1-integrins, a set of adhesion molecules that can bind to collagen and laminin.

Once neutrophils reach a site of inflammation, they phagocytose foreign particles and release enzymes (see Chapter 9). Leucocytes can release proteases and metabolites during chemotaxis and phagocytosis, which are potentially harmful to the host. Neutrophils die during this process, creating pus.

CLINICAL NOTES

Pus is created during acute infections with certain bacteria, termed pyogenic bacteria. These include *Staphylococcus* (causing skin abscesses, septic arthritis, etc.), *Streptococcus* (causing purulent sputum) and *Neisseria gonorrhoeae* (causing genital discharge) amongst many others.

Molecular mediators of inflammation

A variety of molecular mediators are produced during an inflammatory response. They usually have short half-lives and are rapidly inactivated by a variety of systems, enabling a timely offset of inflammation once the cause has been removed. A summary of their actions is given in Table 11.1.

Cell membrane phospholipid metabolites

Prostaglandins (PGs) and leukotrienes (LTs) are derived from the metabolism of arachidonic acid, a constituent of cell membranes. PG metabolism is the target of nonsteroidal antiinflammatory drugs (see Chapter 13). Platelet-activating factor (PAF) is also an important mediator of inflammation.

Cytokines

Cytokines are molecular messengers between cells. In inflammation they attract and stimulate various different cell types, coordinating the inflammatory response. The cytokine response is generated by CD4$^+$ T cells and macrophages or eosinophils.

Cytokines such as IL-8, IL-1 and tumour necrosis factor-α (TNF-α) act to:

- induce expression of CAMs on the endothelium, thus enhancing leucocyte adhesion
- attract neutrophils to the area of injury
- induce prostacyclin (PGI$_2$) production
- induce PAF synthesis
- mediate the development of the acute-phase response
- stimulate fibroblast proliferation and increase collagen synthesis

The complement system

The function of complement in acute inflammation includes attracting and activating white cells and directly attacking pathogens. This is discussed in Chapter 9.

The kinin system

Bradykinin is released following activation of the kinin system by clotting factor XII, which occurs in trauma. Bradykinin increases vascular permeability and mediates pain by modulating afferent neurones.

The coagulation system

The coagulation system is activated at sites of vascular injury (see Chapter 6) so its role in mediating inflammation relates to its activation in tissue damage. Fibrinopeptides produced during coagulation are chemotactic for neutrophils and increase vascular permeability. Thrombin also promotes fibroblast proliferation and leucocyte adhesion.

The fibrinolytic system

Plasmin (see Chapter 6) has several functions in the inflammatory process, including:

- Activation of complement via C3
- Cleavage of fibrin to form 'fibrin degradation products', which may increase vascular permeability.

Results of acute inflammation

There are several possible outcomes resulting from acute inflammation. These include:

- Regrowth and resolution of tissue following trauma or infection
- Healing by collagenous scar formation if the tissue cannot regenerate, e.g., myocardium
- Abscess formation: a pyogenic bacterial infection within a tissue
- Chronic inflammation

Chronic inflammation

Chronic inflammation arises as a result of prolonged acute inflammation, usually when the causative agent cannot be eliminated so antigenic persistence occurs. This may be due to deficiencies in the host response to certain pathogens or the nature of the pathogen itself, for example *Mycobacterium tuberculosis*, which has evolved to evade the immune response. Chronic inflammation also occurs in persistent autoimmune disease such as rheumatoid arthritis; the body is incapable of fully clearing autoantigens.

HEPATITIS B

Hepatitis B is an example of an infection that causes acute inflammation but has the potential to progress to chronic inflammation. Hepatitis B is a blood-borne viral infection that can be transmitted horizontally (e.g., sharing IV drug needles, infected tattoo needles, sexually) or vertically (mother to foetus via the placenta). Around 90%–95% of healthy adults that are infected horizontally will clear the virus after a period of acute hepatitis. Virally infected cells are destroyed by cytotoxic T cells. Antibodies against surface and core viral antigens, called anti-HBs and anti-HBc respectively, are also produced and can help prevent reinfection. Anti-HBs is also produced in isolation after a hepatitis B vaccination. However, if the host has a weakened or ineffective immune system, for example if they also suffer from HIV coinfection and develop AIDS or if they are on chemotherapy, then the virus is not cleared entirely. **Persistence** of the hepatitis B virus surface antigen in the serum for longer than 6 months is an indication of chronic hepatitis B infection. This results in chronic inflammation of the liver, which can potentially lead to cirrhosis and hepatocellular carcinoma. Other factors that affect the likelihood of developing chronic hepatitis B include the HLA alleles of the host, as certain alleles present hepatitis B viral peptides differently, and the subtype of the hepatitis B virus. Babies who are infected vertically have a much poorer prognosis—90% of cases will develop a chronic hepatitis B infection.

The key cells of chronic inflammation are macrophages, lymphocytes and plasma cells. This is in marked contrast to acute inflammation, which is characterized primarily by a neutrophilic inflammation. Ongoing inflammation is associated with tissue destruction, as well as healing.

In chronic inflammation, macrophage numbers are increased because they are recruited by chemotactic factors [e.g., platelet-derived growth factor (PDGF) and C5a] and are prevented from leaving by migration inhibition factor. The overall maintenance of inflammation at a local level is thought to be due to TNF, secreted by macrophages.

When it is secreted at high levels, it has systemic effects, including weight loss (through fat catabolism and appetite inhibition) and fatigue. Other macrophage secretory products mediate characteristic features of chronic inflammation:

- Tissue damage via proteases and oxygen radicals
- Revascularization via angiogenic factors
- Fibroblast migration and proliferation via growth factors (e.g., PDGF) and cytokines (IL-2, TNF-α)
- Collagen synthesis via growth factors (e.g., PDGF) and cytokines (IL-1, TNF-α)
- Tissue remodelling via collagenases
- Simulation of T cell activity by secretion of IL-12

Lymphocytes and plasma cells are also present at the site of inflammation. In the case of chronic infections, both macrophages and T cells are required to control infection. An overview of chronic inflammation is given in Fig. 11.1.

Inflammation in disease

Inflammation is intended to protect the host but can, under certain circumstances, prove destructive. Antigenic persistence results in the continued activation and accumulation of macrophages and T cells. Macrophages develop into epithelioid cells (modified macrophages) and in turn this forms a granuloma (Fig. 11.2).

TNF-α is required for granuloma formation and maintenance. Interferon-γ (IFN-γ), secreted by activated T cells, is also required for the transformation of macrophages into epithelioid cells. IFN-γ also stimulates the production of multinucleate giant cells, which arise from the fusion of several macrophages. The granuloma is surrounded by a cuff of lymphocytes and the subsequent migration of fibroblasts results in increased collagen synthesis.

Granuloma formation is the immune response to 'frustrated' or ineffective phagocytosis; the nature of the damaging stimulus determines the type of granuloma formed. Examples of granulomatous disease include:

- Microorganisms such as *M. tuberculosis*: these induce a persistent, delayed-type hypersensitivity response (see Chapter 12: Type IV hypersensitivity), resulting in granuloma formation in the lung. While harmful to the host, this prevents the spread of infection. Caseous necrotic areas (dry, 'cheese-like' white mass of degenerated tissue) might be present in the centre of a *M. tuberculosis* granuloma.
- Foreign body inhalation (e.g., silica): this induces a granuloma that is predominantly surrounded by macrophages.
- Sarcoidosis: this is an idiopathic multisystem granulomatous disorder, most commonly affecting the lungs.

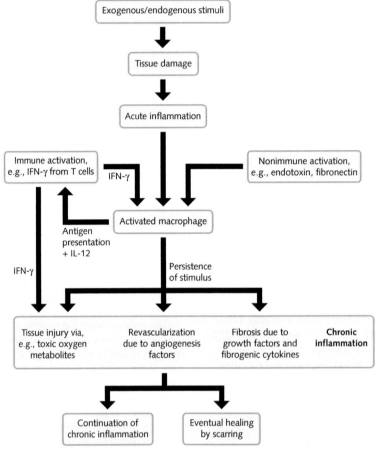

Fig. 11.1 Overview of chronic inflammation. Macrophages can be activated by T cells or by nonimmune mechanisms. Activated macrophages persist at sites of chronic inflammation because of persistent stimulation. They release a number of molecules, which produce the characteristic features of chronic inflammation. Macrophages act as antigen-presenting cells to T cells, which can then activate further macrophages.

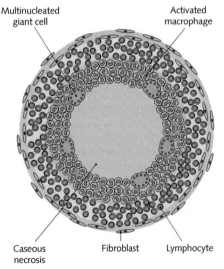

Fig. 11.2 A granuloma, showing typical focal accumulation of lymphocytes and macrophages around a central area of caseous necrosis.

IMMUNE RESPONSE TO PATHOGENS

Immune response to viral infection

Viruses do not always kill host cells but budding and release of new viral particles often causes the cells to lyse. The immune system can act to prevent infection or the spread of infection or to eliminate an intracellular target once infection has occurred.

Humoral immunity to viruses

The humoral response is involved in preventing entry to, and viral replication within, cells.

Antibody

Antibodies can:

- Bind to free virus, preventing their attachment and entry into cells. This is referred to as neutralization of free virus particles. For example, IgG neutralizes the hepatitis

B virus on entering the blood stream and IgA neutralizes the influenza virus entering the nasal mucosa.
- Bind to viral proteins, which are expressed on the surface of infected cells as a result of viral replication within the cells. Antibodies bound to infected cells can initiate antibody-dependent cell-mediated cytotoxicity (ADCC), mediated mainly by natural killer (NK) cells, and complement activation and also act as an opsonin (see Chapter 9).

Responses directed against free virus are considered to be the most important in vivo. Antibodies are important early in the course of infection to prevent the spread of virus between cells.

Interferon

IFNs are produced by virally infected cells. IFN-α and IFN-β act on neighbouring uninfected cells by inhibiting transcription and translation of viral proteins. IFN-γ activates macrophages and NK cells and enhances the adaptive immune response by upregulating expression of major histocompatibility complex (MHC) class I and class II molecules.

Cell-mediated immunity to viruses

Cell-mediated mechanisms are important for eliminating a virus once infection is established. The cells involved include:
- NK cells: these are cytotoxic for virus-infected cells and participate in ADCC.
- Cytotoxic CD8$^+$ T cells: viral peptides are presented to CD8$^+$ T cells on the surface of infected cells in association with MHC class I molecules. CD8$^+$ T cells can destroy these infected cells.
- CD4$^+$ T cells: T helper (Th) cells coordinate the generation of antibody and cytotoxic T cell responses and the recruitment and activation of macrophages.

An overview of the immune response to viruses is given in Fig. 11.3.

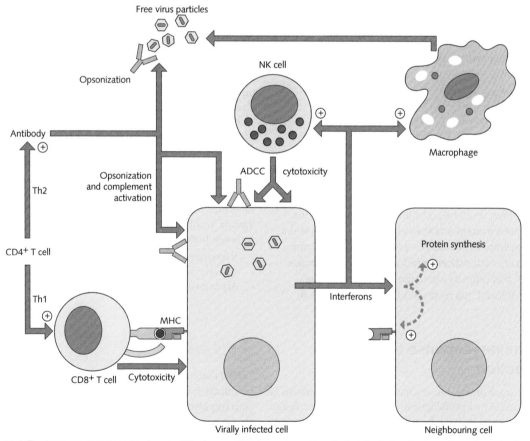

Fig. 11.3 The immune response to viruses. Interferons (IFNs), produced by virally infected cells, have three important actions: induction of an antiviral state in neighbouring cells (IFN-α and IFN-β), macrophage and natural killer (NK) cell activation and major histocompatibility complex (MHC) molecule upregulation (IFN-γ). NK cells kill virally infected cells, macrophages phagocytose opsonized free virus and cell fragments and produce further IFN. CD8$^+$ (cytotoxic) T cells sense viral peptides presented by MHC class I molecules and destroy the cell. CD4$^+$ (helper) T cells help to activate macrophages and are involved in the generation of antibody and cytotoxic T cell responses. *ADCC*, Antibody-dependent cell-mediated cytotoxicity.

Examples of viral infection strategies

Viral infections are common, and most are self-limiting. Some, particularly those that can evade the immune response, can be chronic and are potentially fatal (e.g. HIV, see Chapter 12: HIV, and hepatitis B, see Clinical notes earlier in this chapter). Different viruses use different strategies to evade the host's immune response:

- Antigenic shift and drift: e.g., influenza. These are mechanisms of genetic and therefore antigenic variation. This circumvents immunological memory because the virus expresses different immunological targets over time.
- Polymorphism: e.g., adenovirus, rhinovirus. This also causes antigenic variation.
- Latent virus: e.g., herpes simplex virus (HSV), varicella zoster (see Clinical notes)
- Modulation of normal immune effector functions, principally MHC class I. downregulation: e.g., cytomegalovirus (CMV), adenovirus, Epstein–Barr virus (EBV), HSV, HIV. Viruses can also interfere with IFN or produce inhibitory cytokines.
- Infection and subsequent death of lymphocytes, e.g., HIV, measles, CMV, EBV. This reduces the ability of the immune system to combat viral infection.

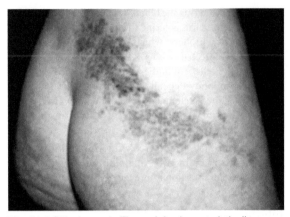

Fig. 11.4 Shingles rash. The rash is characteristically erythematous and vesicular. Its spread is limited to the area that the affected nerve supplies. In this case, it is a dermatome in the lower back/buttock.

extracellular bacterial pathogens include *Staphylococcus aureus*, *Streptococcus* spp., *Haemophilus influenzae* and *Pseudomonas aeruginosa*.

Humoral immunity to extracellular bacteria

Complement—Bacteria activate complement via the lectin or alternative pathways (see Chapter 9). Activated complement products play a role in the elimination of bacteria, especially C3b (an opsonin), C3a and C5a (anaphylatoxins that recruit leucocytes) and the membrane attack complex (MAC), which can perforate the outer lipid bilayer of Gram-negative bacteria such as *H. influenzae*.

Antibody—This is the principal defence against extracellular bacteria. Initially, sIgA binds to bacteria and prevents their binding to epithelial cells, e.g., in the respiratory mucosa. If this response is sufficient, sIgA can prevent the pathogen from entering the body. Antibodies also:

- Neutralize bacterial toxins
- Activate complement
- Act as an opsonin

Immune response to bacterial infection

Bacteria are prokaryotic organisms. Their cell membrane is surrounded by a peptidoglycan cell wall. Many bacteria also have a capsule of large, branched polysaccharides. Bacteria attach to cells via surface pili, but only some bacteria enter host cells. Different immune mechanisms operate, depending on whether the bacteria are extracellular or intracellular.

Extracellular bacteria

The majority of pathogenic bacteria do not require the intracellular environment to replicate and spread. Common

Cell-mediated immunity to extracellular bacteria

Phagocytic cells, predominantly neutrophils, kill most bacteria; C3b and antibody enhance phagocytosis. Bacterial antigens are processed and presented in conjunction with MHC class II to CD4+ T cells. Th17 T cells recruit and activate neutrophils to the site of an extracellular bacterial infection. This is alongside the function of Th2 cells (discussed in the Hints and tips).

An overview of the immune response to extracellular bacteria is given in Fig. 11.5.

Intracellular bacteria

Humoral immunity to intracellular bacteria

The humoral mechanisms that are employed against extracellular bacteria may be used to try to prevent bacteria causing intracellular infection. However, they will not be effective once the infection is intracellular.

Cell-mediated immunity to intracellular bacteria

Cell-mediated immunity is very important in the defence against intracellular bacterial infections, such as those caused by *M. tuberculosis*:

- Macrophages attempt to phagocytose the bacteria. If the organisms persist, chronic inflammation will ensue, as shown in Fig. 11.2. This can lead to delayed (type IV) hypersensitivity (see Chapter 12)

- Cells infected with bacteria can activate NK cells, which cause cytotoxicity and can activate macrophages.
- CD4+ T cells release cytokines that activate macrophages. This is predominantly Th1 cells, in contrast to the chiefly Th2 cell response to extracellular bacteria.
- CD8+ T cells recognize bacterial antigens presented in conjunction with MHC class I molecules on the surface of any infected nucleated cell and lyse these cells.

Examples of bacterial strategies to avoid immunity

Bacterial strategies to avoid the immune response must allow one of the following:

- Avoidance of phagocytosis. This is achieved in a number of ways. Some bacteria have capsules that inhibit phagocytosis, e.g., *S. pneumoniae*, *Haemophilus* spp. Others kill phagocytes with toxins or neutralize IgG, preventing opsonization, e.g., *Staphylococcus* spp.
- Survival within phagocytes, e.g., *M. tuberculosis*, *Mycobacterium leprae*, *Toxoplasma* spp.
- Prevent complement activation, e.g., *Staphylococcus* spp., *Streptococcus* spp., *Haemophilus* spp., *Pseudomonas* spp.
- Avoid recognition by the immune system. This can be done through polymorphism, e.g., *S. pneumoniae*, *Salmonella typhi*.

Like viruses, bacteria can be highly polymorphic. Bacteria of the same species can appear to be entirely different to the immune system.

Immune response to protozoal infection

Protozoa are microscopic, single-celled organisms. Fewer than 20 types of protozoa infect humans, although malaria, trypanosomes and *Leishmania* cause significant morbidity and mortality globally. Protozoa cause intracellular infection, have marked antigenic variation and are often immunosuppressive. They have complex life cycles with several different stages and, therefore, present the immune system with a variety of challenges. Protozoal infection is often chronic, as the immune system is not very efficient at dealing with these organisms. Most of the pathology of protozoal disease is caused by the immune response.

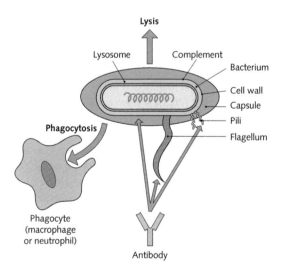

Fig. 11.5 The immune response to extracellular bacteria. The first line of host defence against bacteria is lysozyme. This, together with complement, leads to bacterial lysis. Antibody is produced against flagella (immobilizing the bacteria) and pili (preventing attachment). Capsular polysaccharides can induce T-cell-independent antibody. Antibodies aid complement activation and phagocytosis of bacteria.

Humoral immunity against protozoa

Complement and antibody are important during the extracellular stage of infection. This opsonizes the protozoa and can cause lysis or prevent infection.

Cell-mediated immunity against protozoa

- *Phagocytosis* by macrophages, monocytes and neutrophils is an important part of the immune response against protozoa.
- *CD4$^+$ T cells* are activated in response to protozoal infection. Th1 cytokines, such as IL-2, IFN-γ and TNF-β, are considered protective.
- *Cytotoxic CD8$^+$ T cells* are important in destroying protozoa that replicate within cells, e.g., the sporozoite stage of *Plasmodium falciparum* (which causes malaria).
- *NK cells and mast cells* are often activated in protozoal infection.

Examples of protozoal infection and evasion of the immune response

Protozoa have good mechanisms to prevent the initiation of an immune response. Strategies include:

- Escape into the cytoplasm following phagocytosis, e.g., *Trypanosoma cruzi*
- Prevention of complement actions, e.g., *Leishmania* spp.
- Gene switching to create antigen variation, e.g., trypanosomes
- Immunosuppression, e.g., trypanosomes

CLINICAL NOTES

Systemic protozoal infection normally presents with nonspecific symptoms: *Plasmodium* infection (malaria) can present with malaise, fever (classically in bouts on alternating days), headache, vomiting and diarrhoea. The key feature of the history is recent travel to regions in which malaria is endemic, highlighting the importance of taking a comprehensive history!

Immune response to worms

Multicellular parasites and worms pose a different problem to the immune system, as they are too large to be phagocytosed by macrophages and neutrophils. These worms tend to live on mucosal surfaces and the immune system tries to dispose of these parasites by facilitating their expulsion. The immune system does this by secreting toxic chemicals onto mucosal surfaces, stimulating an increase in mucus secretion and smooth muscle contraction, which together result in expulsion of the worm.

Mast cells are stationed in tissues and have a similar sentinel purpose as macrophages for other types of infection. Mast cells contain preformed granules and when they recognize parasitic infection through cross-linkage of IgE or possibly Toll-like receptors, they degranulate, releasing their preformed granules. They also release proinflammatory cytokines that recruit eosinophils and basophils.

Mast cell preformed granules contain:

- Histamine: causes smooth muscle in the walls of the gut to contract (expel the worm) and smooth muscle of blood vessels to relax.
- Proteolytic enzymes: activate the complement system including anaphylatoxins.

Mast cells also rapidly synthesize chemicals including prostaglandins and leukotrienes, both of which cause vasodilatation and contraction of smooth muscle in gut and bronchial walls.

Eosinophils secrete chemicals similar to those secreted by mast cells, excluding histamine. In addition, they secrete:

- Peroxidase, which generates hypochlorous acid
- A cationic protein, which damages the worm's outer layers and paralyses its nervous system
- A basic protein that also attacks the outer layers of the worm

Mast cells can be activated by IgE and, although this likely evolved to deal with worm infections, it mediates allergy (type I hypersensitivity).

CLINICAL NOTES

When viewing the results of a full blood count, the white cell count (WCC) is often used as a gross marker of infection or inflammation in disease. The WCC differential, detailing the levels of each type of white blood cell, can give further information on the nature of the disease. For example, a raised neutrophil count (neutrophilia) in the presence of an acute illness would point to a bacterial infection, particularly a pyogenic infection (see Clinical notes on pyogenic infection in this chapter). A raised eosinophil count could be due to a parasitic infection or allergy. It is therefore important to remember the context of the illness in question.

● Chapter Summary

- Acute inflammation is triggered in response to physical/chemical damage or the detection of pathogens. It involves multiple cells and molecules, with the aim of healing and removal of the stimulus.
- Chronic inflammation occurs following incomplete resolution of acute inflammation, with the persistence of antigen. The cells involved are different from acute inflammation and can result in an array of chronic inflammatory diseases.
- The immune system prevents viruses entering body cells (humoral immunity) and kills virally infected body cells (cell mediated immunity, humoral immunity aids in detection of infected cells).
- The immune response to bacterial infection depends on the nature of the pathogen. Extracellular bacteria are predominantly killed by humoral components and phagocytes. Intracellular bacteria require greater macrophage and T cell involvement.
- Both humoral and cell-mediated branches of the immune system are involved in responding to protozoal infection, due to both intracellular and extracellular lifecycle stages.
- Multicellular parasites require a more specialised immune response, with a greater involvement of mast cells and eosinophils.

Immune dysfunction 12

HYPERSENSITIVITY

Hypersensitivity is an excessive and, therefore, inappropriate inflammatory response to any antigen. This inflammatory response results in tissue damage.

Hypersensitivity can occur in response to:

- An infection that cannot be cleared, e.g., tuberculosis
- A normally harmless exogenous substance, e.g., pollen, resulting in allergy
- An autoantigen, e.g., thyroid stimulating hormone (TSH) receptors in Graves disease, resulting in autoimmune disease

Classification of hypersensitivity

Hypersensitivity reactions have been classified, by Gell and Coombs, into four types: I, II, III and IV. Types I, II and III are antibody-mediated; type IV is cell-mediated. In this system, the different types of hypersensitivity are classified by their time of onset after exposure to antigen.

TYPE I HYPERSENSITIVITY (IMMEDIATE HYPERSENSITIVITY)

Type I hypersensitivity is mediated by IgE, with resultant and immediate degranulation of mast cells and basophils. Overproduction of IgE in response to an innocuous environmental antigen occurs in type I hypersensitivity and hence it is the underlying mechanism of allergy.

COMMON PITFALLS

Allergy is synonymous with type I hypersensitivity, but not all hypersensitivity reactions are allergies, e.g., type II, III and IV hypersensitivities are not allergies.

Type I hypersensitivity reactions require an initial antigen exposure in order to sensitize the immune system. When allergic individuals are exposed to an allergen they produce lots of IgE specific for that antigen. Mast cells have membrane receptors specific for the fragment crystallisable (Fc) portion of IgE, so that mast cells become coated in IgE. The immune system is now said to be sensitized to the allergen. Subsequent exposure to the same antigen, cross-linking the mast cell surface IgE, causes the release of preformed mediators of inflammation (degranulation). Short-lived basophils with IgE receptors are recruited and also degranulate in response to the antigen.

Mast cells and basophils release their contents within minutes of exposure to an allergen; this is the early phase response. The late phase response, mediated by eosinophils, responds to the same stimulus. This delay occurs because eosinophils have to be mobilized from the bone marrow. Clinically this can manifest itself as an increase in the severity of symptoms several hours after initial exposure.

The immune mechanisms and development of type I reactions are illustrated in Fig. 12.1. Examples of type I reactions include:

- Allergic rhinitis (hay fever): pollens
- Allergic asthma: house-dust mite
- Systemic anaphylaxis: penicillin, peanuts or insect venom

CLINICAL NOTES

Atopy is a genetic predisposition to produce IgE in response to many common, naturally occurring allergens, especially inhaled allergens and food allergens. It has a prevalence of 10%–30%. Atopic patients can suffer from multiple allergies. Although atopy tends to run in families, the genetic basis of atopy is not currently known.

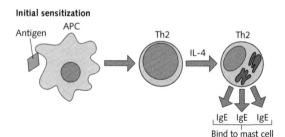

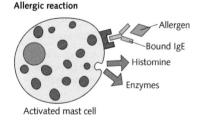

Fig. 12.1 The development and mechanisms of type I hypersensitivity reactions. APCs present antigen to Th2 cells, which in turn stimulate B cells to produce large amounts of IgE for that antigen. This IgE then binds to cell surface receptors on mast cells and basophils. Cross-linkage of this bound IgE results in degranulation. *APC,* Antigen-presenting cell; *Th,* T helper

When diagnosing type I hypersensitivity, the most important part of the history is the timing of allergic symptoms in response to a trigger, as the effects of allergy occur rapidly—within minutes. Allergy can result in a wide spectrum of symptoms, the most severe being anaphylaxis. Common allergens are shown in Table 12.1. Allergy most often produces symptoms local to the site of allergen entry:

- Skin: results in an urticarial rash or allergic eczema
- Nasal mucosa: results in rhinitis, e.g., hay fever
- Lungs: can result in asthma

For an allergic reaction to occur, IgE against that specific allergen needs to be present. This can be tested for by using skin prick testing, where a small amount of the suspected allergen is inoculated into the skin together with a positive and a negative control (see Fig. 12.2). A positive reaction will result in an itchy red lesion with a wheal at the centre; the reaction is strongest after 15–20 minutes, indicating that the patient produces IgE to the tested allergen. Serum IgE can also be directly measured using a blood test.

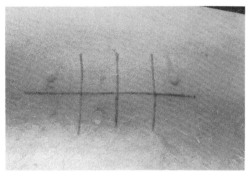

Fig. 12.2 Skin prick testing. The appearance of an itchy wheal, within a short period of time, indicates a positive result. Reading clockwise from the top right: Positive control, negative control, hazelnut, peanut, soya, peas, almond, cashew nut. This patient is allergic to peanut, soya, peas, almonds but not to hazelnut or cashew nut. Skin prick testing is not advisable in severe allergy. (reprinted with permission from Bolognia et al. Dermatology 3rd edition, Elsevier.)

Diseases caused by type I hypersensitivity reactions

Asthma

Asthma is a chronic inflammatory disorder of the airways, characterized by reversible airflow obstruction. The airways become hyper-responsive and exaggerated bronchoconstriction follows a wide variety of nonimmunological stimuli, e.g., exercise or cold air. The symptoms of asthma are dry cough, wheeze, chest tightness and shortness of breath, which tend to be worse at night. Asthma is a common disease and is diagnosed in 5%–10% of children. The incidence has risen over the last few decades, particularly in more economically developed countries.

Pollens, house-dust mite faeces and airborne proteins from domestic animals are the most common allergens in asthma. These cause chronic inflammation of the bronchial wall, resulting in the characteristic airway hyper-responsiveness and bronchoconstriction. Histological findings include:

- Infiltration by eosinophils, mast cells, lymphocytes and neutrophils
- Oedema of the submucosa
- Smooth muscle hypertrophy and hyperplasia
- Thickening of the basement membrane
- Mucous plugging
- Epithelial desquamation

Asthma is diagnosed clinically by the presence of the above symptoms, supported by the finding of a reversal in airway obstruction of ≥15% (measured by peak expiratory flow

Table 12.1 Summary of allergic reactions

Allergic condition	Common allergens	Features
Systemic anaphylaxis	Drugs (e.g., antibiotics, anaesthetics) Bee and wasp venoms Peanuts	Oedema with increased vascular permeability leads to tracheal occlusion, circulatory collapse and possibly death
Allergic rhinitis	Pollen (hay fever) Dust-mite faeces (perennial rhinitis)	Sneezing, oedema and irritation of nasal mucosa
Allergic asthma	Pollen Dust-mite faeces	Bronchial constriction, increased mucus production, airway inflammation
Food	Shellfish Milk Eggs Fish Wheat	Itching, urticaria and potentially anaphylaxis
Atopic eczema	Pollen Dust-mite faeces Some foods	Itchy inflammation of the skin

rate or 'peak flow'), either spontaneously or after the administration of an inhaled short-acting β2-adrenoreceptor agonist (SABA) such as salbutamol. Advice should be given, including avoidance of triggers and how to manage an attack. SABAs are used, as required, for the short-term improvement of symptoms and inhaled corticosteroids (such as beclomethasone dipropionate) are started as a regular preventative therapy. Other immunosuppressive/antiinflammatory drugs can be considered if symptoms persist or if SABAs are used regularly. This is according to the British Thoracic Society's step-wise approach.

Allergic rhinitis

Nasal congestion, watery nasal discharge and sneezing occur after exposure to allergen. The most common allergens are grass, flower, weed or tree pollens, which cause a seasonal rhinitis (hay fever), and house-dust mite faeces, which can cause a more perennial (year-round) rhinitis. Allergic attacks usually last for a few hours and are often accompanied by itching and watering of the eyes. Skin prick tests can identify the allergen.

The most important treatment is topical (nasal) antihistamines or steroids, additionally systemic antihistamines such as loratadine are used. Avoidance of allergens is advised but is often difficult. Grass pollen immunotherapy is increasingly being used to treat severe seasonal rhinitis (see Chapter 10).

Atopic/allergic eczema

Eczema (dermatitis) is a skin rash that is a result of superficial skin inflammation. It can be triggered by allergens, hence a type I hypersensitivity response, or through sustained contact with other substances, commonly nickel. The latter is termed 'contact dermatitis' and is a type IV hypersensitivity response, it is not considered here (see later section on type IV hypersensitivity).

True atopic eczema is most commonly the result of exposure to pollen or house-dust mite faeces. About 10% of children are diagnosed with eczema. The pathophysiology of atopic eczema is thought to be a breakdown in the skin's barrier function, allowing the entry of allergens; atopic eczema is linked to mutations in the filaggrin gene (see later section on development of hypersensitivity). Eczema commonly affects the flexural creases and the fronts of the wrist and ankles. In infancy, the face and trunk are often also involved. Eczematous skin lesions are itchy, erythematous (red), sometimes vesicular and might be dry (see Fig. 12.3). Because of itching, the skin is often excoriated, which can lead to lichenification (thickening of the skin). Eczema is often complicated by superinfection with bacteria, particularly *Staphylococcus aureus*.

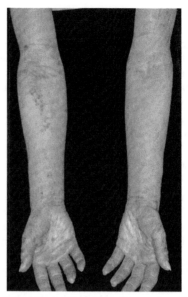

Fig. 12.3 Appearance of an eczematous rash on the arms of an adult. Note the erythematous, raised patches with some excoriation, suggesting itchiness.
(reprinted with permission from Bolognia et al. Dermatology 3rd edition, Elsevier.)

The diagnosis of atopic eczema is usually clinical, based on the atopic history and appearance of the rash. Total serum IgE, specific IgE levels and skin prick testing with common allergens are occasionally performed to confirm the diagnosis of atopic eczema. Treatment of eczema is mainly topical, except in more severe cases, when systemic steroids and immunosuppressants are used. Therapies include:

- Emollients: moisturizes dry skin, replacing the lost barrier against allergens
- Topical steroids: antiinflammatory
- Topical antibiotics or antiseptics: in infected eczema
- Oral antihistamine: reduces itching
- Ciclosporin: resistant cases may require immunosuppression

Anaphylaxis

Anaphylaxis is a life-threatening, generalized hypersensitivity reaction. It caused by a systemic response to an allergen that is either intravenous or quickly absorbed. This results in distributive shock and laryngeal occlusion; increased vascular permeability and dilatation lead to a large amount of fluid moving from the circulation into tissues. The subsequent rapid fall in blood pressure and airway occlusion through oedema can be fatal. Many allergens can cause anaphylaxis, but more common environmental causes include bee stings and peanuts. Many cases of anaphylaxis take place in hospital where they may be triggered by antibiotics, latex or anaesthetic drugs. The signs of anaphylaxis are principally the same as those of shock. Signs include:

- Hypotension with tachycardia
- Warm peripheral temperature
- Signs of airway obstruction such as stridor (a harsh and loud sound heard during exhalation)
- Facial oedema and urticaria (often seen)

The management of anaphylaxis, as per the Resuscitation Council (UK) guidelines, should be known by all medical professionals. The initial management of anaphylaxis is resuscitation, i.e., attend to life-threatening airway, breathing and/or circulatory problems. Allergens should be removed if possible, e.g., by stopping drug infusion. Adrenaline (epinephrine) should be given intramuscularly (IM) as soon as possible. The dose for adults is 500 µg (0.5 mL of 1:1000) and should be repeated after 5 minutes if there is no improvement. Adrenaline should be given intravenously only by a specialist and in environments where monitoring is possible and at a low dose. An intravenous (IV) fluid challenge of between 500 and 1000 mL should be given next to correct hypotension. Chlorphenamine (an antihistamine) and hydrocortisone are also given later. Mast cell tryptase, an enzyme released from degranulating mast cells, is elevated after anaphylaxis. Blood samples taken after an attack can have mast cell tryptase levels measured to confirm the diagnosis of anaphylaxis.

The National Institute for Clinical Excellence requires that any patient who suffers from a proven or suspected anaphylactic reaction should be seen in an allergy clinic by a specialist. They should receive advice regarding future attacks, as well as training on how to administer intramuscular adrenaline. They should carry a preloaded adrenaline syringe for such occasions.

TYPE II HYPERSENSITIVITY

Type II hypersensitivity occurs when antibody specific for cell surface antigens is produced, hence it is said to be antibody mediated. Cell destruction then results via mechanisms discussed in Chapters 9 and 10, including:

- Complement activation
- Antibody-dependent cell-mediated cytotoxicity (ADCC)
- Phagocytosis

The immune mechanisms of type II hypersensitivity reactions are summarized in Fig. 12.4.

Some foreign antigens are too small to stimulate an immune response themselves and need to bind to a host protein first. These antigens are called haptens. An example of a hapten involved in type II hypersensitivity is penicillin-induced haemolysis. Penicillin is too small to induce antibodies alone and binds to the surface of red cells. It now acts as a hapten, inducing IgG production in patients with this type of hypersensitivity. The IgG then binds to the red cells, which leads to their destruction in the spleen.

Diseases caused by type II hypersensitivity reactions

Examples of nonautoimmune type II hypersensitivity reactions in which complement is activated and cells destroyed are:

- Incompatible blood transfusions: ABO mismatch
- Haemolytic disease of the newborn: if a mother is rhesus –ve and her fetus is rhesus +ve, maternal antibodies against the rhesus antigen can cross the placenta and destroy fetal red blood cells.

Antibodies that are specific for self-antigen bind to tissues or cells, causing type II hypersensitivity mediated autoimmune disease. Autoimmunity can result from a variety of mechanisms, including:

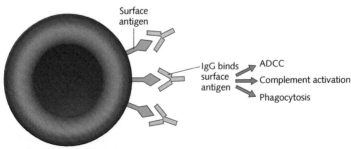

Fig. 12.4 The immune mechanisms of type II hypersensitivity reactions. Antibodies bind to antigen found on the surface of cells resulting in cell death via (1) complement, (2) phagocytes or (3) natural killer cells (ADCC). Note that this can also stimulate the cell, as in Graves disease.
ADCC, Antibody-dependent cell-mediated cytotoxicity; *NK,* natural killer; *RBC,* red blood cell.

- Opsonization: e.g., in autoimmune haemolytic anaemia, IgG binds to red blood cells, which are phagocytosed by macrophages in the spleen. This is commonly triggered by infection or drugs.
- Complement activation: e.g., in severe autoimmune haemolytic anaemia, IgM antibodies bound to red blood cells activate complement, resulting in lysis within the circulation.

Neutralization and ADCC can also occur in response to self-antigen.

Graves disease

Graves disease is the most common cause of hyperthyroidism. It arises as a result of IgG autoantibody production against TSH receptor in the thyroid gland. The anti-TSH receptor antibody activates the receptor, resulting in increased thyroxine production.

Graves disease affects 1%–2% of females. The female:male ratio is 5:1. There is a strong association with human leucocyte antigen (HLA) DR3 in Caucasian people.

CLINICAL FEATURES OF GRAVES DISEASE

Graves disease is associated with the symptoms and signs of hyperthyroidism, as well as some eye signs that occur exclusively in Graves disease (secondary to periorbital inflammation):

- Exophthalmos
- Lid retraction
- Lid lag
- Ophthalmoplegia

These are shown in Fig. 12.5.

TYPE III HYPERSENSITIVITY (IMMUNE COMPLEX)

Type III hypersensitivity reactions are also antibody mediated. However, the antigen is soluble. Antibodies react to soluble (free) antigen by forming lattices of antibody and antigen, termed immune complexes. This is a physiological response and is useful, for example, in the removal of soluble bacterial exotoxin. These immune complexes are broken up by complement and transported to the spleen, where they are phagocytosed. If there is a rapid influx in soluble antigen or if there is a significant amount of antigen, the clearance mechanisms can become overwhelmed. The remaining immune complexes are deposited in tissues, triggering inflammation: this is a type III hypersensitivity reaction (Fig. 12.6).

Diseases caused by type III hypersensitivity reactions

COMMON PITFALLS

Type II hypersensitivity is based on antibodies (IgG) binding to cell-surface antigens, resulting in cell destruction. However, type III hypersensitivity occurs when antibodies bind free antigen. They form immune complexes that can cause tissue damage if present in excessive amounts.

Type III hypersensitivity can occur locally or systemically. Examples of (nonautoimmune) local type III hypersensitivity reactions include:

- Farmer's lung: inhalation of mould spores
- Pigeon fancier's disease: repeated inhalation of dried pigeon faeces

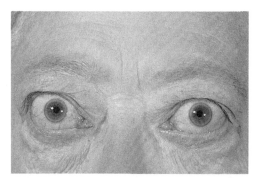

Fig. 12.5 The eye signs associated with Graves disease: lid retraction and exophthalmos.

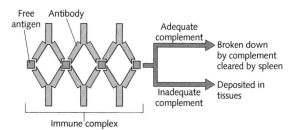

Fig. 12.6 The immune mechanisms of type III hypersensitivity reactions. Immune complexes that are normally broken down by complement and cleared in the spleen are deposited in blood vessels or tissues resulting in severe damage via complement and neutrophils.

Mould spores found in hay can be inhaled, forming immune complexes in the lungs. Symptoms may be cough, breathlessness, fatigue and malaise, made worse after exposure to the hay mould.

If left untreated, the IgG based complexes can cause chronic interstitial lung disease, resulting in fibrosis. Key points in the history are the exposure itself (social history – agricultural) and timing from exposure to symptoms (longer than in an allergic asthma).

Systemic type III hypersensitivity reactions occur when there is a large amount of antigen present throughout the body; this can occur when antigens such as antibiotics are injected into the circulation or if the antigen is an autoantigen (an autoimmune reaction).

POSTSTREPTOCCAL GLOMERULONEPHRITIS

Post-streptococcal glomerulonephritis is an important, systemic non-autoimmune type III hypersensitivity reaction. Antigen produced by β-haemolytic *Streptococcus* forms antigen-antibody complexes. These complexes are deposited in the glomeruli, producing an acute glomerulonephritis. This classically presents in children, 1-2 weeks after a sore throat (the source of the *Streptococcus* antigen), with oedema, hypertension, haematuria and proteinuria.

Systemic lupus erythematosus

An example of a systemic type III autoimmune disease is systemic lupus erythematosus (SLE). Patients with SLE have autoantibodies directed against DNA, histone proteins, red blood cells, platelets, leucocytes and clotting factors. These autoantibodies are also found in other autoimmune conditions; the most specific autoantibody for SLE is anti-double stranded DNA (anti-dsDNA). The sheer amount of corresponding autoantigen in the body means the production of large numbers of immune complexes is inevitable.

Deposition of immune complexes leads to the varied clinical features of SLE, including:

- Arthralgia (pain due to deposition in small joints)
- Rashes in sun-exposed areas
- Glomerulonephritis

Nonspecific systemic features such as fever, malaise and depression are often also present.

Diagnosis is by antinuclear antibody testing. Serum complement levels (C3 and C4) are low in active disease, secondary to their role in breaking apart immune complexes. It is most commonly diagnosed in women in the second or third decade of life.

The aetiology is unknown, but the vast array of autoantibodies present suggests a breakdown in self-tolerance. Genetic factors predispose to the disease; there is an association with HLA-DR2 and HLA-DR3 and with deficiencies of complement proteins, especially C2 or C4 (reduced complement levels result in a decreased ability to clear immune complexes). Other relevant aetiological factors include drugs such as hydralazine, exposure to ultraviolet light and oestrogens.

SLE is treated with immunosuppression (aimed at reducing auto-antibody production), steroids, NSAIDs or other antiinflammatory drugs.

The more common clinical features of systemic lupus erythematosus (SLE) can be remembered with the mnemonic 'A RASH POINts MD':

Arthralgia in the small joints, e.g., metacarpophalageal

Renal disease, e.g., glomerulonephritis

ANA (anti-nuclear antibody): ANA positivity is a nonspecific indicator

Serositis such as pericarditis, pleural effusion

Haematological abnormality: anaemia, lymphopaenia

Photosensitivity: burn easily after UV exposure

Oral ulcers, frequent

Immunological markers such as anti-dsDNA +ve

Neurological disorder such as epilepsy, migraine, ataxia, meningism, psychosis

Malar rash across the cheeks and nose, sparing the nasolabial folds

Discoid rash: erythematous, scaly, round patches

Four or more of these features in a history would be suggestive of SLE.

TYPE IV HYPERSENSITIVITY (DELAYED-TYPE HYPERSENSITIVITY)

Type IV hypersensitivity describes a reaction that takes place days after exposure to antigen. It is chiefly mediated by CD4+ T cells, predominantly Th1, as well as other lymphocytes. Upon first contact with antigen, macrophages present the antigen to Th cells, which are then activated and clonally expanded (this takes 1–2 weeks). Upon subsequent encounter with the same antigen, the sensitized Th cells secrete cytokines. These attract and activate macrophages, which account for more than 95% of the cells involved in type IV hypersensitivity reactions. The type IV reaction peaks at 48–72 hours after subsequent contact with the antigen (time taken for the recruitment and activation of the macrophages), hence it is also termed delayed-type hypersensitivity. An overview of the immune mechanisms involved is given in Fig. 12.7.

Type IV reactions are important for the clearance of intracellular pathogens. However, if antigens persist, the response can be detrimental to the individual, as the lytic products of the activated macrophages can damage healthy tissues. Examples of exogenous antigens that induce a type IV response are:

- Contact dermatitis to antigens such as nickel
- Intracellular pathogens such as *M. tuberculosis*

As with type I reactions, skin testing is used to detect type IV reactions. Instead of a skin prick, however, patch testing is used to diagnose antigens causing delayed hypersensitivity in contact dermatitis. A selection of sensitizing antigens are normally tested at the same time. They are usually placed in a grid pattern on the upper back and then dressed. Patients are then seen, sometimes more than once, over the next 48–72 hours to assess the response. The response varies from no response to an extreme reaction.

The tuberculin skin test can be used to determine whether a person has been exposed to *M. tuberculosis*. An intradermal injection of purified protein derivative (PPD) is given to the individual. Previous exposure to *M. tuberculosis* or bacille Calmette–Guérin (BCG) vaccination results in a positive response. This is apparent as a firm, red (due to the intense infiltration of macrophages) lesion at the injection site 48–72 hours after the injection. The skin lesions in both contact dermatitis and tuberculin testing are composed of macrophages and T cells.

Diseases caused by type IV hypersensitivity reactions

Numerous organ-specific and systemic autoimmune conditions are mediated by type IV hypersensitivity reactions. Organ-specific conditions include type I diabetes mellitus and Hashimoto thyroiditis. Rheumatoid arthritis (RA) is an example of a systemic type IV hypersensitivity reaction.

Type I diabetes mellitus

Type I diabetes mellitus (TIDM) occurs as a result of the destruction of the insulin-producing β cells of the islets of Langerhans of the pancreas. One in 300 people in Europe and the USA are affected. An autoimmune aetiology is very likely. Over 90% of patients with the disease carry either HLA-DR3 or HLA-DR4 or both. HLA-DQ2 is also implicated–this variant appears to prevent pancreatic islet cell autoantigen from binding correctly. Therefore, self-reactive T cells cannot be negatively selected in the thymus and tolerance breaks down. Since not everyone with these HLA alleles develops TIDM, external triggers must also be involved. It is thought that infection may be one of these triggers, causing a degree of inflammation in the pancreatic islets, attracting macrophages and sensitizing self-reactive T cells. This knowledge of the immune basis for TIDM has not previously been useful, but in the next few years it is likely to play a role in the prevention of the disease.

Hashimoto thyroiditis

Hashimoto thyroiditis is the most common cause of hypothyroidism in the developed world. Antigen-specific cytotoxic T cells attack the thyroid gland, leading to progressive destruction of the epithelium. Due to unregulated T-helper cell interaction with B cells, autoantibodies are produced against thyroid antigens such as thyroid peroxidase. Marked lymphocytic infiltration (mainly by B cells and CD4$^+$ T cells) of the thyroid gland is accompanied by migration of large numbers of macrophages and plasma cells, resulting in the formation of lymphoid follicles and germinal centres within the thyroid. Middle-aged females are most commonly affected (female:male ratio as high as 20:1). The disease is associated with the HLA-DR5 haplotype.

Rheumatoid arthritis

Rheumatoid arthritis (RA) is a chronic systemic disease that primarily involves the joints, resulting in inflammation of the synovium and destruction of the articular cartilage (Fig. 12.8). Initially, the disease affects the small joints of the hands and feet symmetrically, later spreading to the larger

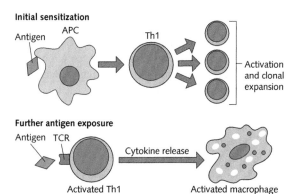

Initial sensitization

Antigen   APC   Th1   Activation and clonal expansion

Further antigen exposure

Antigen   TCR   Cytokine release

Activated Th1   Activated macrophage

Fig. 12.7 The immune mechanisms of type IV hypersensitivity reactions. Antigens are first presented to Th1 cells, which are then activated. These Th1 cells can then activate macrophages. Type IV hypersensitivity reactions take several days to be initiated because of the various cells that are involved.
APC, Antigen-presenting cell; *Th,* T helper.

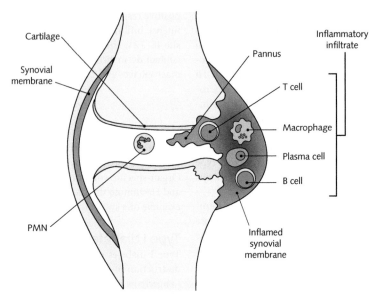

Fig. 12.8 Rheumatoid joint showing pannus formation and cartilage destruction. The synovial membrane is infiltrated by inflammatory cells and hypertrophies forming granulation tissue known as 'pannus'. This eventually erodes the articular cartilage and bone. T cells and macrophages in the inflamed synovium secrete tumour necrosis factor. *PMN,* Polymorphonuclear leucocyte.

joints. A typical history of RA is joint pain and stiffness on waking, lasting at least 30 minutes and progressive over time. RA also has extraarticular pathology in the lungs, eyes and skin. RA affects approximately 1%–2% of the world's population and is most common between the ages of 30 and 55 years. The female:male ratio is 3:1.

A central feature in the immunopathogenesis of RA is the citrullination of proteins. This is the conversion of the amino acid arginine to citrulline in proteins that may not normally contain citrulline. It is thought that citrullinated proteins become a target for autoreactive T and B cells. Additionally, anticyclic citrullinated peptide (anti-CCP) antibodies are found in the serum of most RA patients and in people who will develop RA. Citrullination may occur as a result of inflammation, triggered for reasons such as smoking, which is associated with the development of RA. The overall immunopathogenesis of RA is outlined in Fig. 12.9.

A key event in the pathogenesis of RA is the secretion of tumour necrosis factor (TNF) by T cells and macrophages, which coordinates the neutrophil mediated joint inflammation and osteoclast-mediated bone erosion.

Once RA is suspected clinically, prompt referral is essential to minimize morbidity associated with this chronic condition. Management is based on the early use of steroids and nonsteroidal antiinflammatories (NSAIDs). Specific antirheumatic drugs that modulate the immune response, known as biological disease-modifying antirheumatic drugs (DMARDs), are also used. These biological DMARDs usually target TNF (e.g., infliximab and adalimumab). The anti-B cell monoclonal antibody rituximab and the anti-IL-6

receptor monoclonal antibody tocilizumab can also be used (see Chapter 13).

RHEUMATOID ARTHRITIS INVESTIGATIONS

The blood tests in RA reflect its inflammatory nature; C-reactive protein and erythrocyte sedimentation rate are raised, indicating an acute phase response. Rheumatoid factor (IgM anti-IgG autoantibodies) is present in approximately 80% of patients and indicates a poorer prognosis than those who are rheumatoid factor negative. Anti-CCP antibodies can also be measured and are thought to be more selective and specific for RA than rheumatoid factor. The overall diagnosis of RA is clinical.

Radiographic features include:

- Soft tissue swelling
- Juxta-articular osteoporosis
- Joint space narrowing
- Joint destruction and erosions (see Fig. 12.10)
- Subluxation

A summary of the four types of hypersensitivity is shown in Table 12.2 and a summary of important autoimmune diseases is given in Tables 12.3, 12.4 and 12.5.

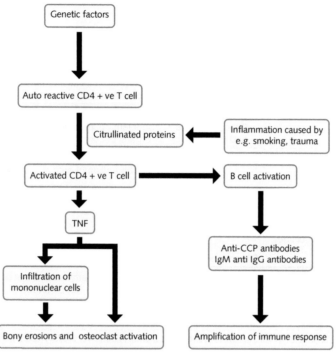

Fig. 12.9 Pathogenesis of rheumatoid arthritis. Autoreactive CD4$^+$ T cells, which target citrullinated peptides, mediate the pathological changes. Synovial T cells produce a number of cytokines including tumour necrosis factor (TNF). These stimulate the acute phase response, synovial inflammation and bone erosion. Activation of B cells can result in the production of anti-CCP antibodies and rheumatoid factor. *CCP*, cyclic citrullinated peptide; *RA*, rheumatoid arthritis.

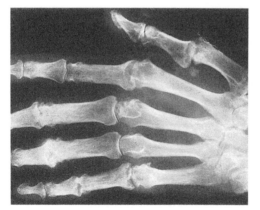

Fig. 12.10 An X-ray of a hand showing joint destruction and erosion due to rheumatoid arthritis.

DEVELOPMENT OF HYPERSENSITIVITY

Allergy

The incidence of allergies has increased dramatically in recent decades and the prevalence is also very high, with up to 40% of the population reporting some form of allergy. This led to the belief that our urban, 'clean' life style has contributed to allergy formation, supported by the fact that allergies are less prevalent in rural populations. It is not clear why this is the case; current theories are that micro-organism exposure during certain points of development reduces the incidence of allergy (an advance on the 'hygiene

Table 12.2 Summary of the different types of hypersensitivity

Type of hypersensitivity	Immune mediators	Time of onset	Examples
Type I	IgE, mast cells, eosinophils	Immediate (if IgE is preformed)	Anaphylaxis, asthma, atopic eczema
Type II	Antibody (normally IgG), complement, phagocytes	Rapid (if IgG is preformed)	Haemolytic disease of the newborn, ABO incompatibility
Type III	IgG, complement and neutrophils	Hours	SLE, farmer's lung
Type IV	Th cells, macrophages	48–72 hours	Contact dermatitis, tuberculin skin test

SLE, Systemic lupus erythematosus; Th cells, T helper cells.

Table 12.3 Other autoimmune diseases of connective tissues

Disease	Autoantigen	Autoantibodies	Features
Sjögren syndrome	Exocrine glands	Anti-Ro and La	Reduced lacrimal and salivary gland secretion, causing dry eyes and mouth
Myositis	Muscle	ANA (Jo-1)	Muscle weakness and atrophy; mild arthritis and rashes are common
Systemic sclerosis	Nucleoli	ANA (topoisomerase 1 and centromere)	Increased collagen deposition in skin; usually runs an indolent course, but eventual involvement of internal organs occurs in most patients
MCTD		ANA (RNP)	Features of SLE, RA, scleroderma and polymyositis; may not be a distinct entity

ANA, Antinuclear antigen; MCTD, mixed connective tissue disease; RA, rheumatoid arthritis; RNP, ribonucleoprotein; SLE, systemic lupus erythematosus.

Table 12.4 Autoimmune vasculitides

Disease	Diagnostic test[a]	Features
Polyangiitis	pANCA (myeloperoxidase)	Necrotizing inflammation of medium-sized arteries. Any organ or tissue can be affected
Granulomatosis with polyangiitis (previously Wegener granulomatosis)	cANCA (proteinase 3)	Presents with respiratory tract lesions, typically in the lungs and nose, in association with glomerulonephritis

[a] *Antineutrophil cytoplasmic antibodies (ANCA) are specific antibodies against neutrophils. pANCA reacts with neutrophil myeloperoxidase and gives a perinuclear pattern on immunofluorescence; cANCA reacts with proteinase 3 in the cytoplasm and gives a diffuse cytoplasmic pattern in immunofluorescence.*

Table 12.5 Summary of organ- or cell-specific autoimmune diseases

Disease	Autoantigen	Features
Myasthenia gravis	Acetylcholine receptor	Muscle weakness and fatigue due to impaired neuromuscular transmission; 70% of patients have thymic hyperplasia, 10% have thymic tumour
Goodpasture syndrome	Type IV collagen in the basement membrane of kidney and lung	Pulmonary haemorrhage and acute glomerulonephritis; peak incidence in men aged in their mid-20s
Pernicious anaemia	Intrinsic factor	See Chapter 3: Pernicious anaemia
AI haemolytic anaemia	Erythrocyte membrane antigens	See Chapter 3: Autoimmune haemolytic anaemia
AI thrombocytopenia	Platelet glycoproteins	See Chapter 6: Thrombocytopenia
Hashimoto thyroiditis	Thyroid peroxidase	See earlier in this chapter
Graves disease	TSH receptor	See earlier in this chapter
Type I diabetes mellitus	Islet cell antigens	See earlier in this chapter
Coeliac disease	Tissue transglutaminase	Malabsorption due to villous atrophy in the small bowel. Diarrhoea and anaemia are common. Patients can present at any age. Treated with a gluten-free diet.

The organ-specific autoantibodies are caused by similar genes, usually in the HLA complex. Family members therefore tend to have different organ-specific diseases.
AI, Autoimmune; HLA, human leucocyte antigen; TSH, thyroid stimulating hormone.

hypothesis'). Allergies run in families, suggesting a genetic influence, but no single genetic polymorphism has emerged that is common to all allergy sufferers. One gene implicated in some cases of allergy codes for the protein filaggrin. This protein normally maintains the skin's barrier function; polymorphisms in the filaggrin gene are highly associated with atopic eczema and allergy.

Ultimately, allergy forms when the initial exposure to an antigen, e.g., grass pollen, results in a Th2-cell-biased response, leading to IL-4 production and subsequent IgE overproduction for that antigen. A breakdown in tolerance also contributes to allergy development (see Chapter 10).

Autoimmune disease

Autoimmunity is a state in which the body exhibits immunological reactivity to itself. The need for 'self-tolerance' and the mechanisms of central and peripheral tolerance have already been discussed in Chapter 10: Tolerance. If tolerance breaks down, autoimmunity can develop. Tolerance can break down in the thymus (usually for genetic reasons) or in the periphery (usually as a result of environmental factors such as infection). Autoimmunity is multifactorial; a defect in at least one of the regulatory mechanisms is required before disease develops.

Role of human leucocyte antigen

Many autoimmune diseases have a familial component. The HLA haplotype is the main identified genetic factor. If an individual has inherited an HLA allele that does not bind well to self-antigen in the thymus, reactive T cells are not deleted during development, leading to a loss of 'self-tolerance'. Certain HLA alleles are linked to specific autoimmune processes, e.g., HLA-DR4 in rheumatoid arthritis, and HLA-DQ8 in coeliac disease. However, a certain HLA haplotype does not automatically result in the development of an autoimmune disease; 95% of patients with ankylosing spondylitis have HLA-B27, but only 5% of the population with HLA-B27 have ankylosing spondylitis.

Role of infection

Many infections are able to activate T and B cells in a non-specific fashion. This results in the proliferation of several T and B cell clones, which can produce autoreactive autoantibody or mediate autoimmunity.

IMMUNE DEFICIENCY

Immune deficiency predisposes individuals to infections from opportunistic pathogens (those that do not normally cause disease) as well as normal pathogens and may increase the risk of developing certain malignancies. Although the cause of the deficiency can be primary or secondary, the part of the immune system that is deficient will determine the sort of infection to which the individual is predisposed. For example, antibody deficits result in extracellular bacterial infection while T cell deficiencies can result in viral, fungal and intracellular bacterial infections.

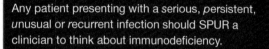

RED FLAG

Any patient presenting with a serious, persistent, unusual or recurrent infection should SPUR a clinician to think about immunodeficiency.

Primary immunodeficiencies

Primary immunodeficiencies are intrinsic, usually inherited, defects of the immune system. They can be caused by single gene mutations, genetic polymorphisms or by the interaction of several genes (polygenic). Different components of the immune system can be affected, including:

- Antibodies (Table 12.6)
- T cells (Table 12.7)
- Phagocytes (Table 12.8)
- Complement (Table 12.9)

It is important to recognize primary immunodeficiencies early. Patients with an antibody deficiency will develop severe lung infections that lead to chronic structural changes

Table 12.6 Primary antibody deficiencies

Disorder	Features
Transient physiological agammaglobulinaemia of the neonate	See Fig. 12.11
X-linked agammaglobulinaemia of Bruton	X-linked recessive disorder with defective B cell maturation. Low serum immunoglobulin levels result in recurrent pyogenic infections (seen after about 6 months). Treatment is with immunoglobulin replacement.
Common variable hypogammaglobulinaemia	Heterogeneous group of disorders with normal lymphocyte numbers but abnormal B cell function; late onset (15–35 years of age) presenting with recurrent pyogenic infections. Treatment is with immunoglobulin replacement.
Selective IgA deficiency	Occurs in 1 in 700 Caucasians but is rarer in other ethnic groups; can be asymptomatic or produce recurrent infections of the respiratory and gastrointestinal tracts.

Pyogenic infections are common due to infections with encapsulated bacteria such as streptococci and staphylococci (not selective IgA deficiency).

Table 12.7 Primary lymphocyte deficiencies[a]

Disorder	Features
DiGeorge syndrome (thymic hypoplasia)	Intrauterine damage to the third and fourth pharyngeal pouches results in failure of development of the thyroid and parathyroid glands. This results in a decrease in the number and function of T cells. Clinical features include abnormal facies, cardiac defects, hypoparathyroidism and recurrent infections.
Severe combined immunodeficiency disease (SCID)	Lymphocyte deficiency and failure of thymic development due to inherited abnormalities: • X-linked SCID is due to defects in the γ-chain of the IL-2 receptor. The γ-chain forms part of several cytokine receptors including IL-7, which is needed for T cell maturation. • Autosomal recessive SCID is caused by defects in adenosine deaminase (ADA) or purine nucleoside phosphorylase in more than 50% of cases. Both are involved in purine degradation and deficiency results in accumulation of toxic metabolites and inhibition of DNA synthesis. Recombinase defects also lead to SCID. In both types of SCID, treatment should be by bone marrow transplant, usually before the age of 2 years. Trials using gene therapy to treat X-linked SCID were stopped due to an increased risk of leukaemia.
Wiskott–Aldrich syndrome	X-linked recessive condition characterized by normal serum IgG, low IgM and high IgA and IgE. Defective T cell function is seen, which worsens as the patient ages. Patients tend to get recurrent infections, eczema and thrombocytopenia.

[a] Primary lymphocyte deficiencies include infections with opportunistic pathogens such as Pneumocystis carinii. T cell deficiency can cause an antibody deficiency due to lack of T-helper-cell activation of B cells.

Table 12.8 Primary phagocyte deficiencies

Disorder	Features
Neutropenia	See Chapter 4: Leucopenia
Leucocyte adhesion deficiency	Lack of β$_2$-integrin molecules results in impaired adhesion and extravasation of phagocytes.
Chronic granulomatous disease	Most commonly X-linked (can be autosomal recessive) inheritance. Lack of NADPH oxidase impairs killing of ingested pathogens, which therefore persist.

NADPH, Nicotinamide adenine dinucleotide phosphate.

Table 12.9 Primary complement deficiencies[a]

Disorder	Features
Deficiency of classical pathway components	Tendency to develop immune complex disease such as SLE
C3 deficiency	Prone to recurrent pyogenic infections
Deficiency of C5, C6, C 7, C8, factor D, properdin	Increased susceptibility to Neisseria infections
C1 inhibitor deficiency	Causes hereditary angioedema

[a] Deficiencies of almost all complement components have been described.
SLE, systemic lupus erythematosus.

in the lungs (bronchiectasis) unless given immunoglobulin. Children with T cell defects can be killed by opportunistic infections or from live vaccines such as BCG.

Neonates do not possess a fully developed immune system at birth. In the neonatal period, infants are normally protected by maternal IgG that crosses the placenta in utero, but this is metabolized during the first months of life. In the first 6 months of life, there is a trough in immunoglobulin levels that makes infants prone to infection. IgA in breast milk can compensate. Babies born prematurely are deprived of maternal IgG and suffer exaggerated neonatal antibody deficiency. Infants normally begin production of their own IgG by the age of 3 months (Fig.12.11). In some individuals, IgG production might not start for up to 9–12 months, possibly due to the lack of help from T cells.

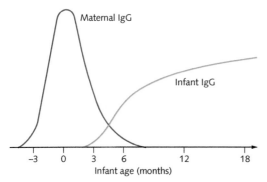

Fig. 12.11 Plasma levels of maternal and neonatal immunoglobulin in the normal-term infant.

NOD2 AND CROHN DISEASE

Polymorphisms in the gene for the pattern recognition molecule nucleotide-binding oligomerization domain containing 2 (NOD2) are found in many cases of Crohn disease. Normally, NOD2 activates the innate immune response in gut epithelial cells. Therefore, the theory is that Crohn disease is caused by repeated bacterial infection resulting from immunodeficiency rather than autoimmunity.

Secondary immunodeficiencies

Secondary immunodeficiency is acquired, through disease, drugs or malnutrition.

Malnutrition and disease

It is rare that the lack of dietary protein and certain elements (e.g., zinc) predisposes patients to secondary immunodeficiency. Infections such as malaria and measles can also result in immunodeficiency.

Malignancy

Secondary immunodeficiency is particularly common with tumours that arise from the immune system, such as myeloma, lymphoma and leukaemia (see Chapter 5). Many other tumours are immunosuppressive. This is likely to provide the tumour cells with a selective advantage, because they evade destruction by cytotoxic cells.

Steroids, other drugs and radiation

Iatrogenic causes of immunosuppression are common. Immunosuppressive drugs can be given to suppress inflammatory or autoimmune disease or to prevent rejection of transplanted material (see Chapter 13: Transplantation).

Radiation and cytotoxic drugs can be used to treat malignancies and frequently cause immunosuppression.

Acquired immunodeficiency syndrome

Acquired immunodeficiency syndrome (AIDS) is caused by severe human immunodeficiency virus (HIV) infection. HIV is a retrovirus, containing a small amount of RNA, that codes three important viral genes: the envelope, reverse transcriptase and protease (Fig. 12.12).

The envelope is composed of gp120, which binds to CD4 receptors and chemokine receptor 5 (CCR5). A conformational change causes gp41 to be expressed on the virus, which penetrates the host cell. This process allows HIV to infect:

- CD4+ve T cells
- Monocytes and macrophages
- Dendritic cells (epithelial antigen presenting cells)

Reverse transcriptase is an enzyme that catalyses the production of HIV DNA from viral RNA, using host cellular machinery.

Protease is an enzyme that cleaves proteins into their component peptides and is important for viral assembly and activity.

Transmission of HIV

Sexual transmission is the most important route for the spread of HIV; it infects mucosal macrophages and dendritic cells via CD4 and CCR5. These professional antigen presenting cells (APCs) then aid in the evolution of the HIV

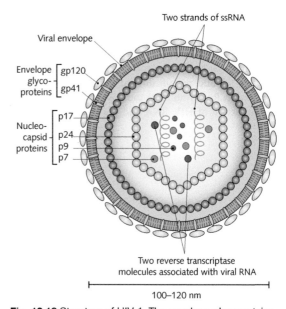

Fig. 12.12 Structure of HIV-1. The envelope glycoproteins gp120 and gp41 are hypervariable. gp120 binds CD4, while gp41 enables entry of the virus into the cell. The viral envelope is a lipid bilayer containing both viral glycoprotein antigens and host proteins.
ssRNA, Single stranded ribonucleic acid.

infection by transporting it to the lymph nodes, where HIV can gain easy access to CD4 +ve T helper (Th) cells.

Transmission can also occur through infected blood (such as via blood transfusions), intravenous drug abuse and needlestick injury (0.3% risk from a single exposure). These routes do not require HIV to gain access through mucous membranes and hence CCR5 receptors.

Vertical transmission is especially important in developing countries, occurring transplacentally during labour (approximately 25% of cases) or through breast milk. It is possible to minimize the risk of vertical transmission by delivering the baby via Caesarean section, feeding with formula milk rather than breast milk and the early use of antiretrovirals (see Treatment of HIV later).

Immune response to HIV

Most individuals exposed to HIV sexually become chronically infected. Infected individuals produce antibodies, but this is largely ineffective against intracellular virus. T cells inhibit HIV by interferon secretion or by killing infected cells. Individuals infected with HIV develop symptoms as their body starts to produce antibodies to HIV. This is called HIV seroconversion illness. The patient experiences fever, rash, malaise, sore throat, diarrhoea and arthralgia; lymphadenopathy may also be present. Not all patients experience seroconversion illness and it is often diagnosed retrospectively.

How does HIV progress to AIDS?

HIV can evade the immune system by mutating its DNA; reverse transcriptase makes an error for roughly 1 in every 10,000 bases. Some of these mutations provide a selective advantage to HIV because cells of the immune system may no longer recognize the mutated virus and another immune response has to start afresh. Even if the immune system manages to clear the entire free virus, HIV can hide in host DNA and remain dormant for many years—the latent phase. Reactivation of the host cell then results in the production of HIV RNA and the infection therefore continues.

Crucially, HIV infects and destroys the cells that are responsible for the immune response. As the CD4 +ve T cell count declines, cytotoxic T lymphocytes become less effective as they are receiving less support from Th cells. This leads to the development of AIDS.

HINTS AND TIPS

Each infected individual contains many hundreds of slightly different strains following infection with a single virus, reflecting the ongoing mutation of the virus.

Diagnosis and monitoring of an HIV infection

Screening for HIV infection is performed using enzyme-linked immunosorbent assays (ELISAs) to detect anti-HIV antibodies (see the section on ELISA). If the ELISA is positive, confirmatory tests must be carried out, e.g., a Western blot, which detects antibodies against specific HIV proteins. False positives may occur with the HIV ELISA in those with recent influenza vaccination, hepatic disease or a recent viral infection. As seroconversion (production of antibodies) might not take place until 3 months after infection, there is a window period when ELISA will be negative. This is a potential problem in blood donation and transfusion.

In infants, anti-HIV IgG can be maternally derived and persist for up to 18 months, making diagnosis of HIV by ELISA unreliable. Detection of HIV by polymerase chain reaction (PCR) is used to confirm HIV infection in neonates.

Determinations of CD4 +ve T cell counts and measurement of the viral load (serum HIV RNA) are useful in assessing response to treatment and the prognosis.

CD4 counts provide a guide of the current immunological status of the patient (Fig. 12.13), whereas HIV RNA levels predict what will happen to the patient over the next few months and years.

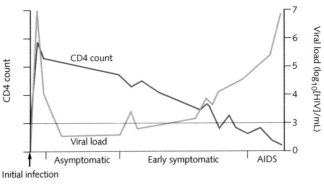

Fig. 12.13 Variation in CD4 count and viral load during the course of HIV infection.

Table 12.10 Clinical infections at different CD4 counts

CD4 count	Infection
<400	Tuberculosis
<300	Kaposi sarcoma. Oesophageal candidiasis
<200	*Pneumocystis carinii* pneumonia Toxoplasmosis
<100	*Mycobacterium avium intracellulare* Cytomegalovirus retinitis

During the latent phase of the infection, T cells are constantly battling with the HIV and gradually the CD4 count falls. With the falling CD4 count, individuals become increasingly susceptible to infections. Initially, these include virulent organisms such as *Candida albicans* and *Mycobacterium tuberculosis*. However, as the CD4 count continues to fall, the individual is more susceptible to opportunistic infections (Table 12.10). When the CD4 count drops to <200 cells/μL or the individual begins to suffer from an infection indicative of AIDS (an 'AIDS-defining condition'), they are said to be suffering from AIDS (as opposed to just being HIV +ve).

Treatment of HIV

The treatment of HIV is now very successful. Although the infection cannot be cured, survival and the quality of life of sufferers have been greatly increased, with the life expectancy of patients in the UK thought to match that of HIV − ve individuals. The drugs used to combat the virus are called antiretrovirals (ARVs) and include classes of drug that work on the three main elements of the virus (Fig. 12.14):

- Fusion inhibitors prevent attachment to the envelope.
- Reverse transcriptase inhibitors (RTIs) inhibit the production of DNA. There are both nucleotide analogue RTIs (NARTIs) and nonnucleotide RTI (NNRTIs).
- Protease inhibitors prevent the production of viral peptides.

When treating HIV, it is important to remember its ability to mutate and that antiretrovirals could provide a selective advantage for a more resistant strain to develop. For this reason, a combination of a least two classes of drug are used and they are not started until there is evidence of CD4 + ve T cell decline. This combination of more than one drug is known as highly active antiretroviral therapy (HAART).

For individuals who have been diagnosed when there is already immune system damage (indicated by a low CD4 count), antibiotic prophylaxis against infections such as *Pneumocystis carinii* and *Toxoplasma gondii* is effective and usually given (if the CD4 count is <200/μL). It has been shown that antibiotic prophylaxis can be safely stopped following immune restoration using treatment with antiretroviral therapy.

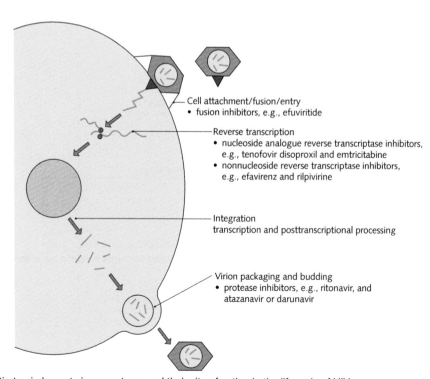

Fig. 12.14 Antiretroviral agents in current use and their site of action in the lifecycle of HIV.

Postexposure prophylaxis (PEP) has long been offered to any person that has recently been exposed to HIV in a high-risk manner, such as unprotected sexual intercourse or exposure to infected bodily fluids in a health care setting. PEP involves a 28-day course of antiretroviral drugs and should ideally be started within 72 hours of exposure.

Preexposure prophylaxis is the regular, long-term use of antiretroviral drugs in populations that are HIV –ve but are at high risk of infection. It aims to prevent the virus from establishing in the host after inoculation.

INVESTIGATION OF IMMUNE FUNCTION

Immunoassays

This is a technique that uses antibodies to identify and to quantify antigen or biological molecules.

Enzyme-linked immunosorbent assay

ELISA is a sensitive test that allows quantitative analysis of the amount of a specific antigen or antigen/antibody complex in a sample.

In an ELISA, the antigen or antibody being studied is linked to an enzyme. This enzyme catalyses the conversion of a colourless substrate to a coloured product; the amount of coloured end-product is proportional to the amount of antigen or antibody and can be measured using a spectrometer.

ELISAs are commonly used to measure specific antibody in a patient's serum, as in HIV. Using this as a working example:

- A plate containing the HIV glycoprotein gp120 is exposed to the patient's serum; any of the appropriate antibodies present in the serum will bind the antigen on the plate.
- A monoclonal antibody that is specific for the Fc portion of the anti-HIV antibody in the patient's serum is added. This antibody is labelled with the enzyme that catalyses the colour conversion (see Fig. 12.15).
- The enzyme substrate is then added and the colour conversion occurs.

Each of these steps is incubated for a consistent period of time with any excess being washed before the next substance is added.

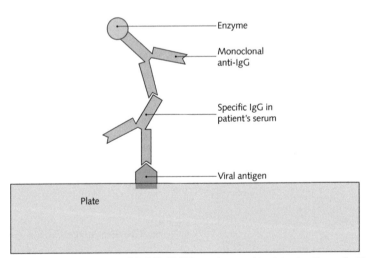

Fig. 12.15 Enzyme-linked immunosorbent assay (ELISA). ELISA can be used to detect antigens but is most commonly used to measure antibody to specific antigen (e.g., a virus).

● Chapter Summary

- Hypersensitivity is an excessive immune response to any antigen. Its causes are multifactorial and involve a breakdown in tolerance. It can be classified by type of immune response:
- Type I hypersensitivity involves IgE mediated mast cell degranulation. Examples include food and pollen allergy, asthma and eczema.
- Type II hypersensitivity is mediated by other immunoglobulins, often followed by complement activation and antibody-dependent cell-mediated cytotoxicity. Examples include Graves disease and ABO mismatch reactions in blood transfusion.
- Type III hypersensitivity is caused by tissue deposition of antigen-antibody complexes. Examples include systemic lupus erythematosus and Farmer's lung.
- Type IV hypersensitivity is coordinated and mediated by T cells. Examples include contact dermatitis and rheumatoid arthritis.
- Hypersensitivity is generally managed by avoidance of triggers (if possible), local or systemic immunosuppression, or targeted therapy.
- Immunodeficiency can be intrinsic (primary) or acquired (secondary). Primary immunodeficiency can involve one or many components of the immune system. Secondary immunodeficiency has many causes, including immunosuppressive drugs and infection.
- Acquired immune deficiency syndrome (AIDS) is caused by severe human immunodeficiency virus (HIV) infection, a virus that infects antigen-presenting cells and CD4 + T cells. Treatment aims to reduce the viral load and restore the CD4 + T cell count.

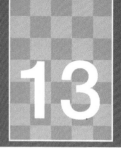

Medical intervention 13

The immune system can be manipulated in various ways, either to enhance its beneficial actions (vaccination) or to supress any adverse reactions (immunosuppression, antiinflammatory drugs).

IMMUNIZATION

Immunity can be achieved by passive or active immunization (Table 13.1).

Passive immunization

This is a temporary immunity that results from the transfer of exogenous antibody from one person to another. It occurs without prior exposure to the specific antigens. Passive immunity is seen in the foetus when maternal IgG crosses the placenta and in breast-fed babies due to the IgA content of breast milk. Passive immunity can be conferred to individuals who have been exposed to a pathogen to which they are not immune by the injection of immunoglobulins to the antigen specific to that pathogen. These are taken from blood donors immune to the pathogen.

Examples where passive immunity is used include:

- Open fracture management: if tetanus vaccination history is uncertain or incomplete, anti-tetanus immunoglobulin is given.
- Hepatitis B post exposure prophylaxis: hepatitis B immunoglobulin can be given to unvaccinated individuals, for example after a contaminated needlestick injury.
- Management of digoxin toxicity with Digibind (immunoglobulin that binds and neutralizes digoxin molecules).

Active immunization

Active immunization results from contact with antigens, either through natural infection or by vaccination. Individuals exhibit a primary immune response with clonal expansion of B and T cells and formation of memory cells. Subsequent exposure to the same antigen will induce a secondary immune response (see Chapter 10).

Vaccination

Vaccination is a form of active immunization that induces specific immunity to a particular pathogen. The aim is to produce a rapid, protective immune response on re-exposure to that pathogen. An ideal vaccine is:

- Safe, with minimal side-effects and free from contaminating substances
- Immunogenic, activating the required branches of the immune system, inducing long-lasting local and systemic immunity
- Heat stable because there are difficulties with refrigeration, particularly in tropical countries
- Inexpensive, an important consideration, especially in developing countries

Types of vaccine

The types of vaccine in current use are listed in Table 13.2. Vaccines can be live attenuated (weakened) organisms, killed organisms or subunit; the features of each are compared in Table 13.3. In general, live vaccines are more potent but risk greater side-effects than subunit vaccines. The vaccination schedule changes from time to time as new vaccines become available. For the UK, the Government's website is a good place to look for the most up-to-date schedule and details of individual vaccines: www.gov.uk/government/collections/immunisation. Each country has its own version. It is not necessary to memorize this schedule, but it is worth having a rough idea of what is given and when. A condensed version of the UK's vaccination schedule is given in Table 13.4.

CLINICAL NOTES

A healthy immune system can cope with live attenuated vaccines. However, these vaccines are contraindicated in immunocompromised patients as they can cause severe infection. Anaphylaxis to a certain vaccine is also a contraindication to future treatment. Some vaccines, for example measles, yellow fever and BCG, are contraindicated in pregnancy.

Vaccines are not 100% efficacious. A small proportion of individuals receiving vaccination will not respond adequately. However, by immunizing the majority of the population, nonresponders are unlikely to come into contact with the virus because the viral reservoir is reduced (herd immunity).

You will notice that a number of vaccinations are given simultaneously; this is not just for convenience. Given alone, some of the subunit vaccines would not

Table 13.1 Comparison of passive and active immunity

	Features	Examples
Passive	Preformed immunoglobulins transferred to individual Large amounts of antibody available immediately Short lifespan of antibodies	Anti-tetanus toxin antibody
Active	Contact with antigen induces adaptive immune response Takes some time to develop immunity Long-lived immunity induced: includes T cells, B cells and antibody	Natural exposure Vaccination

Table 13.2 Different types of vaccine in use in the UK today

Vaccine	Features	Examples
Live attenuated	Attenuation achieved by repeated culture on artificial media or by serial passage in animals; immunogenicity is retained, but virulence is significantly diminished	Oral polio (Sabin), BCG, measles, mumps, rubella (MMR)
Killed	Intact organisms killed by exposure to heat or chemicals, e.g., formalin	Intramuscular polio (Salk), pertussis, influenza
Subunit	Purified, protective immunity-inducing antigenic components; often surface antigens	Nonconjugated pneumococcal, acellular pertussis
Recombinant	Genes encoding epitopes, which elicit protective immunity, are inserted into pro- or eukaryotic cells; large quantities of vaccine are produced rapidly	Hepatitis B surface antigen (produced in yeast cells), human papilloma virus (HPV) vaccines
Toxoids	Bacterial toxins inactivated by heat or chemicals	Diphtheria, tetanus
Conjugates	Polysaccharide antigen is linked to protein carrier to enhance immunogenicity	*Haemophilus influenzae* type B (Hib), meningococcal, pneumococcal

BCG, Bacille Calmette–Guérin.

Table 13.3 Features of live versus killed vaccines

Feature	Live attenuated vaccine	Killed vaccine
Level of immunity induced	High: organism replicates at site of infection (mimicking natural infection)	Low: nonreplicating organisms produce a short-lived stimulus
Cell-mediated response	Good: antigens are processed and presented with MHC molecules	Poor
Local immunity	Good	Poor
Cost	Expensive to produce and administer	Cheaper than live vaccines
Reversion to virulence	Possible but rare	No (therefore safe for immunocompromised and pregnant patients)
Stability	Heat labile	Heat stable
Risk of contamination	Possible, e.g., by virus in cell media	N/A

The genes of attenuated organisms can differ from the wild type by just a few base pairs. It is relatively easy for them to mutate back to the disease-causing strain.
MHC, Major histocompatibility complex; N/A, not applicable.

Table 13.4 Routine immunisation schedule used in the UK

Age	Vaccine
8 weeks	Diphtheria, tetanus and pertussis (DTaP), polio (IPV), *Haemophilus influenzae* type b (Hib), hepatitis B (HepB). These are known as the 6-in-1.
	Pneumococcal conjugate vaccine (PCV) Meningococcal group B (MenB) Rotavirus
12 weeks	DTaP/IPV/Hib/HepB
	Rotavirus
16 weeks	DTaP/IPV/Hib/HepB
	PCV MenB
1 year	Measles, mumps, rubella (MMR)
	PCV
	Hib/MenC MenB
3 years 4 months	DTaP/IPV
	MMR
12–13 years (girls only)	Human papillomavirus (HPV) types 6, 11, 16 and 18
14 years	DT/IPV MenACWY
>65 years	Annual influenza
	Pneumococcal polysaccharide vaccine (PPV): one-off Shingles
Any age	Occupation, e.g., Hep A, Hep B
	Travel, e.g., Yellow fever

CLINICAL NOTES

Vaccination against toxins such as tetanus does not provide immunity against the toxin-producing bacterium (*Clostridium tetani*). Its benefits come from preventing the sequelae associated with the tetanus toxin, i.e., tetanus of the masseter muscles (lock jaw).

TRANSPLANTATION

Mechanisms of solid organ transplant rejection

HINTS AND TIPS

Autologous grafts are grafts moved from one part of the body to another, e.g., skin grafts.
Syngeneic grafts are between genetically identical individuals, e.g., monozygotic twins.
Allogeneic grafts are between individuals of the same species.
Xenogeneic grafts are between different species.

The immune system presents a challenge for the long-term survival of organ and tissue transplants. Unless the donor and recipient are immunologically identical, the recipient will mount a rejection response against 'foreign' antigens expressed by the graft. The graft antigens responsible for most of the immune response in the recipient are the major histocompatibility complex (MHC) molecules (see Chapter 10: The major histocompatibility complex). However, even when the donor and recipient are genetically identical at the MHC loci, graft rejection can occur due to differences at other loci, which encode minor histocompatibility antigens. A rejection response can lead to loss of a graft. There are three types of graft rejection:

1. Hyperacute: occurs within hours as a result of preformed antibodies against the donor tissue, a type II hypersensitivity reaction often due to ABO mismatch.
2. Acute: takes several days to develop, a type IV hypersensitivity reaction that develops against incompatible donor MHC and other molecules. It can be reduced by human leucocyte antigen matching and managed with antirejection therapy.
3. Chronic: occurs months to years after transplantation. It can be caused by a variety of mechanisms. It cannot be treated.

evoke a sufficient immune response in order for immunity to develop. For example, the diphtheria, tetanus, pertussis (DTaP) vaccination relies strongly on the danger signal produced in response to the killed pertussis organism to develop immunity to the diphtheria and tetanus toxoids.

It is also possible to enhance the immune response to subunit vaccines by using adjuvants. Adjuvants, e.g., aluminium salts and *Bordetella pertussis*, are nonspecific stimulators of the pattern recognition molecules of the innate immune system. When these are present, the innate immune system transmits a 'danger signal' to the adaptive immune system to promote a good response.

Strategies for preventing rejection

Human leucocyte antigen typing

Considering that MHC is the main antigen in foreign tissue rejection, the ideal donor tissue would have identical human leucocyte antigen (HLA) molecules as the recipient. The perfect donor would be a monozygotic twin because they would have the same HLA genes. In all other situations, there will be some genetic disparity between donor and recipient. The aim of HLA matching is to minimize genetic differences between donor and recipient. Both donors and recipients are HLA typed and the closest match is used.

Antirejection therapy

Immunosuppressive drugs can be used to prevent rejection by suppressing antibody and T cell responses. Examples of drugs used include:

- Steroids: these have antiinflammatory effects, as well as directly affecting T cell and phagocyte function (see below)
- Antiproliferative drugs (reduce cell division): azathioprine, mycophenolate mofetil and methotrexate
- T cell signalling inhibitors (calcineurin inhibitors): tacrolimus and ciclosporin

Immunosuppression can also be induced by using monoclonal antibodies against components of the immune system, for example, the anti-IL-2 receptor antibody basiliximab. Due to its potency, basiliximab tends to be used in the short term, such as in treatment of acute transplant rejection.

Table 13.5 Common transplants

Transplant	Notes
Kidney	Live or cadaveric donor; the fewer the MHC mismatches, the greater the success rate; must be ABO compatible.
Heart	Matching is beneficial, but often time is a more pressing concern.
Liver	No evidence to suggest that matching affects graft survival; rejection less aggressive than for other organs.
Skin graft	Most grafts are autologous, but allografts can be used to protect burns patients.
Corneal graft	Matching (MHC class II) is required only if a previous graft was vascularized.
Stem cell	Host-versus-graft (HVG) or graft-versus-host (GVH) responses possible. The transplant must be well matched and antirejection therapy used. Host immune cells are destroyed by irradiation prior to transplant (avoids HVG). T cells are depleted from the graft (avoids GVH) using monoclonal antibody and complement.

MHC, Major histocompatibility complex.

The disadvantage of immunosuppressive therapy is that the recipient is at increased risk of opportunistic infections (e.g., cytomegalovirus) and certain malignancies. Most transplant patients will stay on these drugs for life as rejection can still take place many years after transplantation.

Common types of transplantation performed today are summarized in Table 13.5.

Stem cell transplantation

Stem cell transplants are used in the treatment of some cancers and primary immunodeficiencies. Haematopoietic stem cells are obtained from bone marrow or blood. Imperfectly matched stem cells can be rejected by the recipient. In addition, stem cells give rise to lymphocytes, which can attack the host, causing acute or chronic graft-versus-host disease.

ANTIINFLAMMATORY DRUGS

Antiinflammatory drugs are commonly used for inflammatory pain, as well as the treatment of a variety of hypersensitivity reactions. Antiinflammatory drugs may be used alongside immunosuppressive drugs, such as ciclosporin, azathioprine or methotrexate.

Different types of antiinflammatory drug are available, including:

- Corticosteroids
- Nonsteroidal antiinflammatory drugs
- Biologic antiinflammatory drugs

Clinical trials have developed evidence-based guidelines for the use of these drugs. In rheumatoid arthritis, nonsteroidal antiinflammatory drugs (NSAIDs), paracetamol or corticosteroid injections into joints are used for the treatment of symptoms, while methotrexate is started as a long-term disease-modifying antirheumatic drug (DMARD). If this fails or is contraindicated, biologic antiinflammatory drugs are the next choice. Systemic corticosteroids are only used in short bursts, for example while waiting for the above drugs to work or to treat acute flare-ups.

Corticosteroids

The adrenal cortex releases several steroid hormones into the circulation. Glucocorticoids affect carbohydrate and protein metabolism and also affect the immune system, acting as immunosuppressive and antiinflammatory agents. Glucocorticoids act primarily on phagocytes. By binding to intracellular receptors and modifying gene expression, they inhibit the production of mediators of inflammation (prostaglandins, cytokines) and prevent antigen presentation. At higher doses they have a direct effect on lymphocytes. Several corticosteroids are available therapeutically, including:

- Hydrocortisone: can be given intravenously in status asthmaticus or topically for inflammatory skin conditions.
- Prednisolone: oral preparations are given in many inflammatory, rheumatological and allergic conditions, as well as in exacerbations of chronic obstructive pulmonary disease.
- Beclomethasone: used as an aerosol in asthma or topically for eczema.

Adverse effects and contraindications

Glucocorticoids cause many adverse effects at the high doses required to produce an antiinflammatory effect and many patients find them difficult to put up with. The clinical features are that of Cushing syndrome. Some important adverse effects are shown in Table 13.6.

Steroids are contraindicated if there is evidence of systemic infection. Long-term high-dose steroid therapy is usually avoided. When they are used long term, there should be regular checks on blood pressure, blood sugar and bone density. Care should be taken when finishing a course of corticosteroid therapy, as endogenous corticosteroid production is suppressed by long term (>3 weeks) or high dose therapy. The dose of corticosteroids should be gradually reduced over weeks if a long course or high dose has been used. Failure to do so could result in an Addisonian crisis.

Table 13.6 Some adverse effects of glucocorticoids and their prevention or treatment

Adverse effect	Prevention or treatment
Diabetes	Regular blood sugar measurements
Osteoporosis	Bone density should be regularly monitored during steroid treatment. Patients, especially the elderly, may need bisphosphonates and calcium supplements.
Peptic ulcer	Proton pump inhibitors may be required.
Thin skin, easy bruising and poor wound healing	No treatment, but early and intensive intervention of wounds is necessary to prevent chronic morbidity.
Adrenal insufficiency	Prevent sudden decreases in dose, increase dose when ill and carry a steroid card. Treatment is resuscitation and steroid replacement.

RED FLAG

ADDISONIAN CRISIS (ACUTE ADRENAL INSUFFICIENCY)

This develops when a patient cannot mount an effective steroid response, for example due to adrenal suppression from exogenous corticosteroids. Symptoms and signs are mainly those of shock. They may have hyperkalaemia with hyponatraemia, as well as hypoglycaemia.

Initial treatment is with IV hydrocortisone and IV fluid resuscitation. Patients on long-term corticosteroids should carry a steroid card, informing medical personnel of their requirement for corticosteroids.

Nonsteroidal antiinflammatory drugs

NSAIDs include a large number of drugs that can be bought over the counter, e.g., aspirin, ibuprofen and naproxen. They are chemically diverse but all act to inhibit cyclooxygenase (COX; Fig. 13.1). This attenuates, but does not abolish, inflammation. As well as their antiinflammatory effects, NSAIDs have analgesic and antipyretic actions. They are used primarily in conditions where pain is accompanied by inflammation, such as ligament damage or rheumatoid arthritis.

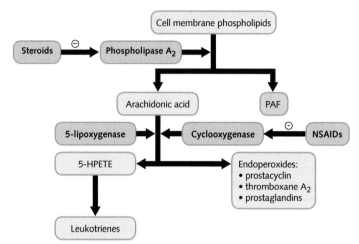

Fig. 13.1 The actions of nonsteroidal antiinflammatory drugs (NSAIDs) in arachidonic acid metabolism. *COX,* Cyclooxygenase; *PAF*, Platelet-activating factor; *5-HPETE*, Arachidonic acid 5-hydroperoxide.

COX mainly occurs as two isoenzymes: COX-1 and COX-2. COX-1 is constantly produced and is responsible for the production of physiological prostaglandins that protect the gastric mucosa and protect renal function. COX-2 is produced in inflammation and is important for the formation of proinflammatory prostaglandins. Most NSAIDs block both COX isoenzymes, but some are more active against one or the other. Selective COX-2 inhibitors (e.g., celecoxib) were released in the hope of having antiinflammatory effects without gastric and renal side-effects. However, because they were found to increase cardiovascular and cerebrovascular risk, the use of traditional NSAIDs versus selective COX-2 inhibitors is tailored to the patient's risk profile.

Aspirin

Acetylsalicylic acid (aspirin) is an antiinflammatory that causes a lot of adverse effects. As a consequence of this, newer NSAIDs (e.g., ibuprofen) are usually preferred for the treatment of inflammatory conditions because they exhibit fewer side-effects. Aspirin is far more efficient at inhibiting COX-1 (hence the side-effects) and is therefore used prophylactically in low doses in people who have had strokes or have ischaemic heart disease because of its ability to inhibit platelet function (see Chapter 6: COX inhibition)

Adverse effects and contraindications

Adverse effects with NSAIDs are common and occur mainly as a result of COX-1 inhibition. NSAIDs often cause damage to the mucosa of the gastrointestinal tract because they remove the cytoprotective effects of prostaglandins in the gut; the mucosa becomes ulcerated because of the damaging effects of stomach acid. NSAIDs can be nephrotoxic and cause bronchospasm, which can also be due to the role of COX-1-produced prostaglandins in renal and respiratory function. The side-effects of aspirin include nausea, vomiting, epigastric pain and tinnitus.

Biologics

Biologics are drugs manufactured in a living system and are very large, complex molecules. Biologics can be designed to block specific parts of the immune system. Typically, they are either monoclonal antibodies against cellular receptors, monoclonal antibodies against cytokines, or soluble receptor molecules (Fig. 13.2). There are many different biologics

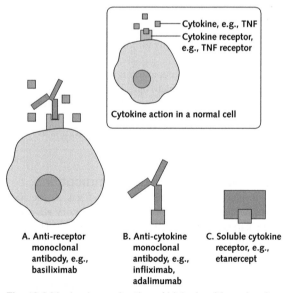

Fig. 13.2 Mechanisms of action of biologics. Monoclonal antibodies can be employed to block receptors, altering cellular function (A). Monoclonal antibodies can also be designed to bind to cytokines directly, attenuating the action of the cytokine (B). Similarly, soluble receptors can be produced, which bind to cytokines, reducing their action on cells (C). While the mechanism of action of anti-cytokine monoclonal antibodies and soluble cytokine receptors is similar, their molecular components are distinct.

Table 13.7 Examples of biologic agents and their uses

Examples of drugs	Target and mechanism	Examples of use
Infliximab, adalimumab	Binds to circulating TNF-α, preventing it from binding to TNF receptors on immune cells.	Inflammatory arthropathies (e.g. RA, psoriatic arthritis), inflammatory bowel disease
Ipilimumab	Binds to and blocks CTLA-4. Cancer cells stimulate CTLA-4 receptors on T cells, preventing a T cell response to cancer antigens. Blocking CTLA-4 allows T cells to respond to cancer antigens.	Melanoma
Basiliximab	Binds to and blocks IL-2 receptors on T cells, preventing their clonal expansion and subsequent B cell activation/antibody production.	Induces immunosuppression for organ transplantation, treats acute transplant rejection
Rituximab	Binds to CD20 receptor on B cells, which are then killed by ADCC.	Autoimmune disease (RA, SLE, myasthenia gravis), non-Hodgkin lymphoma, chronic lymphocytic leukaemia
Pembrolizumab	Blocks PD-1 receptors on T cells. PD-1 activation by cancer cells provides an immune tolerance to the cancer, blocking PD-1 removes this tolerance.	PD-L1-positive non-small-cell lung cancer

ADCC, Antibody-dependent cell-mediated cytotoxicity; CTLA-4, cytotoxic T-lymphocyte-associated protein 4; PD-1, programmed cell death protein 2; PD-L1, programmed death ligand 1; RA, rheumatoid arthritis; SLE, systemic lupus erythematosus; TNF-α, tumour necrosis factor α.

and their use is specialized. It is useful to understand that they also have specific side-effects. For example, drugs that block tumour necrosis factor (TNF) are widely used and include infliximab, adalimumab (both monoclonal antibodies against TNF) and etanercept (a soluble TNF receptor). However, TNF-blocking drugs can cause the reactivation of TB. Some biologics boost the immune response to cancers, e.g., ipilimumab. Other biologics bypass the immune system entirely and interact with cancer cells directly. For example, trastuzumab (Herceptin) interacts with the human epidermal growth factor receptor 2 on some breast cancer cells.

Due to their cost, many of these drugs are used as second or third line therapy. Some examples of immunological biologic therapy and the targets involved are detailed in Table 13.7. The field of biologics is rapidly expanding and this is by no means a comprehensive list.

ADVANCED IMMUNOTHERAPY

Immunotherapy is the manipulation of the immune response in order to treat or prevent a disease. The use of vaccines to prevent infection by provoking an immune response is an example of immunotherapy. Immunotherapy is increasingly used to provoke an immune response against cancer cells.

On the other hand, immunotherapy is also used to restore tolerance to allergens, such as in insect venom, pollen and food allergies (see Chapter 10: Clinical notes on tolerance). In general, this is performed by exposing the patient to very small doses of antigen by injection or by mouth and slowly increasing the dose.

Immunotherapy is also being researched as a treatment for autoimmunity, for example attempting to restore tolerance to pancreatic islet cell antigen in type I diabetes mellitus.

● Chapter Summary

- Immunization is active or passive: each type of immunization can be used in appropriate settings.
- Vaccination is an important form of active immunization; there are different types of vaccine depending on the pathogen targeted.
- Organ transplantation presents an immunological challenge, which can be mediated by HLA matching and using antirejection therapy (which itself presents problems).
- Antiinflammatory drugs are widely used and have important side-effects. Steroids cause a range of problems, including cushingoid effects.
- Biologics and immunotherapy have an important role in the future of medicine and allow us to target or change aspects of the immune system.

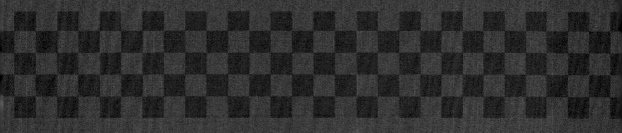

SELF-ASSESSMENT

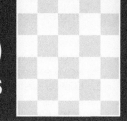

Single best answer (SBA) questions

Chapter 1 Principles of haematology

1. Which of the following is a progenitor cell of the lymphoid lineage?
   A. BFU-E
   B. CFU-Meg
   C. CFU-GEMM.
   D. CFU-Eos
   E. Pre-B cell

2. Which of the following is a mature cell of myeloid lineage origin?
   A. Natural killer (NK) cell
   B. T lymphocyte
   C. Platelet
   D. CFU-Eos
   E. CFU-Meg

3. Which of the following statements most accurately describes the spleen?
   A. The major site of haematopoiesis in adults
   B. The main site of blood filtration
   C. The organ responsible for detoxification of ingested molecules
   D. An organ accounting for ~5% of body weight
   E. The organ responsible for the majority of erythropoietin synthesis

4. Which of the following diseases is not associated with splenomegaly?
   A. Falciparum malaria
   B. Primary myelofibrosis
   C. Thalassaemia major
   D. Portal vein thrombosis
   E. Pernicious anaemia

5. Which of the following is a common cause for generalized lymphadenopathy?
   A. Mumps virus infection
   B. Lyme disease (borreliosis)
   C. Left ventricular failure
   D. Polycythaemia rubra vera
   E. Sickle cell anaemia

6. Which of the following cells does the following description apply to? 'A myeloid lineage cell, derived from the CFU-GM progenitor, which contains granules, has a large reniform nucleus and is ~20 µm in diameter?'
   A. Eosinophil
   B. Neutrophil
   C. Monocyte
   D. Platelet
   E. Erythrocyte

7. Regarding the management of asplenic patients, which of the following interventions is of lowest priority?
   A. Pneumococcal vaccination
   B. Annual influenza vaccinations
   C. Haemophilus influenza vaccination
   D. Testing for cytomegalovirus and Epstein-Barr Virus status
   E. Prophylactic daily oral antibiotics

8. Which of the following growth factors stimulates CFU-Meg and megakaryocytes?
   A. Interleukin 1
   B. Erythropoietin
   C. Granulocyte-colony stimulating factor
   D. Thrombopoietin
   E. Interleukin 6

9. Which of the following would be appropriate in the clinical management of a severely neutropenic 18-year-old?
   A. Erythropoietin
   B. Thrombopoietin
   C. Interferon
   D. Granulocyte-colony stimulating factor
   E. Pegylated interferon

10. A 35-year-old patient with end-stage renal failure (awaiting renal transplant) complains to his nephrologist of breathlessness and palpitations on exertion. He is noted to be very pale. His lung function is normal. The nephrologist feels a regular subcutaneous injection of a synthetic growth factor would be appropriate. Which of the following is appropriate?
    A. Thrombopoietin
    B. Erythropoietin
    C. Granulocyte-colony stimulating factor
    D. Levemir
    E. Fragmin

Chapter 2 Red Blood cells and haemoglobin

1. Regarding red cell structure, which of the following options describes the structure most accurately?
   A. Highly variable 3D structure
   B. A biconcave discoid

C. Irregularly polygonal
D. Nearly spherical
E. Elliptical (stretched ovoid)

2. Regarding physiological iron levels, which of the following statements is most accurate?
   A. All iron intake accumulates over the lifespan of a person since there is no mechanism for iron to leave the body.
   B. The primary regulation mechanism for iron excretion is via variable blood loss, since 1 mL blood contains 0.5 mg iron.
   C. Hepcidin, via downregulation of the iron exporter, represents the main regulation mechanism, affection iron absorption.
   D. Most absorbed iron is removed from the body by fecal elimination.
   E. Iron elimination is mediated by albumin binding, then hepatic conjugation to glucuronide and finally biliary secretion.

3. Regarding the mature red cell metabolism, which of the following pathways contributes most to adenosine triphosphate (ATP) generation?
   A. The tricarboxylic acid (TCA) cycle
   B. Oxidative phosphorylation
   C. Glycolysis
   D. The pentose phosphate pathway
   E. Fatty acid oxidation

4. A 35-year-old patient is having elective complex hand surgery under regional anaesthesia. Using anatomical landmarks, the anaesthetist infiltrates a large volume of prilocaine. Ultimately, the operation proceeds under general anaesthesia, as adequate numbness to the operating zone cannot be achieved. Shortly after induction, the patient becomes a deep cyanosed blue and the pulse oximetry oxygen saturation falls to 85% despite an inspired oxygen of 100%. Surprisingly, her heart rate, blood pressure and end-tidal CO_2 are unaffected. Which of the following is most likely to be the cause of the cyanosis?
   A. An elevated proportion of haemoglobin with oxidized (ferric) iron
   B. Anaphylaxis to local anaesthetic infiltration
   C. Hypoxia secondary to massive pulmonary embolism
   D. Hypoxia secondary to tension pneumothorax
   E. Hypoxia secondary to pulmonary aspiration

5. Which of the following sequences correctly describes part of haem metabolism?
   A. Separation into protoporphyrin and iron components, protoporphyrin conjugation to bilirubin
   B. Protoporphyrin conversion to bilirubin, bilirubin conjugation to acetyl groups

C. Conjugated bilirubin is secreted (in bile) into the gastrointestinal (GI) lumen, conversion to urobilinogen
D. Urobilinogen reabsorption from the GI lumen, intravascular metabolism to stercobilinogen
E. Bilirubin conversion (in hepatocytes) to urobilinogen for renal excretion

6. In which of the following scenarios would the patient be most likely to suffer from inadequate erythropoietin production?
   A. Iron deficiency anaemia
   B. End-stage renal failure awaiting transplant
   C. Chronic haemolytic anaemia
   D. Athlete following 2 months training at altitude
   E. Patient with metastatic renal cell carcinoma

7. Regarding the oxygen dissociation curve, which of the following options is accurate?
   A. A left shift in the curve describes a decrease in the affinity of haemoglobin (Hb) for oxygen.
   B. The presence of elevated levels of methaemoglobin shifts the curve towards the right.
   C. Under conditions of high pCO2, low pH and high [2,3-DPG], the dissociation curve shifts to the left.
   D. A right shift means that a particular % of Hb oxygen saturation, e.g. 50%, will occur at a higher pO2 value.
   E. Fetal Hb has a dissociation curve positioned to the right of that of adult Hb.

8. Which of the following diseases is least likely to carry a risk of iron overload?
   A. Thalassaemia
   B. Sickle cell anaemia
   C. B12 deficiency
   D. Haemochromatosis
   E. Prolonged oral iron ingestion

Chapter 3 Red blood cell disorders

1. In pyruvate kinase deficiency, what is the best description of the biochemical disturbance in the red cell?
   A. Increased susceptibility to oxidative stress due to inadequate availability of glutathione
   B. Increased structural fragility due to insufficient adenosine triphosphate (ATP) generation due to failure of glycolysis
   C. Abnormal precipitation of oxidized, denatured haemoglobin intracellularly
   D. Abnormal tetramerization of spectrin dimers resulting in abnormal structure and reduced integrity

E. Loss of normal membranal expression of phosphatidylinositol glycan protein A (PIG-A) leading to complement-mediated lysis

2. In clinical features associated with glucose-6-phosphate dehydrogenase (G6PD) deficiency, which of the following is true?
   A. Chronic background haemolysis results in a mild but permanent normocytic anaemia.
   B. Haemolysis is primarily extravascular; the spleen and reticuloendothelial system remove red cells prematurely.
   C. In the African subtype, sufferers must avoid eating fava beans as this provokes haemolysis.
   D. Insufficient glutathione regeneration occurs due to failure of the pentose phosphate pathway.
   E. If this diagnosis is suspected, a sample drawn during active haemolysis is of greatest diagnostic use.

3. Which diagnosis best accounts for the following findings? A 6-month-old baby with Portuguese parents presents with failure to thrive and is found to have: Hb 35 g/L, MCV 62 fL; and electrophoresis showed HbF to be predominant and HbA to be absent.
   A. Beta thalassaemia minor (trait)
   B. Alpha thalassaemia major (no alpha globin genes)
   C. Haemoglobin H disease (one alpha globin chain)
   D. Beta thalassaemia major (two abnormal beta genes)
   E. Sickle cell anaemia (two sickle variant beta genes)

4. Which of the following is more likely to be associated with iron than vitamin B12 deficiency?
   A. Peripheral paraesthesia and numbness
   B. Subacute combined degeneration of the cord
   C. Angular stomatitis and glossitis
   D. Megaloblastic anaemia
   E. Diffuse hair loss and koilonychia

5. In B12 deficiency, what is the correct statement regarding the effect on folate metabolism?
   A. B12 deficiency impairs folate absorption leading to secondary deficiency
   B. B12 deficiency impairs tetrahydrofolate regeneration from methylfolate
   C. B12 and folate deficiency symptoms are identical
   D. B12 deficiency is less potentially dangerous than folate deficiency
   E. B12 promotes folate absorption, so deficiency of B12 leads to folate deficiency

6. Which of the following statements best describes a megaloblastic anaemia?
   A. A reduced haemoglobin (Hb), accompanied by a raised mean cell volume (MCV) and mean cell haemoglobin (MCH)
   B. A raised MCV, low Hb and megaloblasts visible on blood film
   C. A normal MCV, raised Hb and red cell count, erythropoietin (EPO) elevated
   D. Low Hb, raised MCV, megaloblasts seen on bone marrow examination
   E. A reduced Hb and MCV, basophilic stippling of red cells

7. Which of the following sets of investigation results is consistent with iron deficiency?
   A. Haemoglobin (Hb) 85 g/L, mean cell volume (MCV) 50 fL, total iron binding capacity (TIBC) 70 µmol, ferritin 280 µmol, transferrin 2.8 g/L
   B. Hb 75 g/L, MCV 110 fL, bone marrow iron stores increased, TIBC 80 µmol, transferrin 3.0 g/L, ferritin 350 µmol
   C. Hb 100 g/L, MCV 115 fL, TIBC 55 µmol, transferrin 2.9 g/L, red cell folate: low
   D. Hb 90 g/L, MCV 69 fL, TIBC 95 µmol, transferrin 5.5 g/dL HI, ferritin 5 µmol
   E. Hb 140 g/L, MCV 82 fL, TIBC 50 µmol, transferrin 3 g/dL, ferritin 300 µmol, red cell folate: normal

8. A 22-year-old patient complains of fatigue. On investigation, she has a macrocytic, megaloblastic anaemia, haemoglobin of 9.5 g/dL and both low serum folate and low red cell folate. She is adamant she cannot be iron or folate deficient since as a vegan she eats so many dark leafy green vegetables. Which of the following options represents the best treatment strategy?
   A. B12 by intramuscular injection, oral folate supplements
   B. Iron supplementation for at least 4 months
   C. Oral B12 supplementation
   D. Oral folate supplementation
   E. Two units red cell transfusion

Chapter 4 White blood cells

1. Which myeloid lineage leucocyte is the macrophage precursor?
   A. Lymphocyte
   B. Neutrophil
   C. Basophil
   D. Monocyte
   E. Eosinophil

2. Which of the following conditions is most likely to be associated with lymphopenia?
   A. Ancylostoma (hookworm) infection
   B. Human immunodeficiency virus (HIV) infection

C. Epstein–Barr virus infection
D. Acute lymphoblastic leukaemia (ALL)
E. Toxoplasmosis

3. Which of the following neutrophil precursors is most likely to be present in the peripheral blood in 'left shift'?
A. Band cell
B. Metamyelocyte
C. Promyelocyte
D. Myelocyte
E. Myeloblast

4. A 35-year-old female patient with rheumatoid arthritis and significant hepatosplenomegaly due to amyloidosis is being treated for septic shock on ITU with vancomycin for a suspected methicillin-resistant *Staphylococcus aureus* infection of a recent total hip replacement. Her latest full blood count indicates that she is profoundly neutropenic. Which of the factors revealed by this history is most likely to be responsible for her neutropenia?
A. Recent surgery
B. Vancomycin treatment
C. Hypersplenism
D. Rheumatoid arthritis
E. Severe infection

Chapter 5 Haematological malignancies

1. Which of the following statements most accurately describes the myelodysplastic syndromes?
A. A clonal proliferation of abnormal plasma cells in bone marrow and blood.
B. Accumulation of abnormal lymphoid cells in nodal and extranodal tissues.
C. Replacement of normal marrow with dysplastic haemopoietic precursors.
D. Neoplastic proliferation of a myeloid precursor resulting in hypercellular marrow.
E. Accumulation of abnormal neoplastic white cells in bone marrow.

2. A 6-year-old boy with trisomy 21 presents with fever and recurrent infections. His mother states that he has been extremely tired recently, becoming breathless on minor exertion. On examination he is pale and has numerous bruises and palpable hepatosplenomegaly. Investigation results are shown below:
Full blood count (FBC): Haemoglobin 8.5 g/dL, platelets 35 × 109/L, white cell count (WCC) 25.0 × 10^9/L
Bone marrow biopsy: Hypercellular, with large numbers of lymphoblast cells seen

Cytogenetics: MLL gene rearrangement
What is the most likely diagnosis?
A. Nonaccidental injury
B. Acute lymphoblastic leukaemia
C. Chronic myeloid leukaemia
D. Primary myelofibrosis
E. Non-Hodgkin lymphoma

3. A 35-year-old patient with known acute myeloid leukaemia (AML) who has recently completed consolidation chemotherapy presents with a fever. He is acutely confused and is sweating profusely. Clinical findings are:
Blood pressure   65/20 mm Hg
Heart rate   140, sinus rhythm
Respiratory rate   30/min
Temperature   38.2°C
Blood gas:
pH   7.15
pO_2 8.0 kPa
pCO_2 2.5 kPa
Lactate   6.5 mM
Investigations:
Haemoglobin   6.5 g/Dl
Platelets   23 × 10^9/L
White cell count   0.5 × 10^9/L
Neutrophils   0.05 × 10^9/L
Uric acid   300 µmol (normal range 180–420 µmol/L)

Of the following actions, which is the first priority in managing this patient?
A. Perform urgent red cell transfusion
B. Administer granulocyte-colony stimulating factor (G-CSF) and discuss with haematology
C. Administer intravenous (IV) crystalloid and broad-spectrum antibiotics
D. Administer allopurinol and rasburicase
E. Arrange urgent plasmapheresis

4. A 25-year-old man presents with night sweats, fever and weight loss of 15 kg over the last 6 months. On examination, he has widespread, painless, nontender lymphadenopathy and moderate splenomegaly. Lymphoma is suspected, and a superficial lymph node is biopsied. Which of the historical features below would provide the best chance of discriminating between Hodgkin lymphoma (HL) and non-Hodgkin lymphoma (NHL) while waiting for the biopsy result?
A. Past Epstein–Barr virus (EBV) infection
B. Complaint of fever, weight loss and night sweats
C. Known immunodeficiency
D. A complaint of severe itching
E. The patient's age

5. A 75-year-old female patient presents acutely with back pain and lower limb neurological symptoms. She reports recurrent chest infections, fatigue, weight loss, polydipsia and polyuria, but she attributed this to a recent diagnosis of depression. On examination she is pale and has widespread petechiae. Findings are as follows:
Full blood count: Haemoglobin 9.5g / dL, platelets 50×10^9/L, white cell count 1.9×10^9/L
Erythrocyte sedimentation rate: Raised
Film: Rouleaux present
Serum electrophoresis: Prominent monoclonal immunoglobulin noted
Corrected calcium: 3.5 mM
Urine dip: +++ protein
Lumbar spine X-ray: Multiple vertebral body collapse fractures
Skeletal survey: Multiple healed fractures and lytic lesions
Bone marrow: 30% clonal plasma cells
What is the most likely diagnosis?
   A. Monoclonal gammopathy of uncertain significance (MGUS)
   B. Acute myeloid leukaemia
   C. Chronic myeloid leukaemia
   D. Multiple myeloma
   E. Solitary plasmacytoma

6. A patient complains of nausea, vomiting, muscle cramps and widespread severe joint pains. He is 24 hours post commencement of R-CHOP chemotherapy for a high-grade non-Hodgkin lymphoma, and the haematologist supervising his treatment informs you he had a particularly high neoplastic burden. His electrocardiogram (EKG) shows tall, peaked T waves and flattening of the P wave. Which of the biochemical findings correspond to the likely diagnosis?
   A. K+ 3.5 mM, Ca++ 1.9 mM, PO42-0.5 mM, uric acid 800 µmol/L
   B. K+ 7.2 mM, Ca++ 1.2 mM, PO42-4.5 mM, uric acid 1500 µmol/L
   C. K+ 5.0 mM, Ca++ 3.5 mM, PO42-1.2 mM, uric acid 220 µmol/L
   D. K+ 6.5 mM, Ca++ 1.9 mM, PO42-3.5 mM, uric acid 250 µmol/L
   E. K+ 4.5 mM, Ca++ 2.7 mM, PO42-3.5 mM, uric acid 1500 µmol/L

Chapter 6 Haemostasis

1. Which of the following statements most accurately describe the sequence of events in primary haemostasis?
   A. Vasoconstriction, adhesion, aggregation, release reaction, fibrin deposition
   B. Vasoconstriction, transient tethering, release reaction, adhesion, aggregation

   C. Transient tethering, release reaction, vasoconstriction, adhesion, aggregation
   D. Adhesion, release reaction, transient tethering, aggregation, vasoconstriction
   E. Release reaction, transient tethering, vasoconstriction, adhesion, aggregation

2. Which of the following statements most accurately describes a stage in the extrinsic pathway?
   A. FXa unites with FVa and calcium ions to form prothrombinase
   B. Exposed subendothelial tissue factor binds to circulating FVII
   C. FXII is activated by the surface membrane of an activated platelet
   D. FVIIIa and FIXa unite with calcium ions to form 'tenase'
   E. FXIII is activated by thrombin to covalently cross-link fibrin polymers

3. Which of the following statements most accurately summarizes the common pathway?
   A. Products derived from intrinsic and extrinsic pathways integrate via the common pathway which culminates in generation of thrombin
   B. It is activated by exposure to procoagulants such as subendothelial tissue factor
   C. Vasoconstriction, transient tethering, release reaction, adhesion, aggregation
   D. It commences with activation of factor XII by an activated platelet and ultimately generated activated factor X.
   E. Tissue plasminogen activator binds to fibrin-bound plasminogen, forming plasmin which degrades fibrin.

4. A 15-year-old patient with easy bruising presents to his general practitioner. He wonders if he has inherited a bleeding disorder from his mother's side of the family, but unhelpfully cannot remember the name of the disorder. His mother bruises easily and is largely asymptomatic, but has had bleeding complications whenever she has needed surgery and suffers from frequent nosebleeds. Which of the options below gives the most likely diagnosis?
   A. Protein S deficiency
   B. Protein C deficiency
   C. Antithrombin deficiency
   D. Factor V Leiden
   E. Von Willebrand disease (vWD)

5. A 70-year-old gentleman presents to his general practitioner with widespread bruising. His platelet count, which has always been normal, has fallen to 10×10^9/L. All other investigation findings are normal. He had recently had a medication review,

where several new drugs were started. Which of the following is the most likely culprit?

A. Candesartan
B. Paracetamol
C. Codeine
D. Quinine
E. AdCal (a combined calcium and vitamin D supplement)

6. A 45-year-old black female presents to the Emergency Department with a right hemiplegia, aphasia and a low-grade fever (37.9°C). On examination by the haematology registrar, she is jaundiced, with widespread bruising and petechiae. Surprisingly, her neurologic symptoms have now disappeared. The correct diagnosis is made and she recovers with supportive treatment and plasmapheresis. Investigations are as follows:

Na	137 mM/L
K	5.5 mM/L
Creatinine	150 µm/L
Urea	15 mM/L
C-reactive protein	15 mg/L
Haemoglobin (Hb)	8.5 g/dL
Platelet (Plt)	35×10^9/L
White blood cell count (WCC)	9.0×10^9/L
Bilirubin	230 µm/L
Lactate dehydrogenase (LDH)	500 U/L
Prothrombin time (PT)	13 seconds
Activated partial thromboplastin time (APTT)	35 seconds
Fibrinogen	3.0 g/L
Blood film	microangiopathic haemolysis

Which of the following diagnoses accounts for this clinical presentation?

A. Haemolytic uraemic syndrome (HUS)
B. Disseminated intravascular coagulation (DIC)
C. Transient ischaemic attack (TIA)
D. Thrombotic thrombocytopenic purpura (TTP)
E. Immune thrombocytopenic purpura (ITP)

7. An 85-year-old lady is found by her daughter lying on the bathroom floor. She explains she had tripped up 2 hours earlier on the bathroom mat and couldn't get herself back up. Her left leg is externally rotated and foreshortened. She has numerous extensive subcutaneous haematomas and is pale. She takes warfarin for atrial fibrillation. Admission bloods reveal:

Haemoglobin	9.0 g/dL
Mean corpuscular volume (MCV)	82 Fl
Platelets	425×10^9
White cell count	13.0×10^9
International normalized ratio (INR)	6.0
Activated partial thromboplastin time	36 seconds
Fibrinogen	6.5 g/dL

The orthopaedic registrar diagnoses a fractured neck of femur and lists her for an arthroplasty on the afternoon trauma list. However, he would like her INR to be normalized before surgery (2 hours from now). What would be the best treatment to normalize her clotting parameters in this emergency timeframe?

A. Fresh frozen plasma
B. Intravenous vitamin K
C. Prothrombin complex concentrate (PCC)
D. Recombinant factor VIII
E. Cryoprecipitate

Chapter 7 Transfusion products

1. A 75-year-old man is receiving his third unit of red cells following a revision of his total hip replacement. He complains of breathlessness and chest pain. His heart rate is 110 beats per minute, blood pressure is 155/95 mmHg, respiratory rate is 35 breaths per minute and oxygen saturation is 88% on air. What is the first priority in managing this acute transfusion reaction?

A. Help him to sit up and administer 20 mg of intravenous (IV) frusemide
B. Stop the transfusion and clinically assess the patient
C. Administer intramuscular (IM) adrenaline, 500 µg and elevate his legs
D. Provide reassurance and administer IV paracetamol
E. Take blood cultures and administer urgent IV antibiotics

2. Which of the following descriptions most accurately explains the mechanism underlying an ABO incompatibility reaction?

A. IgG binds to A or B antigens, causing delayed intravascular haemolysis
B. IgM binds to red cell H antigen, causing extravascular haemolysis
C. IgM and complement-mediated acute intravascular haemolysis
D. IgG binds to the red cell H antigen, causing acute intravascular haemolysis
E. IgM and cell-mediated delayed extravascular haemolysis

3. Which of the following blood products is stored at 2–6°C in a saline, adenine, glucose and mannitol solution with a shelf life of 35 days?
   A. Platelets
   B. Clotting factor concentrates
   C. Red cells
   D. Fresh frozen plasma (FFP)
   E. Immunoglobulin

4. Which of the following would represent an additional (i.e., not one of the standard screening investigations) investigation if performed on a blood donation samples?
   A. Human immunodeficiency virus antibodies
   B. Hepatitis C nucleic acid
   C. Human T-lymphotropic virus II antibodies
   D. Hepatitis B core antibody
   E. Hepatitis B surface antigen

5. Regarding ABO compatibility, which of the following transfusions is ABO incompatible and would place the recipient at risk of a haemolytic transfusion reaction?
   A. Red cells: Donor blood group A → recipient blood group AB
   B. Fresh froze plasma (FFP): Donor group AB → recipient blood group O
   C. Platelets: Donor blood group O → recipient blood group O
   D. FFP: Donor group O → recipient group A
   E. Red cells: Donor blood group O → recipient blood group B

6. Which of the following patients are appropriately indicated for a platelet transfusion?
   A. Patient with platelet count 35 awaiting a potentially life-saving laparotomy
   B. Patient with platelet count 110 and ongoing haemorrhage
   C. Patient with platelet count 45 and acute liver failure, no active bleeding
   D. Patient with platelet count 15 during induction chemotherapy, no active bleeding
   E. Patient with platelet count 50 and a resolved gastrointestinal bleed

7. Which of the following is a delayed and usually fatal transfusion reaction defined by lymphocyte implantation in the transfusion recipient?
   A. Posttransfusion purpura
   B. IgM mediated haemolytic reaction
   C. Transfusion-associated graft-versus-host disease (TA-GVHD)
   D. Chronic hepatitis C infection
   E. Transfusion-related lung injury

8. Regarding eligibility for blood donation, which of the following candidates would be permanently ineligible?
   A. A patient who has had unprotected sex with a partner recently immigrated from Uganda, she has no further plans to see him again
   B. A 48-year-old dancer who once worked as a male prostitute
   C. A 22-year-old builder with multiple tattoos and piercings
   D. A 35-year-old lady with a haemoglobin [Hb] of 120 g/dL caused by iron deficiency
   E. A 40-year-old lady weighing 48 kg after a recent bout of gastroenteritis

9. A 6-year-old girl is brought in by ambulance following a road traffic accident. She has a ruptured spleen and haemorrhage is ongoing. She is drowsy, clammy, pale and peripherally cool with prolonged capillary refill time, hypotension and tachycardia. Type O negative blood is prepared and transfusion about to commence when her parents arrive and adamantly refuse to let it go ahead, since they are devout Jehovah's witnesses. Despite clear and frank explanation of the life-threatening consequences of withholding the transfusion by the Emergency Department consultant, the parents will not consent to the transfusion and produce an advanced directive signed by the child. What is the legally and ethically appropriate course of action?
   A. Abandon transfusion, attempt to maintain blood pressure with intravenous crystalloid
   B. Attempt to source a cell salvager for recovery of blood during the child's laparotomy
   C. Seek a court order and proceed with the transfusion in best interests in the interim period awaiting the court order
   D. Continue to attempt to persuade the parents to give their consent, recruiting additional colleagues if necessary
   E. Accept that the decision to refuse transfusion was made by the child herself and respect her wishes

10. Which of the following is least likely to be associated with massive transfusion?
   A. Hypothermia
   B. Hyperkalaemia
   C. Hypercalcaemia
   D. Dilutional coagulopathy
   E. Transfusion-associated circulatory overload

Chapter 9 The innate immune system

1. Concerning the innate immune response, which one of the following is correct?
   A. It is a specific response to a particular antigen.
   B. The response improves with repeated exposure

C. It is composed of phagocytes and complement
D. It is good at combating intracellular pathogens
E. It takes a long time to develop

2. Concerning the adaptive immune system, which one of the following is correct?
   A. It is often the first branch of the immune system to encounter pathogens to which the host has not been exposed before
   B. Each component can target multiple different types of pathogen
   C. It presents antigen to the innate immune system to aid coordination of the immune response
   D. It may respond differently if reexposed to the same pathogen
   E. Acute phase proteins are a molecular component of it

3. A general practitioner starts a patient on ciprofloxacin for a severe urinary tract infection. A few days later the patient develops severe watery diarrhoea and abdominal pain. Which answer best describes the likely cause of these symptoms?
   A. Anaphylaxis caused by an allergy to the antibiotic
   B. Progression of the urinary tract infection to sepsis
   C. Gastric ulceration caused by the antibiotic
   D. Flare up of an inflammatory bowel disease
   E. Disruption of the patient's normal gut flora by the antibiotic, allowing colonization by pathogenic organisms

4. Which one of the following is a phagocyte?
   A. Neutrophil
   B. Basophil
   C. B cell
   D. T cell
   E. The membrane attack complex

5. Which of the following is true of macrophages?
   A. They have shorter lifespan than neutrophils
   B. They are key antigen presenting cells
   C. They express high levels of major histocompatibility complex (MHC) class I molecules
   D. They are smaller than neutrophils
   E. They develop into dendritic cells in epithelia

6. A patient presents with a perianal abscess. Pus is drained; which one of the following types of cells are the major constituents in pus?
   A. Plasma cells
   B. Macrophages
   C. Mast cells
   D. Eosinophils
   E. Neutrophils

7. A patient presents with a cold sore and you diagnose Herpes simplex infection. Which innate immune cell is primarily involved in the killing of Herpes infected body cells?
   A. Neutrophils
   B. Natural killer cells
   C. Macrophages
   D. Basophils
   E. Mast cells

8. The protein and fat catabolism seen in infection is directly mediated by what?
   A. Acute phase proteins
   B. Bacterial antigens
   C. Immunoglobulins
   D. Cytokines
   E. Complement proteins

9. A patient presents with temporal tenderness and jaw claudication, you suspect giant cell arteritis (GCA). Which acute phase response would most support your suspicion?
   A. Raised white cell count
   B. Raised fibrinogen
   C. Raised C-reactive protein (CRP)
   D. Raised erythrocyte sedimentation rate (ESR)
   E. Raised complement levels

10. The classical pathway of the complement system is started by which process?
    A. Microbial surfaces, along with factor B and D, activate C3
    B. Antigen is presented by dendritic cells
    C. Mannan-binding lectin binds to some encapsulated bacteria
    D. Antigen-antibody complexes activate C1
    E. Class I major histocompatibility complex present intracellular antigen

11. The membrane attack complex (MAC) mediates its actions on pathogens by which one of the following mechanisms?
    A. Phagocytosis
    B. Opsonization
    C. Osmotic lysis
    D. Apoptosis
    E. Degranulation

12. A patient presents with a chronic cough. Full blood count shows a raised eosinophil count. Which of the following is the likely diagnosis?
    A. Bacterial infection
    B. Chronic obstructive pulmonary disease (COPD)
    C. Asthma
    D. Parasitic worm infection
    E. Hodgkin disease

Chapter 10 The adaptive immune system

1. Which **one** of the following statements about major histocompatibility complex (MHC) is true?
   A. MHC class II molecules present endogenous antigens.
   B. The haplotype is found on chromosome 6.
   C. CD4 positive T cells bind MHC class I molecules.
   D. MHC class I molecules are only present on antigen-presenting cells.
   E. MHC class I molecules present peptides that are usually longer than MHC class II.

2. What is the name of the process whereby a B cell can produce different types of immunoglobulin with the same specificity?
   A. Junctional diversity
   B. Somatic hypermutation
   C. Affinity maturation
   D. Positive selection
   E. Class switching

3. Which one of the following is **not** a member of the immunoglobulin superfamily?
   A. T cell receptor
   B. CD4
   C. Major histocompatibility complex (MHC)
   D. Immunoglobulin E (IgE)
   E. Toll-like receptor-4 (TLR-4)

4. Regarding B cell activation, which **one** of the following statements is correct?
   A. B cells are activated in the follicles of primary lymphoid organs.
   B. The expression of bcl-2 results in apoptosis.
   C. Somatic hypermutation of immunoglobulin genes occurs in the germinal centres.
   D. B cells are activated following the presentation of antigen by neutrophils.
   E. B cells are able to be activated and produce antibody without help from T cells.

5. Which antibody is important in the antiparasitic response?
   A. Immunoglobulin G (IgG)
   B. IgD
   C. IgM
   D. IgE
   E. IgA

6. Which of the following statements about T cells is correct?
   A. T cells are major histocompatibility complex (MHC)-restricted while developing in the bone marrow.
   B. Th1 cells are involved in the response to intracellular pathogens more than T helper (Th) 2 cells.
   C. Cytotoxic T cells express CD4.
   D. Apoptosis is induced in T cells that bind to self-MHC.
   E. Positive selection occurs in developing T cells that have a high affinity for self-antigens.

7. A healthy man has eaten peanuts his whole life without any ill effects. Epithelial cells in his gut secrete transforming growth factor-β (TGF-β). What best describes the effect of TGF-β in this situation?
   A. Any T cells that react to the peanut antigen are transformed into Tregs specific to the peanut antigen.
   B. Local T helper (Th) 2 cells are recruited and begin secreting IL-4 and IL-10, mounting an allergic response to the peanut antigen.
   C. Peptides in the peanut cross-react with peptides on pathogens and an immune response is triggered.
   D. Macrophages are recruited, these process and present the antigen to T cells.
   E. MHC expression is upregulated on neighbouring epithelial cells.

8. One winter, a 44-year-old surgeon develops a fever, muscle pain, sore throat and vomiting. She self – diagnoses influenza and immediately regrets not having the flu vaccine. After 4 days in bed, she gradually improves. Which of the following is correct?
   A. The reason that she has flu this winter is that she has never encountered the flu virus previously.
   B. She clears the flu virus by secreting large quantities of antibody against it.
   C. Natural killer and CD8+ cytotoxic T cells of the innate and adaptive immune system are responsible for clearing the flu virus.
   D. Her symptoms are caused by the secretion of transforming growth factor-β (TGF-β).
   E. Neutrophils and T helper (Th)17 T cells are required to kill the flu virus.

9. A 25-year-old woman is found unconscious and is taken to the Emergency Department. She is pale and sweaty. She is also found to have a diffuse macular rash. She has a blood pressure of 75/38 and a heart rate of 132. After initial resuscitation, a diagnosis of toxic shock syndrome (TSS) is made. Which of the following is capable of causing TSS?
   A. *Streptococcus pneumoniae*
   B. *Clostridium* enterotoxin
   C. Cholera toxin
   D. Staphylococcal enterotoxin
   E. *Escherichia coli*

Chapter 11 The functioning immune system

1. A child grazes their arm in a park. Shortly after, the graze appears red and swollen and it is painful to touch. Which one of the following processes is occurring within a few hours of the child's injury?
   A. Fibroblasts migrate and lay down new collagen
   B. Decreased vascular permeability.
   C. Homing due to integrin molecules.
   D. Leucocytes leave the tissues.
   E. Release of interferon-γ (IFN-γ)

2. Which of the following is the reason that autoimmune diseases result in chronic inflammation?
   A. Genetic predisposition
   B. Persistence of antigen
   C. Granuloma formation
   D. Prolonged increase in tumour necrosis factor-α (TNF-α)
   E. Inadequate immune response

3. A 56-year-old male presents with a 3-week history of dry cough and weight loss after returning from visiting his family in India. He is treated for suspected tuberculosis infection. Which of the following statements best describes how the immune system manages primary *M. tuberculosis* infection in the lungs?
   A. T helper 2 (Th2) cells release IL-4, activating B cells.
   B. Neutrophils can phagocytose the pathogen directly.
   C. Delayed type hypersensitivity response; the pathogen is surrounded by granulation tissue.
   D. Antibodies can neutralize the pathogen directly, as well as act as an opsonin against infected cells.
   E. CD4 positive T cells are able to destroy infected cells.

4. A 38-year-old female health care worker goes to her general practitioner for her annual flu vaccine. Which of the following correctly describes how her immune system would respond if she later encounters the seasonal flu virus?
   A. Antibodies can neutralize the pathogen directly, as well as act as an opsonin against infected cells.
   B. Interferon gamma (IFN-γ) acts on neighbouring cells by inhibiting transcription and translation of the pathogen.
   C. Neutrophils phagocytose the pathogen directly.
   D. CD4 positive T cells are able to destroy infected cells.
   E. Macrophages fuse to form multinucleate giant cells around the pathogen, creating a granuloma.

5. A young child develops a widespread, itchy rash. Over the first few days the rash develops vesicles, which then rupture. The child has a low-grade fever and feels unwell. Some other children at nursery had the same symptoms. The rash resolves by itself in 2 weeks. Considering the most likely causative organism, how does this pathogen evade the immune system?
   A. Antigenic shift and drift
   B. Polymorphism
   C. Infection of lymphocytes
   D. Becoming latent in neurons
   E. Modulation of major histocompatibility complex expression

6. Which one of the following components of the immune system can prevent bacterial pathogens present at a mucosal surface from entering the body?
   A. Lysozyme
   B. C3b
   C. Neutrophils
   D. Dendritic cells
   E. Secretory immunoglobulin A (sIgA)

7. Which of the following is the hepatitis B virus (HBV) serology result that implies that the patient has previously cleared the virus without vaccination?

   HBsAg, HBV surface antigen; anti-HBc, HBV core antibody; anti-HBs, HBV surface antibody.

	HBsAg	Anti-HBc	Anti-HBs
A	+ve	+ve	+ve
B	−ve	−ve	−ve
C	+ve	−ve	−ve
D	−ve	+ve	+ve
E	−ve	−ve	+ve

8. A 24-year-old medical student presents to his general practitioner (GP) with a 2-week history of headaches and a swinging fever following his medical elective in Colombia. He has no other past medical history and has not been taking any medication recently, despite his GP's advice considering where he was travelling. Which of the following statements is true for the likely causative organism?
   A. The pathogen tends to cause extracellular infections.
   B. The pathogen has a complex lifecycle, which presents the immune system with a variety of challenges.

C. The pathogen causes significant damage selectively to CD4 +ve T cells, reducing the effectiveness of the adaptive immune system.
D. Infections with this pathogen are normally self-limiting.
E. The pathogen is pyogenic.

9. Which white blood cell count differential result would you expect to see in a parasitic worm infection?
   A. Raised neutrophils
   B. Raised eosinophils
   C. Raised lymphocytes
   D. Raise in all cells
   E. No raise in any parameter

Chapter 12 Immune dysfunction

1. Which type of immune dysfunction is characterized, in immunological terms, by IgE-mediated degranulation of mast cells?
   A. Nickel hypersensitivity
   B. ABO incompatibility
   C. Allergic rhinitis
   D. Farmer's lung
   E. Rheumatoid arthritis

2. A young patient is referred to an immunologist after an episode of anaphylaxis at a restaurant. What investigation is the immunologist likely to carry out?
   A. Skin prick testing
   B. Anti-double stranded DNA antibody assay
   C. Rheumatoid factor assay
   D. Patch testing
   E. C-reactive protein measurement

3. Which of the following conditions is caused by the deposition of antibody–antigen complexes in tissues?
   A. Eczema
   B. Farmer's lung
   C. Asthma
   D. Haemolytic disease of the newborn
   E. Nickel hypersensitivity

4. Type IV hypersensitivity is mainly mediated by which cells?
   A. Neutrophils
   B. Plasma cells
   C. CD8 positive T cells
   D. Mast cells
   E. T helper cells

5. A 21-year-old man is brought to Accident and Emergency suffering from breathing problems that he developed after eating a sandwich in a local bakery. He has an audible stridor, is warm to the touch and has obvious facial oedema. Which of the following is the most appropriate next step in his management?
   A. Intravenous fluid challenge
   B. Chlorphenamine IV
   C. Hydrocortisone V
   D. Intramuscular adrenaline (0.5 mL of 1:1000)
   E. C1 inhibitor IV

6. A 42-year-old woman presents to her general practitioner (GP) with a persistent and general weakness in her arms. When the GP asks the patient to gaze upwards, the patient's eyelids droop after a short period. The patient is found to have anti-acetylcholine receptor antibodies in her serum. What is the likely diagnosis?
   A. Coeliac disease
   B. Graves disease
   C. Multiple sclerosis
   D. Myasthenia gravis
   E. Goodpasture syndrome

7. A 23-year-old patient presents to their general practitioner with a 3-week history of intermittent diarrhoea and fatigue. The patient appears pale. The patient is found to have anti-tissue transglutaminase antibodies in their serum. What is the likely diagnosis?
   A. Rheumatoid arthritis
   B. Type I diabetes
   C. Crohn disease
   D. Pernicious anaemia
   E. Coeliac disease

8. A 38-year-old lady presents to her general practitioner with a longstanding history of worsening pain and stiffness in the first and second metacarpophalangeal joints (MCPJs) of both of her hands, worst in the morning. An X-ray radiograph of her hands shows a loss of joint space, bony erosions and subluxation of the affected joints. There is a family history of rheumatoid arthritis. What serum antibodies would confirm the likely diagnosis?
   A. Anti-double stranded DNA antibodies
   B. Anti-cyclic citrullinated peptide antibodies
   C. Anti-Ro antibodies
   D. Anti-nuclear antibodies
   E. IgE anti-IgA antibodies

9. Which cytokine coordinates neutrophil-based inflammation and stimulates osteoclasts to reabsorb bone in rheumatoid arthritis?
   A. Interleukin-8 (IL-8)
   B. Interleukin-17 (IL-17)
   C. Tumour necrosis factor alpha (TNF-α)
   D. Transforming growth factor beta (TGF-β)
   E. Interferon gamma (IFN-γ)

10. Deficiency in complement function can lead to which of the following autoimmune conditions?
    A. Type I diabetes mellitus
    B. Multiple sclerosis
    C. Systemic lupus erythematosus
    D. Graves disease
    E. Coeliac disease

11. A previously healthy 38-year-old is admitted with a serious chest infection. They take longer than expected to recover and are admitted with similar chest infections multiple times over the subsequent year. Which of the following immunodeficiencies is most likely in this patient?
    A. Acquired immunodeficiency syndrome
    B. Chronic granulomatous disease
    C. DiGeorge syndrome
    D. Wiskott-Aldrich syndrome
    E. Severe combined immunodeficiency disease

12. What type of virus is the human immunodeficiency virus HIV?
    A. A double-stranded DNA virus
    B. A single-stranded DNA virus
    C. A single-stranded RNA retrovirus
    D. A double-stranded DNA retrovirus
    E. A single-stranded RNA virus

13. Which of the following HIV +ve patients would be classified as suffering from AIDS?
    A. A patient with a CD4 count of 250 cells/μL
    B. A patient with a malignant melanoma
    C. A patient with a neutrophil count of 2×10^9 cells/L
    D. A patient with oesophageal candidiasis

Chapter 13 Medical intervention

1. A 28-year-old man presents to Accident and Emergency with an open tibial fracture that he sustained in a road traffic collision. There is dirt and debris in the wound. Since he cannot recall if he has had a full course of tetanus vaccinations, you opt to give him anti-tetanus immunoglobulin. Which of the following best describes how this treatment works?
    A. Clonal expansion of reactive B cells
    B. Vaccination booster
    C. Passive immunity
    D. Active immunity
    E. Initial sensitization

2. Concerning vaccinations, which one of the following statements is correct?
    A. An ideal vaccine should not be immunogenic.
    B. The vaccines against measles, mumps and rubella (MMR) are recombinant vaccines.
    C. Killed vaccines are more expensive than live attenuated vaccines.

D. Live attenuated vaccines produce a good cell-mediated response.
    E. Recombinant vaccines can rarely induce disease, especially in the immunocompromised.

3. Concerning transplant rejection, which of the following is correct?
    A. Hyperacute rejection is caused by T cells.
    B. Acute cellular rejection is primarily mediated by natural killer cells.
    C. Chronic rejection responds well to long-term corticosteroids.
    D. Hyperacute rejection is prevented by human leucocyte antigen-matching the organ donor and recipient.
    E. Acute cellular responses take days to develop.

4. A patient on regular corticosteroid therapy is followed up by their general practitioner. Which of the following would be unlikely to be caused by the corticosteroids?
    A. Abnormal liver function tests
    B. Raised blood pressure
    C. Poor glucose tolerance
    D. Poor wound healing
    E. Repeated infections

5. An 89-year-old lady presents to her general practitioner with knee pain related to her osteoarthritis. She also suffers from hypertension and has no known allergies. She does not suffer from asthma. You prescribe her oral naproxen. Which of the following side-effects of nonsteroidal antiinflammatory drugs (NSAIDs) would most concern you in this patient?
    A. Tinnitus
    B. Headache
    C. Bronchospasm
    D. Gastritis
    E. Rash

6. A 54-year-old woman is brought to Accident and Emergency by ambulance. She is confused, generally unresponsive and pale. Initial observations show she is profoundly hypotensive, tachycardic but apyrexial. Initial blood tests show that she is hyperkalaemic and hyponatraemic. Inflammatory markers are normal. You find a card in her bag that says that she is on long-term steroids. What would your immediate management be?
    A. Administer O_2, blood cultures, intravenous (IV) antibiotics, IV fluid challenge, bloods for full blood count/urea and electrolytes/lactate, measure urine output (sepsis 6).
    B. IV hydrocortisone and IV fluids
    C. Oral antibiotics
    D. Oral prednisolone
    E. IM adrenaline (500 μg)

Extended-matching questions (EMQs)

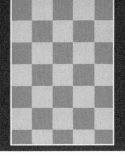

Chapter 1 Principles of haematology

Blood cells

A. Erythrocyte
B. Platelet
C. Macrophage
D. Monocyte
E. Eosinophil
F. Basophil
G. Plasma cell
H. Memory B cell
I. Natural killer cell
J. T cell

For each scenario below, choose the most likely corresponding option from the list given above. Each answer can be used once, more than once or not at all.

1. This cell typically resides in lymph nodes, secretes immunoglobulin and has a diameter of 6–9 μm, nongranular basophilic cytoplasm and a relatively large nucleus:cytoplasm ratio.
2. Of lymphoid lineage, two important subtypes of this cell express CD4 and CD8 glycoproteins at their plasma membranes.
3. This myeloid lineage cell accounts for ≤1% of circulating white blood cells and stains strongly with basic stains.
4. It is derived from the BFU-E progenitor cell, which responds to a growth factor primarily synthesized in the kidney. Gas transport is its primary physiological role.
5. Important for the destruction of multicellular parasitic organisms, the majority of this cell type reside in tissues rather than the bloodstream.
6. The largest type of lymphocyte commonly found in the blood stream, with granular cytoplasm and an important role in innate immunity.
7. An enucleate cell with a prominent role in haemostasis.

Chapter 2 Red Blood cells and haemoglobin

Abnormalities of the blood film

A. Poikilocytosis
B. Echinocytes
C. Howell-Jolly bodies
D. Teardrop cells
E. Target cells
F. Spherocytes
G. Elliptocytes
H. Sickle cells
I. Rouleaux
J. Acanthocytes
K. Anisocytosis
L. Heinz bodies

For each scenario below, choose the most likely corresponding option from the list given above. Each answer can be used once, more than once or not at all.

1. A patient with Child-Pugh C liver disease is admitted to the Intensive Care Unit following a large variceal bleed.
2. A patient with temporal arteritis presents with acute vision loss and throbbing tender temporal pain.
3. A patient has his spleen removed to control haemorrhage following a road traffic accident.
4. A patient with mixed iron and B12 deficiencies has an increased red cell distribution width (RDW) parameter reported on a full blood count.
5. A Greek patient who vigilantly excludes broad beans from his diet experiences an acute fall in his Hb whilst hospitalized. He had an episode of diabetic ketoacidosis, precipitated by the pyelonephritis for which he was admitted. Cotrimoxazole has been effective in reducing his inflammatory markers.

Chapter 3 Red blood cell disorders

Haemolytic anaemia

A. Pyruvate kinase (PK) deficiency
B. Glucose-6-phosphate dehydrogenase (G6PD) deficiency
C. Hereditary spherocytosis
D. Alloimmune haemolysis
E. Paroxysmal nocturnal haemoglobinuria
F. Warm autoimmune haemolytic anaemia
G. Cold autoimmune haemolytic anaemia (AIHA)
H. Drug-induced haemolytic anaemia
I. Microangiopathic haemolytic anaemia (MAHA)
J. Haemoglobin H disease (alpha thalassemia)

For each of the following clinical vignettes and accompanying explanations of the mechanism leading to the haemolytic anaemia, choose the corresponding primary diagnosis from the list above. Each answer can be used once, more than once or not at all.

1. A patient is receiving a blood transfusion for severe anaemia of chronic disease. He becomes extremely

anxious, febrile and hypotensive. Rapid IgM-mediated destruction of the donor red cells, most likely by antibodies specifically against red cell A or B antigen, is occurring intravascularly. The transfusion is stopped and he is transferred to the intensive care unit where he later receives temporary renal replacement therapy for anuric acute kidney injury and cryoprecipitate for disseminated intravascular coagulation (DIC).

2. A 48-year-old Greek patient admitted with a legionella lower respiratory tract infection (LRTI) is noted to be extremely pale several days after admission. His daily full blood count (FBC) shows his Hb has fallen from 130 g/L on admission to 85 g/L. Heinz bodies are found in the blood film. Increased oxidant stress due to the infection has provoked haemolytic anaemia as his red cells were unable to maintain sufficient available glutathione.

3. A 25-year-old lady with hypothyroidism, type 1 diabetes and coeliac disease complains to her general practitioner about cold intolerance. She states her fingers and toes become extremely painful and purple in colour when she is working in the garden. As she has just come in from walking to the surgery without mittens on and the outside temperature is cold, he is able to see for himself. He also notes mild jaundice. A FBC reveals Hb of 95 g/L. She is referred to haematology and an autoimmune haemolytic anaemia, provoked by cold, is diagnosed. Rituximab is effective in treating her symptoms.

4. A patient with severe burns develops disseminated intravascular coagulation. The blood film report highlights schistocytes. Fibrin deposition within the microvasculature is the underlying cause.

5. A patient is started on cefalexin for a streptococcal ear infection. She develops breathlessness and syncope and presents to the emergency department. Haemolytic anaemia is diagnosed. The hapten mechanism, immune complex or autoantibody formation are likely underlying causes of red cell destruction in this patient.

Complications of sickle cell anaemia

A. Acute chest crisis
B. Dactylitis
C. Severe anaemia
D. Septic shock
E. Splenic sequestration crisis
F. Aplastic crisis
G. Haemolytic crisis
H. Increased opiate tolerance
I. Painful infarctive crisis

For each scenario below, choose the most likely corresponding option from the list given above. Each answer can be used once, more than once or not at all.

1. An 8-year-old Senegalese girl is brought from school by the school nurse complaining of extreme pain in her back. She is crying with the pain. Examination is normal. The pain does not respond to paracetamol or ibuprofen and the Senior House Officer in the Emergency Department is reluctant to prescribe opiates to a child with apparently nothing physically wrong. Her parents are contacted and explain that it is known that she has sickle cell anaemia. Under haematology supervision, she receives an exchange transfusion.

2. A 25-year-old man is in recovery following a general anaesthetic for an elective anterior cruciate ligament reconstruction. The nurse is extremely concerned because he has become extremely breathless, complaining of chest pain, coughing and has SpO$_2$ of 91%. A chest X-ray shows diffuse bilateral shadowing. He admits to being homozygous for sickle variant but had concealed this as he feared it might prevent the operation going ahead.

3. An 18-year-old female with known sickle cell anaemia attends the emergency department with her mother. She has suffered from diarrhoea and vomiting for 48 hours. Her mother states that the entire family have had the same thing, but she is the only one so badly affected. On examination she is peripherally cool (CRT 5 s), pale, tachycardic (heart rate 140 beats per minute), tachypnoeic (respiratory rate 30 breaths per minute), drowsy (Glasgow Coma Scale 13) and hypotensive (systolic blood pressure 55 mmHg; diastolic blood pressure unrecordable) despite several IV fluid boluses.

4. A 1-year-old girl is brought in with severe abdominal pain. Her family, recent immigrants from the Ivory Coast, speak no English and cannot provide a history, but they are obviously very worried about her. She is extremely pale with massive splenomegaly palpable in the left iliac fossa and is obviously very unwell. The attending doctor is shocked to discover her Hb is only 30 g/L. She is transfused and resuscitated and, when stable, undergoes a splenectomy.

5. A 14-year-old boy with sickle cell anaemia is brought into the emergency department with bleeding gums and widespread bruising. He is very pale and had been complaining of breathlessness, fatigue and palpitations. He is febrile, but cardiovascularly stable. His FBC reveals pancytopaenia. His mother reports that his little sister, who was adopted and does not have sickle cell anaemia, has recently had a minor illness with runny nose and raised temperature along with a red rash on one cheek that looked as she had been slapped.

Chapter 5 Haematological malignancies
Haematological malignancies

A. Polycythaemia rubra vera
B. Primary myelofibrosis

C. Myelodysplastic syndrome
D. Acute myeloid leukaemia
E. Acute lymphoblastic leukaemia
F. Chronic myeloid leukaemia
G. Chronic lymphocytic leukaemia
H. Multiple myeloma
I. Waldenstrom macroglobulinaemia
J. Hodgkin lymphoma
K. Non-Hodgkin lymphoma

For each patient's presentation, select the most likely underlying malignancy. Each answer can be used once, more than once or not at all.

An 80-year-old man presents with an incidental leucocytosis discovered on a routine preoperative full blood count (white cell count 40). Careful history notes poor appetite and lately some night sweats but nothing else. On examination he has generalised painless lymphadenopathy and palpable splenomegaly. Blood film reveals 'smear cells' and mature lymphocytes.

1. A 50-year-old woman presents to her general practitioner (GP) with fatigue, shortness of breath and palpitations. The GP notes her weight has decreased from 65 kg to 52 kg over the last year. On examination massive splenomegaly is noted. She is therefore referred to haematology for further investigations. The blood film shows nucleated red cell and granulocyte precursors and poikilocytosis, whilst bone marrow aspirate results in a dry tap.

2. An asymptomatic elderly patient is referred to haematology when a routine full blood count indicates anaemia and thrombocytopenia. Bone marrow findings include unilineage dysplasia and ringed sideroblasts.

3. A 30-year-old man presents with 3 months duration of a high cyclical fever. On direct questioning he admits to neck, axillary and groin pain after nights out drinking. On examination he has generalised painless lymphadenopathy and mild. A lymph node biopsy indicates presence of Reed-Sternberg cells.

4. A 45-year-old woman presents with septic shock. She has widespread bruising and her husband reports that she has had a chest infection for 8 weeks despite antibiotics prescribed by the general practitioner. She recovers well in the intensive care unit with broad-spectrum antibiotics, intravenous hydration and vasopressor support. Investigations were notable for anaemia, thrombocytopenia and neutropenia and myeloid blasts were present in the blood. Bone marrow exhibited >20% myeloid blasts.

Chapter 6 Haemostasis

Integrating clinical assessment, full blood count, blood film and coagulation assay investigations

A. Antithrombin deficiency
B. Disseminated intravascular coagulation
C. Haemolytic uremic syndrome
D. Haemophilia A
E. von Willebrand disease
F. Warfarin treatment
G. Heparin-induced thrombocytopenia
H. Factor V Leiden
I. Advanced liver disease
J. Primary biliary cirrhosis
K. Antiphospholipid syndrome

Instructions: For each patient's presentation, investigation results and treatment plan, select the correct diagnosis from the list above. Each answer can be used once, more than once or not at all.

1. A 35-year-old female patient with hypothyroidism and systemic lupus erythematosus (SLE) presents with a swollen, painful right calf. A deep vein thrombosis (DVT) is confirmed by Doppler ultrasound. When her admission history is being taken is notable for having had two DVTs in the past, but that they had been attributed to postoperative immobility and a long-haul flight respectively. She has also been trying to conceive but has experienced five miscarriages. The following investigation results are obtained: prothrombin time 12 seconds, activated partial thromboplastin time 34 seconds, fibrinogen 4.5 g/dL, Haemoglobin 12.5 g/dL, Platelets 325 × 10^9, White cell count 8.5 × 10^9, alkaline phosphatase 100, alanine aminotransferase 25, bilirubin 22, albumin 40, lupus anticoagulant = positive

2. An obese 55-year-old lady is on the orthopaedic ward following a traumatic hip fracture, which was managed with a total hip arthroplasty. She has breast cancer but is otherwise well. Since she avoids low-molecular-weight heparins (LMWHs; because of rash and soreness at site of subcutaneous enoxaparin during a previous admission), the Foundation doctor prescribed subcutaneous unfractionated heparin postoperatively for thromboprophylaxis. She recovers well initially, but on day 6 postoperatively, she complains of abdominal pain and calf pain. On examination, necrotic skin changes are noted at the injection site and her calf is red, swollen and tender. Deep vein thrombosis is confirmed on Doppler ultrasound, and investigations are as follows. Heparin is immediately discontinued, and alternative anticoagulation (bivalirudin) commenced. She recovers well and is discharged 1 week later with advice to avoid heparin and LMWH lifelong.

Preoperative platelet count	350×10^9
Day admission platelet count	365×10^9
Postoperative day 6 platelet count	70×10^9
Postoperative day 13 platelet count	30×10^9
Prothrombin time	12 seconds
Activated partial thromboplastin time	36 seconds
Fibrinogen	5.5 g/dL

3. A young man is admitted following a road traffic accident in which he was the unrestrained driver; the paramedics state his car was struck on the passenger side (as he turned onto the main road) by an oncoming lorry travelling at 50 mph. They report a 'bullseye' impact shatter on the driver's window. He is agitated and confused; the only useful history you can elicit is that he is visiting family in the area, he has a 'really serious bleeding problem' and has 'lost count' of the number of transfusions he has had in the past. On examination, he has a large swelling on the right side of his head. You also note several deformed joint contractures and that venous access is extremely difficult, although he is not haemodynamically compromised. He is managed via ATLS protocols and given fresh-frozen plasma and cryoprecipitate whilst preparing for trauma computed tomography (CT) and awaiting further collateral history. A single historic result [full blood count (FBC), prothrombin time (PT) and activated partial thromboplastin time (APTT)] score is the only information on historic electronic records, from an admission some 10 years previously. A CT is performed, showing a right-sided extradural haematoma. His Glasgow Coma Scale remains stable at 14, with no focal neurology, and once his family arrive they confirm the suspected condition allowing you to treat him with the appropriate recombinant factor, aiming for 100% of normal levels, before neurosurgical evacuation. Platelets 200 × 109/L, PT 13 seconds, APTT 55 seconds.

4. A 25-year-old patient is investigated following prolonged bleeding following a dental extraction. She told the dental surgeon who packed the cavity to reduce the bleeding she has always 'bruised like a peach,' often has nosebleeds and takes mefenamic acid and the oral contraceptive pill (OCP) for menorrhagia. Her mother died in labour from massive obstetric haemorrhage. Haemoglobin 11.0 g/dL, platelets 450 g/dL, prothrombin time 13 seconds, activated partial thromboplastin time 42 seconds, fibrinogen 3.5 g/dL, Factor VIII: C Reduced, Factor IX assay: Normal, vWF antigen concentration: 30% normal levels

5. An obese 18-year-old female who has recently commenced the oral contraceptive pill for

contraception presents breathless with chest pain. Electrocardiogram is normal, but ABG demonstrates type 1 respiratory failure. CT-PA reveals a large pulmonary embolism. She has bilateral extensive DVTs in her lower limbs. Apart from raised cholesterol, which her general practitioner was monitoring and she was addressing with diet, she is generally in good health. She was adopted but knows her biological mother had numerous blood clots and eventually died from complications of a clot. The haematologist explains to the patient that her blood clots too readily because she lacks a protein which inhibits coagulation factors IX, X and XII. He commences warfarin and advises that this is lifelong.

Chapter 7 Transfusion products

Integrating interpretation of laboratory results with decision-making regarding transfusion of blood products, plasma derivatives and recombinant factors

A. Red blood cells, group O, Rh −ve, irradiated
B. Red blood cells, group A, Rh +ve
C. Platelets
D. Platelets (cytomegalovirus [CMV] −ve)
E. Fresh frozen plasma (FFP; donor group O Rh +ve)
F. Prothrombin complex concentrate
G. Cryoprecipitate
H. Granulocyte concentrate
I. Whole blood
J. Anti-D immunoglobulin
K. FFP (donor group A Rh +ve)
L. Red blood cells, group O, Rh −ve, washed
M. Human albumin solution, 4%

For each patient's presentation, investigation results and treatment plan, select the most appropriate product from the aforementioned list to administer as a first priority. Each answer can be used once, more than once or not at all.

1. Following an obstetric haemorrhage of 1.6 L, a 32-year-old female with blood group A Rh +ve is found to have a haemoglobin (Hb) of 78 g/dL. She feels faint and dizzy and looks very pale. Clotting parameters are normal, and platelet count is 125. She reports that she has had severe febrile reactions during previous appropriately matched red cell transfusions.

2. A 35-year-old male with blood group A Rh −ve undergoes a 14-hour laparotomy with extensive tumour debulking and significant haemorrhage. Appropriate intraoperative red cell, platelet, FFP, human albumin solution, calcium and cryoprecipitate are transfused throughout. The patient is received intubated on the intensive care unit (ICU)

postoperatively with no active or ongoing bleeding, but the surgeons warn that he is at high risk for rebleeding. The following laboratory results are then obtained: Hb 95 g /dL, platelets 105×10^9/L, prothrombin time (PT) 27 seconds, activated partial thromboplastin time (APTT) 52 seconds, fibrinogen 1.9 g/dL.

3. A 54-year-old male presented with a severe chest infection. He was found to be HIV positive following investigations during admission. He became hypotensive with severe type 2 respiratory failure and was admitted to intensive care for mechanical ventilation and vasopressor support. His platelet count on admission to the ICU was noted to be 16×10^9/L. His CMV status is negative.

4. A patient with septic shock secondary to urosepsis is admitted to the ICU. The nurse is concerned as his cannula and venepuncture sites have started to ooze, and he has passed a large amount of black tarry stool. He also appears to have several enlarging areas of purplish bruises over his torso and limbs despite no apparent trauma or pressure areas. Urgent blood tests reveal Hb 85 g/dL, Platelets 55×10^9/, PT 20 seconds, APTT 45 seconds, fibrinogen 0.3 g/dL.

5. A woman has just delivered her first baby by spontaneous vaginal delivery with an estimated blood loss of <500 mL. She and the baby are well. She is blood type AB Rh −ve, whilst her partner is blood type O Rh +ve.

Chapter 9 The innate immune system
Concerning innate immunity

A. Mucociliary escalator
B. Mast cells
C. Basophils
D. Normal gut flora
E. Natural killer cells
F. T cells
G. Salivary lysozyme
H. Macrophages
I. Neutrophils
J. Acidic pH

For each scenario described, choose the single most likely match from the list of options. Each option may be used once, more than once, or not at all.

1. A phagocyte that can be found circulating in the blood.
2. A physical barrier component of the innate immune system.
3. Derived from common lymphoid progenitor cells, these innate immune cells participate in antibody-dependent cell-mediated cytotoxicity.

4. An innate immune cell that resides in the tissues and degranulates upon interaction with appropriate immunoglobulin (Ig) E molecules.
5. A chemical component of the innate immune system that prevents infection in the stomach.

Concerning complement

A. Alternative pathway
B. C3
C. Lectin pathway
D. Collectins
E. Anaphylotoxin
F. C1 esterase inhibitor
G. Membrane attack complex
H. C7
I. Classical pathway
J. Complement inhibitors

For each scenario described, choose the single most likely match from the list of options. Each option may be used once, more than once, or not at all.

1. Final set of complement proteins, which form a polymer that punches holes in cell membranes.
2. The initiation of complement proteins by antibodies.
3. Deficient in hereditary angioedema.
4. Causes increased vascular permeability and attracts white blood cells to the site of infection.
5. Regulates the processes involved in the complement cascade.

Chapter 10 The adaptive immune system
Concerning cell surface molecules

A. B cell receptor
B. Toll-like receptor
C. Major histocompatibility complex (MHC) class I
D. FAS ligand
E. T cell receptor
F. Major histocompatibility complex class II
G. Antigen
H. Cell adhesion molecules (CAMs)
I. CD3
J. Collectins

For each scenario described below, choose the **single** most likely match from the above list of options. Each option may be used once, more than once or not at all.

1. Substances recognized by the specific receptors of the adaptive immune system.
2. Pattern recognition molecules found in solution.
3. Molecules that bind and present peptide antigens from intracellular pathogens.

4. Molecule that recognizes intracellular or phagocytosed antigen when it is expressed simultaneously with the MHC in which it is lying.
5. Family of related molecules found on cell surfaces that, upon recognizing a pathogen, activate the innate immune system.

Concerning tolerance

A. Peripheral Tolerance
B. Central Tolerance
C. Costimulation
D. Major histocompatibility complex (MHC) restriction
E. Interleukin-10 (IL-10)
F. IL-4
G. IL-17
H. Interferon-β (IFN-β)
I. IFN-γ
J. Tumour necrosis factor-α

For each scenario below, choose the most likely corresponding option from the list given above. Each answer can be used once, more than once or not at all.

1. The process that occurs in the bone or thymus that prevents any self-reactive developing B or T lymphocytes respectively from maturing and entering the circulation.
2. A key molecular mediator of peripheral tolerance.
3. A 35-year-old athlete presents to his general practitioner (GP) with severe and persistent allergic rhinitis. He has been trialled unsuccessfully on multiple antihistamines, nasal sprays and leukotriene receptor antagonists. His GP refers him for grass pollen desensitization therapy. Through which feature of the adaptive immune system does this therapy work?
4. A feature of the immune system that prevents indiscriminate activation of T lymphocytes by limiting activation to sites of infection.
5. A cytokine that Th1 cells secrete if tolerance has broken down and hypersensitivity develops.

Concerning B and T lymphocytes

A. CD8
B. Myeloid stem cells
C. Plasma cells
D. Basophil
E. Memory B cells
F. T helper cells
G. Cytotoxic T cells
H. Memory T cells
I. CD40
J. Lymphoid stem cells

For each scenario described below, choose the **single** most likely match from the above list of options. Each option may be used once, more than once or not at all.

1. Induces B cells to become fully active and begin releasing antibody.
2. Cells from which B and T lymphocytes originate.
3. Cells with a vast amount of endoplasmic reticulum in order to secrete large quantities of immunoglobulin.
4. Cell marker associated with cytotoxic T cells.
5. Cells that recognize antigen in conjunction with class I major histocompatibility complex (MHC).

Chapter 11 The functioning immune system
Concerning the immune system in action

A. Phagocytes
B. Secretory immunoglobulin A (sIgA)
C. Tumour necrosis factor alpha (TNF-γ)
D. Major histocompatibility complex (MHC) class I
E. Natural killer cells
F. The membrane attack complex (MAC)
G. Mast cells
H. Interferon alpha (IFN- γ)
I. Plasma cells
J. Toll-like receptors

For each scenario below, choose the single most likely match from the list of options. Each option can be used once, more than once, or not at all.

1. The cells that release histamine in response to immunoglobulin E stimulation, for example in parasitic infections.
2. The cells that destroy most extracellular bacteria.
3. The cytokine secreted by virally infected cells to communicate with other cells.
4. Viral peptides are presented to CD8 positive T cells by this molecule.
5. The cytokine involved in granuloma formation and maintenance.
E. A patient with a single episode of *Strep. pneumoniae* pneumonia

Chapter 12 Immune dysfunction
Immune dysfunction

A. Skin prick test
B. C-reactive protein titre
C. Enzyme-linked immunosorbent assay (ELISA)
D. Patch test
E. Polymerase chain reaction (PCR)
F. Flow cytometry
G. Tuberculin skin test.
H. HLA-typing

I. Measurement of IgG, IgA and IgM levels
J. Differential white cell count

For each scenario described below, choose the single most appropriate test from the above list of options. Each option may be used once, more than once, or not at all.

1. The test needed to confirm a primary immunoglobulin deficiency.
2. A test that can help differentiate between acute appendicitis and constipation in acute abdominal pain.
3. The test that involves an intradermal injection of purified protein derivative (PPD).
4. The test that uses labelled antibodies to bind to, and detect, antigens or antigen-antibody complexes.
5. The test used to confirm nickel hypersensitivity.

Concerning hypersensitivity

A. Skin prick test
B. Asthma
C. Post-streptococcal glomerulonephritis
D. Nickel hypersensitivity
E. Type I hypersensitivity
F. Type III hypersensitivity
G. Atopic eczema
H. ABO incompatibility
I. Type IV hypersensitivity
J. Anaphylaxis

For each scenario described below, choose the single most likely match from the above list of options. Each option may be used once, more than once, or not at all.

1. A type of hypersensitivity that results from antibody–antigen complex deposition. Farmer's lung is a form of this hypersensitivity.
2. A medical emergency that requires 0.5 mL of 1:1000 of adrenaline intramuscularly as part of the immediate management.
3. A type of hypersensitivity that results from IgE-mediated mast cell degranulation. Allergic rhinitis is a form of this hypersensitivity.
4. A form of type II hypersensitivity.
5. A form of type III hypersensitivity.

Concerning autoimmunity

A. Hashimoto thyroiditis
B. Graves disease
C. Type II diabetes
D. Rheumatoid arthritis
E. Central tolerance
F. Molecular mimicry
G. Systemic lupus erythematosus (SLE)
H. Ankylosing spondylitis
I. Type I diabetes
J. Peripheral tolerance

For each scenario described below, choose the single most likely match from the above list of options. Each option may be used once, more than once, or not at all.

1. The autoimmune disease caused by the deposition of immune complexes, which often causes a photosensitive rash.
2. In which disease is HLA-DQ2 thought to prevent antigen being presented correctly in the thymus, resulting in breakdown of tolerance?
3. A disease associated with individuals carrying HLA-B27.
4. The process in which self-reactive T cells and B cells are eliminated.
5. A condition that results from stimulatory antibody production.

Chapter 13 Medical intervention

Concerning immunological interventions

A. Nonsteroidal antiinflammatory drugs (NSAIDs)
B. Referral to a rheumatologist
C. Oral prednisolone
D. Adrenaline
E. Tacrolimus
F. Infliximab
G. Rituximab
H. Azathioprine
I. Beclomethasone inhaler
J. Methotrexate

For each scenario described below, choose the single most likely match from the above list of options. Each option may be used once, more than once, or not at all.

1. The drug most likely to cause weight gain, hypertension and osteoporosis if used long term.
2. The most appropriate option for a general practitioner who sees a 34-year-old lady presenting with painful swelling of joints in her hands. An X-ray of the joints shows bony erosions and joint destruction. A blood test shows the patient is positive for rheumatoid factor.
3. The drug for which thiopurine methyltransferase (TPMT) activity levels must be measured before commencing treatment.
4. A drug that causes immunosuppression by inhibiting calcineurin.
5. A monoclonal antibody that targets tumour necrosis factor α.

Concerning the immune system in action

A. Phagocytes
B. Secretory immunoglobulin A (sIgA)
C. Tumour necrosis factor alpha (TNF-α)
D. Major histocompatibility complex (MHC) class I
E. Natural killer cells
F. The membrane attack complex (MAC)
G. Mast cells
H. Interferon alpha (IFN-α)
I. Plasma cells
J. Toll-like receptors

For each scenario described below, choose the single most likely match from the above list of options. Each option may be used once, more than once, or not at all.

1. The cells that release histamine in response to immunoglobulin E stimulation, for example in parasitic infections.
2. The cells that destroy most extracellular bacteria.
3. The cytokine secreted by virally infected cells to communicate with other cells.
4. Viral peptides are presented to CD8 positive T cells by this molecule.
5. The cytokine involved in granuloma formation and maintenance.

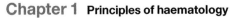

SBA answers

Chapter 1 Principles of haematology

1. E. Option (E) is the only listed example of a lymphoid lineage progenitor. Pre-B cells are derived from the common lymphoid progenitor and ultimately develop into mature B cells. All other options describe myeloid lineage progenitors. BFU-E are destined to become red cells, CFU-Meg differentiates into megakaryocytes to form platelets, CFU-Eos develop into eosinophils, CFU-GEMM is the common myeloid progenitor analogous to the common lymphoid progenitor.

2. C. Options A, B and C are mature cells, but only option C is a mature cell of myeloid lineage origin: NK cells and T lymphocytes are of lymphoid origin. Options D and E are myeloid lineage, but they are progenitor cells, not mature cells.

3. B. Option B is the only listed option describing one of the spleen's physiological roles; destruction of senescent erythrocytes and filtration of particulate matter from the bloodstream, initiation of immune response to blood-borne antigens, fetal haemopoiesis and a storage reservoir for platelets are the main physiological roles of the spleen. Options A and D refer to bone marrow, option C refers to the liver and option E the kidney.

4. E. Option E does not cause splenomegaly; this disorder results from impaired erythropoiesis secondary to B12 deficiency due to a failure of intrinsic-factor mediated gastrointestinal absorption. Options A–D are all causes associated with massive splenomegaly.

5. B. Only option B, Lyme disease, is commonly associated with generalized lymphadenopathy. Mumps (option A) causes local enlargement of the parotid glands and D and E are not associated with generalized lymphadenopathy. C may lead to right ventricular failure, which may result in hepatomegaly and splenomegaly, but not generalized lymphadenopathy. Table 1.4 lists causes of generalized lymphadenopathy.

6. C. The description refers to a monocyte (C). All listed options are of myeloid lineage, but only monocytes (C) and neutrophils (D) are derived from the CFU-GM precursor. Since a neutrophil has a multilobed nucleus and are smaller (12–14 μm diameter) and eosinophils (A) are also smaller than monocytes (20 μm diameter), options A and B can be excluded.

7. D. Options A, B, C and E are all mandatory features of caring for asplenic patients. Option D would not offer any additional benefit to the patient and would be costly. Once these viruses establish latency, they cannot be eliminated.

8. D. Thrombopoietin stimulates both megakaryocyte differentiation from CFU-Meg and megakaryocyte spawning of platelets, therefore option D is the answer. See Table 1.2 for details of the other growth factors' primary roles.

9. D. Option E is most commonly used in the treatment of hepatitis C virus. Option C has applications in multiple sclerosis. The remaining options are growth factors. Option A would promote erythropoiesis in a patient with a failure of endogenous synthesis. Option B could potentially reduce the chance of needing a platelet transfusion. Option D is the correct answer and could raise a dangerously low neutrophil count.

10. B. Options A, B and C are all clinically used growth factors, but only option B is appropriate in this scenario. The patient's symptoms are secondary to a normochromic normocytic anaemia, arising from his renal failure to synthesize erythropoietin. Iatrogenic replacement is therefore appropriate and is commonplace in patients with end-stage renal failure. Option D is a subcutaneous insulin preparation and option E is a low molecular weight heparin.

Chapter 2 Red Blood cells and haemoglobin

1. B. Erythrocytes have a uniform appearance. The 3D structure is that of a thick disc with central depressions on each face: a biconcave disc. B is therefore the correct answer. This shape allows the red cell to enjoy a large surface area: volume ratio for maximum gas exchange, while offering a narrower leading edge for entering narrow vasculature than other high surface area:volume ratio 3D shapes.

2. C. E describes the sequence of events undergone by bilirubin as part of haem (not iron) catabolism. D refers

to unabsorbed iron. There is no specific iron excretion mechanism; however, small continual losses occur via desquamation and background blood loss (making A and B untrue). C represents the major mechanism for limiting uptake of ingested iron, which is the only step in iron metabolism that can be significantly controlled to influence total body iron levels and is therefore the correct answer. Hepcidin reduces expression of the iron exporter molecule at basal surfaces of enterocytes, limiting absorbed iron's access to the portal circulation.

3. C. C and D both occur in mature red cells, but the main role of D in red cells is as a source of NADPH+H+ (i.e., reduced NADP), whilst cytoplasmic glycolysis (C) is the main ATP generation pathway in mature red cells and is the correct answer. Since mature red cells lack mitochondria, A, B and E do not occur in red cells, since these pathways are partially or entirely mitochondrial.

4. A. A, methaemoglobinaemia, is the correct answer. The clue here is the cyanosis fails to improve with increased inspired oxygen developing soon after a predisposing drug. We know the regional anaesthesia was performed without ultrasound or electrostimulation and failed to obtain an adequate block for surgery. A large volume of prilocaine was probably injected intravascularly rather than perineurally. Prilocaine is a known to be a predisposing cause of methaemoglobinaemia, particularly if intravascularly injected. The patient is blue due to methaemoglobinaemia rather than an increased proportion of deoxyHb. Cyanosis due to the latter cause would almost certainly be accompanied by tachycardia and reduced end-tidal CO_2. B, C, D and E all describe potential perioperative catastrophes; B, C and D would be accompanied by cardiovascular collapse and can be excluded. E would cause hypoxia, but the pulse oximetry and cyanosis would be responsive to supplemental oxygen.

5. C. Only option C is accurate. Haem is degraded to its iron and protoporphyrin components. Protoporphyrin is degraded to bilirubin, which travels to the liver bound to albumin. There it is conjugated to glucuronide (not acetylated) and secreted into the GI lumen. Here it is converted to urobilinogen, which is either reabsorbed and renally excreted or further converted to stercobilinogen and stercilin and excreted in the faeces.

6. B. Loss of functional renal mass (B) is the correct answer; since renal tissue synthesizes the bulk of erythropoietin. D and E are associated with raised erythropoietin production; in the case of E, the

resulting polycythaemia can lead to dangerous hyperviscosity complications. A and C would probably have a chronically raised erythropoietin secondary to impaired peripheral oxygen delivery due to reduced haemoglobin.

7. D. Only D is correct. The p50 value (the pO_2 at which oxygen is 50% saturated) is used to compare different haemoglobins or the same haemoglobin under different conditions, since lying on the straight portion of the curve it is least vulnerable to misinterpretation). A rightward shift moves the p50 to a higher corresponding pO_2 value.

8. C. B12 deficiency, C, is not treated with red cell transfusion or iron supplementation, thus it carries no risk of iron overload. It may coexist with an iron deficiency if inadequate diet is the cause. Thalassaemia (A) and sickle cell anaemia (B) are conditions with a high requirement for red cell transfusions. Prolonged oral iron ingestion (E) and haemochromatosis (D) both result in pathological increase in iron absorption.

Chapter 3 Red blood cell disorders

1. B. Option B is the most accurate description. Lacking mitochondria, erythrocytes are dependent on glycolysis. Failure of glycolysis leads to severe restriction of ATP availability. Option A and C describes glucose-6-phosphate dehydrogenase (G6PD) deficiency. Option D refers to hereditary spherocytosis or elliptocytosis. Option E describes paroxysmal nocturnal haemoglobinuria.

2. D. D is the correct answer. Patients are typically asymptomatic but experience bouts of haemolysis (A incorrect). The Mediterranean (not African: C incorrect) subtype of G6PD deficiency renders sufferers at risk of haemolysis episodes when exposed to oxidative stress including fava beans. Haemolysis is primarily intravascular (B incorrect). Blister/bite cells and Heinz bodies are characteristic features of the blood film during a haemolytic episode. Definitive diagnosis is by enzyme assay; but if the blood sample is drawn during active haemolysis, reticulocytosis can confound the assay (as reticulocytes have much higher enzyme levels, a false negative diagnosis may be made). Therefore E is incorrect.

3. D. Option D is correct. The age of presentation is typical for beta thalassaemia major where the individual is homozygous (two copies) for the beta globin mutation. At the time that fetal Hb synthesis would be expected to decline, the failure of normal

HbA synthesis becomes apparent. Electrophoresis has absent HbA and persistence of HbF.

4. E. Option E is classically associated with iron deficiency, which will most likely be accompanied with reduced Hb, mean cell volume and mean cell haemoglobin. All options except E are typical of severe B12 deficiency. Epithelial symptoms predate or accompany haematological symptoms, which themselves precede neurological symptoms.

5. B. B12 does not influence the absorption of folate; however, sufficient B12 must be available in order to maintain the bioavailability of folate. The exact mechanism of this is described in option B: methylcobalamin releases folate from the methylfolate trap. All other options are incorrect.

6. D. Option D is specific for a megaloblastic anaemia. Option A describes macrocytic anaemia, but this could be due to megaloblastic anaemia or any other cause of macrocytosis. Option B is incorrect; the megaloblasts are the abnormal precursors and reside in the bone marrow and are rarely seen in peripheral blood. Option C describes secondary polycythaemia. Option E would be characteristic of lead poisoning.

7. D. Option D shows a microcytic anaemia, low ferritin and raised TIBC/transferrin, which is what you would expect in iron deficiency anaemia. Option A is beta thalassaemia major: microcytosis even more pronounced for the degree of anaemia. Option B is sideroblastic anaemia (acquired – remember that the hereditary form is microcytic): note the increased bone marrow and ferritin (iron status biomarkers). Option C represents B12 deficiency (note the secondary reduction in red cell folate). It could also represent folate deficiency – a B12 serum would be needed to discriminate. Option E is within normal ranges.

8. A. The low serum folate and red cell folate inform us that the patient has long-term folate deficiency. However, this may be functional, i.e., due to folate remaining trapped as methylfolate due to inadequate B12 availability. From the available information, a B12 deficiency cannot be ruled out. The safest and best option is to treat both in combination, i.e., option A. Iron supplementation (B) and red cell transfusion (E) are inappropriate (no evidence of iron deficiency and she is not acutely unwell from her anaemia nor is it particularly extreme). Option D, treatment of presumed isolated folate deficiency with folate supplements alone, risks correcting the anaemia but allowing neurodegeneration secondary to an occult B12 deficiency to progress unchecked. Option C (B12 alone), risks failing to address a potentially deficient

folate status, which could easily reflect true depletion of folate stores. Both folate and B12 are water soluble and nontoxic in excess. Vegans are at particular risk of both B12 deficiency.

Chapter 4 White blood cells

1. D. Only the monocyte is a macrophage precursor, even though neutrophils, basophils, and eosinophils are also of myeloid lineage. Monocytes are derived from CFU-M, which is derived from CFU-GM, derived from CFU-GEMM. They circulate in the bloodstream, and when they leave the circulation to enter the tissues, they undergo further differentiation and acquire additional features, when they are referred to as macrophages. Lymphocytes are of lymphoid origin

2. B. Only HIV infection would cause lymphopenia. Ancylostoma (hookworm) infection would be expected to cause eosinophilia. Epstein-Barr virus infection would likely cause mononucleosis and lympocytosis. ALL and toxoplasmosis would cause a lymphocytosis.

3. D. The band cell is most likely to be seen in 'left shift,' where immature neutrophil precursors are released into peripheral blood from bone marrow. The more severe the factor that provoked premature release of neutrophil precursors, the earlier the developmental stage of the immature cells released, so essentially what this question is asking is what precursor is immediately prior to a mature neutrophil. Band cells are most likely to be seen, then metamyelocytes, then myelocytes and so on (see Fig. 4.6).

4. B. The most common cause of neutropenia is drugs; therefore, vancomycin is the correct answer. Recent surgery would be most likely to cause a neutrophilia. Hypersplenism results in increased splenic sequestration of neutrophils, and so may cause neutropenia by reducing neutrophil lifespan in the circulation. Rheumatoid arthritis is an autoimmune disease; recall that neutropenia may arise via immune-mediated neutrophil destruction that can be idiopathic or associated with existing autoimmune disease. Severe infection would be most likely to cause a neutrophilia, but it could also possibly result in neutropenia due to extortionately high 'demand' created by overwhelming bacterial infection.

Chapter 5 Haematological malignancies

1. C. Cytopenias result from invasion of normal marrow by the dysplastic haemopoietic precursors. Clonal proliferation of abnormal plasma cells in bone marrow and blood describes multiple myeloma. Accumulation

of abnormal lymphoid cells in nodal and extranodal tissues defines lymphoma. Neoplastic proliferation of a myeloid precursor resulting in hypercellular marrow defines myeloproliferative disorders. Accumulation of abnormal neoplastic white cells in bone marrow defines the leukaemias.

2. B. The clinical presentation and examination findings in this example are nonspecific in terms of haematological malignancy, but acute lymphoblastic leukaemia should be forefront in the practioner's mind because it is the most common childhood cancer. The elevated WCC and cytopenias suggests a leukaemia, but bone marrow biopsy is only consistent with a lymphoid leukaemia. The MLL gene rearrangement is also common in acute lymphoblastic leukaemia. Chronic myeloid leukaemia would exhibit myeloid lineage cells with the defining translocation 9:22 and anaemia and thrombocytopenia are not typical features of chronic myeloid leukaemia. Furthermore, this would be a very unusual diagnosis in a child. Nonaccidental injury should always be considered when bruising is noted in a child, but would not present with the investigation results above, nor the reported symptoms. Primary myelofibrosis is not a childhood diagnosis nor does it present with lymphoblasts. Non-Hodgkin lymphoma similarly does not show lymphoblasts

3. C. This patient presents with septic shock secondary to neutropenic sepsis with type 1 respiratory failure and metabolic acidosis. Urgent resuscitation via an ABC approach, with early input from critical care is the only appropriate action in a patient presenting with septic shock. He requires urgent large-bore IV access and vigorous IV hydration to address the distributive shock, and immediate broad-spectrum antibiotics (ideally after taking blood cultures, but not if this would cause a delay). Because it lists two components of urgent resuscitation, 'Administer IV crystalloid and broad-spectrum antibiotics' is correct. Performing an urgent red cell transfusion as well as administering G-CSF and discussing with haematology are inappropriate. The cytopenias are only a component of this patient's current status, although these options may be appropriate under haematologist supervision after acute resuscitation has been effectively implemented. Administering allopurinol and rasburicase would be appropriate in tumour lysis syndrome, but the uric acid is in the normal range, refuting this diagnosis. Arranging urgent plasmapheresis would be appropriate if symptoms were secondary to leucostasis, which the low white cell count precludes.

4. E. The patient's age would provide the best chance of discriminating between Hodgkin and non-Hodgkin lymphoma while waiting for the biopsy result because almost all subtypes of NHL present at older age (median age, 60 years). Alcohol-induced painful lymphadenopathy and cyclical fever are also features of HL and are not seen in NHL, but are extremely rare. Past EBV infection and known immunodeficiency are nondiscriminatory because they predispose to both HL and NHL. Likewise, fever, weight loss, night sweats or pruritus can be presenting features of either HL or NHL.

5. D. The polydipsia and polyuria are secondary to hypercalcaemia and renal involvement. The urine dip represents proteinuria from tubular damage and Bence-Jones protein. The depression may be incidental or secondary to the hypercalcaemia. The serum electrophoresis and presence of clonal plasma cells in the bone marrow excludes a leukaemia but suggests a plasma cell dyscrasia. Widespread system involvement excludes solitary plasmacytoma and MGUS, as does the high percentage of clonal cells in the marrow.

6. B. This patient would be at high risk of tumour lysis syndrome, given his high burden of lymphoma cells. The biochemical abnormalities 'K+ 7.2 mM, Ca++ 1.2 mM, PO42-4.5 mM, uric acid 1500 µmol/L' would correspond with this acute complication secondary to his treatment. The joint pain arises from acute crystal deposition of uric acid, and the hypocalcaemia the other symptoms. The high potassium accounts for the EKG changes and would warrant emergency intravenous 10% calcium gluconate and potassium-lowering treatments.

Chapter 6 Haemostasis

1. B. Vasoconstriction is the most immediate event. Transient tethering then promotes the platelet release reaction, which allows more stable adhesion to occur. Finally, aggregation follows.

2. B. Option B correctly describes the first step of the extrinsic pathway. The events in options A, C and D are accurate, but refer to stages of the intrinsic pathway. Option E describes a stage in fibrin formation, which only occurs after the common pathway.

3. A. Only option A summarizes the common pathway. Statement B describes the extrinsic pathway. Option C describes primary haemostasis; the common pathway is an element of secondary haemostasis. Option D describes the intrinsic pathway. Option E describes fibrinolysis.

4. E. Only option E describes a bleeding disorder. vWD is associated with mucocutaneous bleeding and prolonged bleeding after major trauma or surgery, as evidenced by his mother. vWD comes in three subtypes: type 1, 2 and 3. Types 2 and 3 are more severe and are managed in specialist centres. Options A–D all describe hereditary thrombophilias, which would manifest with thromboses secondary to hypercoagulability.

5. D. D is the most common culprit for drug-induced immune thrombocytopenic purpura, where platelets are destroyed by a drug-dependent immune mechanism, reducing their survival in the circulation and manifesting on with thrombocytopenia. Remember that direct myelosuppression is another important mechanism of reduced platelet synthesis, which similarly manifests as a thrombocytopenia developing in response to a drug.

6. D. She presents with the traditional pentad of symptoms suggesting TTP, although often not all five symptoms (fever, transient neurologic deficit, renal impairment, MAHA (see Microangiopathic haemolytic anaemia and thrombocytopenia section) are present. Whilst all options (excluding C) would present with bruising, the jaundice suggests haemolysis, which is not a feature of either option C or option E. The LDH is raised and the Hb low because of this haemolysis, which the film helpfully informs you is microangiopathic in origin—this tells you MAHA is present, and in combination with low platelets should suggest DIC, HUS or TTP. HUS (option A) would not present with transient neurologic symptoms and in an adult would usually be preceded by an infection, usually gastrointestinal, as well as most likely having a more dramatically raised urea and creatinine. DIC (option B) would be associated with a critically ill patient, prolonged PT and APTT and low fibrinogen. Option C would not exhibit the biochemical and haematologic derangements revealed by the investigations, nor would jaundice and bruising be present. Option E would not include haemolysis, nor the fever and neurologic features.

7. C. Options A–C all reverse warfarin, but for emergency reversal of warfarin, only option C would achieve this in the stated timeframe. Since the patient has likely lost a large amount of blood into her thigh (the femur is highly vascular) and will be at risk of further blood loss whilst the hip prosthesis is surgically implanted, her INR needs lowering. Dosage of PCC is best discussed with the on-call haematologist. Different surgeons will accept different maximum INRs perioperatively and thus communication with the operating surgeon is

important. Option D would only be appropriate in an acute bleeding scenario in a patient with haemophilia A–factor VIII is not a vitamin-K dependent coagulation factor and thus would not address warfarin-induced deficiency of factors II, VII, IX and X. Option E (cryoprecipitate) only contains factors VIII, XIII, vWF and fibrinogen and thus would not be useful in this scenario.

Chapter 7 Transfusion products

1. B. Answer B is the safest and most competent answer: failure to do both these things would potentially result in a wrong diagnosis and incorrect management, and certainly failing to pause the transfusion could massively worsen the outcome. Option A would be appropriate for transfusion-associated circulatory overload, however without assessing the patient and making the diagnosis it would be inappropriate to take this action. Option C would be appropriate if anaphylaxis was suspected, but this is unlikely with a higher-than-normal blood pressure. Option D is part of the treatment for a nonhaemolytic febrile transfusion reaction, but inappropriate without fully assessing the patient. Option E is the treatment for septic shock secondary to bacterially contaminated blood products, but also inappropriate without assessing the patient.

2. B. Only option C is entirely correct. IgM binds to A or B antigens, causing complement-mediated intravascular haemolysis. This is the underlying mechanism of an ABO incompatibility acute transfusion reaction.

3. C. Option C is correct. Please see table 7.1 for storage solutions and shelf lives of the other major blood products.

4. D. Option D is a valid investigation into a patient with current or historic suspected hepatitis B infection and is not part of the standard battery of tests performed on all donation samples. The hepatitis B test included within the standard screening instead is option E: surface antigen, not an antibody enzyme-linked immunoassay. The other options are all performed on all donation samples (see Table 7.2).

5. D. Option D is the correct answer. FFP from a group O donor will contain anti-A and anti-B antibodies, which would bind to the group AB recipient's red cell A and B antigens. Remember that for FFP, AB is the universal donor, in contrast to red cells where AB represents the universal recipient.

6. A. A platelet count below 50 would potentially place a patient at risk of catastrophic bleeding during major abdominal surgery. If the surgery is urgent and cannot be safely delayed, the patient in option A should be transfused with one adult therapeutic dose of platelets. The other options as presented are not indications for platelet transfusion.

7. C. Options A, C and D are all delayed transfusion reactions, however the correct answer is option C as the question describes the underlying mechanism of this much-feared complication. Leucodepletion is routinely performed to minimize the likelihood of TA-GVHD, and patients with impaired cell-mediated immunity that are at higher risk are transfused with irradiated blood products for the same reason. B and E represent acute transfusion complications.

8. B. Option B permanently excludes the dancer from donation. The lady in option A would be able to donate once 12 months had elapsed from the encounter. The patient in option C would be able to donate if their body modifications were all performed at least 12 months earlier. The patients in D and E would be able to donate in the future if their [Hb] and weight increased respectively.

9. C. The correct legal, ethical and clinical course of action is option C. Option A will not stabilize the child and the haemodilution may hasten her demise. Option B is not appropriate; this child is in haemorrhagic shock and will not survive waiting for a cell saver to be brought in from offsite. Furthermore, she is far too unstable and would almost certainly arrest on induction of general anaesthesia if not before. Option D wastes time and even if successful could be too late to save her. Option E is not acceptable as a child cannot refuse lifesaving treatment and an advance directive is not valid in the life-threatening circumstances with a child as young as 6 years of age.

10. C. All the aforementioned options are complications of large volume transfusions, except option C. Hypocalcaemia, not hypercalcaemia is a complication of massive transfusion. Hypocalcaemia exacerbates myocardial dysfunction in haemorrhagic shock and causes platelet dysfunction and impaired coagulation.

Chapter 9 The innate immune system

1. C. It is composed of phagocytes and complement. The other options describe traits of the adaptive immune system.

2. D. It may respond differently if reexposed to the same pathogen. After primary exposure, secondary exposure usually elicits a faster, stronger adaptive immune system response. A, B and E are true for the innate immune system. C is true the other way around—the adaptive immune system coordinates the response according to antigen presentation by the innate immune system.

3. E. Disruption of the patient's normal gut flora by the antibiotic, allowing colonization by pathogenic organisms. This frequently happens with the use of broad spectrum antibiotics, such as ciprofloxacin. Progression of a urinary tract infection to sepsis is unlikely to present with diarrhoea, neither would anaphylaxis. However, a nonanaphylactic allergic reaction to the antibiotic could present with diarrhoea.

4. A. Neutrophil. None of the other answers phagocytose pathogens.

5. B. They are key antigen presenting cells. Macrophages present antigen to the adaptive immune system in association with MHC class II molecules, activating further immune responses. Dendritic cells have a similar role in the epithelia, however they are distinct cells to macrophages. Macrophages live longer and are larger than neutrophils.

6. E. Pus is formed in some bacterial infections and contains many dead neutrophils. Pus in an enclosed space is an abscess.

7. B. Herpes simplex downregulates major histocompatibility complex I on infected cells so natural killer cells are no longer inhibited from killing these infected cells.

8. A. While cytokines increase acute phase protein synthesis and bacterial antigens may cause cytokine release, it is the direct effect of acute phase proteins on metabolism that cause this catabolism.

9. D. While a raised CRP is also seen in GCA, the raised ESR is more indicative of the chronic inflammatory process behind the condition and raised CRP may have many other causes.

10. D. Antigen-antibody complexes activate C1. (A) describes the alternative pathway, while (C) describes the lectin pathway. (B) describes the activation of B cells. (E) describes the activation of cytotoxic T cells.

11. C. The MAC, made up of multiple complement proteins, punches a hole in the pathogen's cell membrane, allowing water to enter and lyse the pathogen.

12. C. Whilst answers D and E commonly cause eosinophilia, parasitic worms and Hodgkin disease are not associated with chronic cough. Eosinophilia is classically more associated with asthma than COPD and reflects the hypersensitivity underlying the disease.

Chapter 10 The adaptive immune system

1. B. The haplotype is found on chromosome 6. MHC class I molecules present endogenous antigen, CD8 positive T cells bind MHC class I, MHC class II are only present on antigen-presenting cells and there is no difference in peptide length that MHC class I and II present.

2. E. Class switching. Somatic hypermutation and affinity maturation are different names for the same process that increases the affinity of an antibody for its antigen. Junctional diversity refers to the increased variability in antibodies due to the formation of junctions between the various gene segments. Positive selection refers to the process in which T cells that are able to recognize self-major histocompatibility complex (MHC) survive, whereas those that cannot recognize self-MHC do not survive.

3. E. These are not members of the immunoglobulin superfamily, but they are pattern-recognition molecules. The remaining molecules all contain immunoglobulin domains and are therefore members of the immunoglobulin superfamily.

4. C. Somatic hypermutation of immunoglobulin genes occurs in the germinal centres. B cells are activated in the follicles of secondary lymphoid organs. The expression of bcl-2 prevents apoptosis of the B-cell. B cells are activated after dendritic cells present antigen. Activated T helper cells aid B cells in producing antibody by producing cytokines.

5. D. IgE.

6. B. Th1 cells secrete IL-2, IFN-γ and TNF-β, all of which enable them to combat intracellular pathogens. Th2 cells are more concerned with extracellular bacteria and parasites. MHC restriction takes place in the thymus. Cytotoxic T cells express CD8. T cells are required to bind to self-MHC for their function, but any T cells that bind self-MHC in association with self-antigens undergo apoptosis (this is **negative** selection).

7. A. The role of TGF-β in oral tolerance is to transform any T cells that react to harmless antigen into Tregs, which in turn secrete TGF-β to inhibit other reactive T cells. Because the secretion of TGF-β is to promote oral tolerance, the answers referring to the production of an immune response against the antigen (B, D and E) are incorrect.

8. C. This combination of cytotoxic cells (as well as Th1 lymphocytes) is crucial to eliminating the influenza virus from the body, which is why B and E are incorrect. It is likely that she will have encountered the flu virus before, but the strain mutates annually. The flu symptoms are mainly due to interferon as opposed to TGF-β.

9. D. Staphylococcal enterotoxin causes cross-linking of the V-β domain of the TCR and a MHC class II molecule on an antigen-presenting cell, resulting in large and indiscriminant activation of the adaptive immune system. This results in the presentation in the question. A, B, C and E all pertain to infectious diseases but none acts as a superantigen.

Chapter 11 The functioning immune system

1. C. Homing due to integrin molecules. This is required for leucocytes to enter the tissue for the acute inflammatory response (described here as rubor, tumor and dolor of the child's arm). Fibroblast migration and proliferation tends to happen later, resulting in scar formation or chronic inflammation (resolutions of the acute inflammatory response). Vascular permeability is increased, hence tumor. IFN-γ is a mediator more associated with chronic inflammation and frustrated phagocytosis.

2. B. Persistence of antigen. This is the main factor in the progression of all inflammation from acute to chronic. While TNF-α is raised in chronic inflammation and is targeted in autoimmune disease, it is mediator rather that the cause of the chronic inflammatory response.

3. C. Delayed type hypersensitivity response; the pathogen is surrounded by granulation tissue. *M. tuberculosis* is an intracellular pathogen: phagocytes cannot easily manage the infection by engulfing the bacteria and antibodies can neither neutralize nor opsonize it. Th2 cell release of IL-4 is more concerned with extracellular pathogens and allergic responses. CD4 positive T cells do not directly destroy infected cells. Primary tuberculosis infection, in an immunocompetent patient, is managed by granulation tissue forming caseous necrosis.

4. A. Antibodies can neutralize the pathogen directly, as well as act as an opsonin against infected cells. IFN-γ

activates macrophages and natural killer cells: it does not directly affect viral transcription or translation. Neutrophils can phagocytose bacteria, not viruses. CD8 positive T cells destroy infected cells, not CD4. Granuloma formation is not classically associated with flu infection.

5. D. Becoming latent in neurons. The infection described is chicken pox, caused by *Varicella zoster* virus. This evades complete elimination by becoming a latent virus in neurons, with the potential to reactivate later (causing shingles). See the section on examples of viral infection strategies in this chapter for more detail on the strategies used by other viruses to evade immunity.

6. E. sIgA can bind to bacteria and prevent them from binding to epithelial cells.

7. D. HBsAg −ve, anti-HBc +ve, anti-HBs +ve. If the virus has been cleared, HBsAg will be −ve (there is no antigenic persistence and the disease has not become chronic). Vaccinated immunity will only produce anti-HBs because vaccinations use the surface antigen. If a patient gains immunity through exposure to the virus, as in this case, then they will produce antibodies to the core and surface antigens (anti-HBc and anti-HBs).

8. B. The pathogen has a complex lifecycle, which presents the immune system with a variety of challenges. While the patient's symptoms are fairly vague, his recent travel to a malaria endemic area without any malaria prophylaxis makes *Plasmodium* infection more likely. This is an intracellular protozoon with a complex lifecycle, making immune response difficult. Most of the symptoms are due to the immune response rather than the pathogen directly. It causes a chronic infection.

9. B. Raised eosinophils. Mast cells and eosinophils interact with parasitic worms on mucosal surfaces and are chiefly responsible for the immune response to parasitic worms. While a raised eosinophil count may be found in parasitic worm infections, it does not imply infection and may also indicate an allergy.

Chapter 12 Immune dysfunction

1. C. IgE-mediated degranulation of mast cells is the cause of type I hypersensitivity reactions. Nickel hypersensitivity and rheumatoid arthritis are type IV hypersensitivities and are cell mediated. ABO incompatibility is a type II hypersensitivity, which is antibody mediated but not IgE mediated. Farmer's lung is a type III hypersensitivity, involving immune complex deposition in tissues.

2. A. Because anaphylaxis is the result of a systemic type I hypersensitivity response, skin prick testing is used. A small amount of each of the likely allergens is injected into the skin in order to determine which caused the allergic reaction and hence should be avoided. The response is compared to a histamine control.

3. B. This is a hypersensitivity pneumonitis (a type III hypersensitivity reaction). Eczema and asthma are due to IgE mediated mast cell degranulation (type I hypersensitivity). Nickel hypersensitivity is cell mediated (type IV) and haemolytic disease of the newborn is antibody mediated, with red blood cell destruction secondary to complement activation and antibody-dependent cell-mediated cytotoxicity (type II hypersensitivity).

4. E. These cells secrete cytokines on contact with the antigen resulting in the attraction and activation of macrophages. This process takes 24-72 hours to peak, hence the name delayed-type hypersensitivity.

5. D. This dose should be known by all medical professionals. A, B and C are all used but later in the management. C1 inhibitor is used in hereditary angioedema.

6. D. This disease is characterized by muscle weakness and fatigue. It is a type II hypersensitivity, with antibodies formed against postsynaptic acetyl choline receptors at neuro-muscular junctions, leading to receptor loss.

7. E. The antitissue transglutaminase test is very sensitive and specific for coeliac disease but confirmation may be needed with a duodenal biopsy, which would show villous atrophy.

8. B. Given the clinical history, family history and radiographic features, the most likely diagnosis is rheumatoid arthritis. You would therefore expect to find anti-CCP antibodies in the patient's serum. There may also be IgM anti-IgG antibodies (rheumatoid factor) in the serum.

9. C. TNF-α is central to the pathogenesis of rheumatoid arthritis and hence is the target of some of the biological disease modifying antirheumatic drugs, such as infliximab or etanercept (see Chapter 13).

10. C. There is an association between genetic deficiencies in complement proteins and SLE; reduced complement function may lead to reduced immune complex breakdown and hence increased immune complex deposition, as seen in SLE.

11. A. Immunodeficiency should be suspected because the patient has a serious, persistent and recurrent infection, but considering their age and previous normal health, a secondary immunodeficiency is much more likely. AIDS is the only secondary immunodeficiency listed.

12. C. HIV possesses reverse transcriptase, which allows it to manufacture double-stranded DNA, which is incorporated into host cells genetic material.

13. D. This is an AIDS defining infection. AIDS can also be diagnosed with a CD4 count of less than 200 cells/µL. The other conditions, in isolation, do not indicate that the patient has progressed to AIDS.

Chapter 13 Medical intervention

1. C. The immunoglobulin administered does not directly stimulate the immune system and therefore it is not active immunity. No immunological memory is created, therefore once the immunoglobulin is excreted no immunity will be conferred. Another example of passive immunity is the passage of maternal IgG to babies via breast milk.

2. D. Vaccines should be immunogenic if they are going to stimulate a host response. The MMR vaccines are live attenuated vaccines. Live attenuated vaccines are more expensive than killed vaccines.

3. E. Hyperacute rejection is rapid because antibodies have been induced prior to transplantation, e.g., by blood transfusion. It is prevented by cross-matching the donor cells and recipient serum. Chronic rejection is not well understood and if it occurs, it cannot be treated. Acute cellular rejection is mediated by T cells (as it is type IV hypersensitivity reaction).

4. A. Raised blood pressure is seen due to mineralocorticoid activity of the steroids. The glucocorticoid action of the steroids means they act as an anti-insulin and promote gluconeogenesis, affecting glucose tolerance. Wound healing is attenuated directly by systemic steroids and the immunosuppressive action of them also predisposes patients to infections.

5. D. While all side-effects can cause concern, you should pay particular attention to the risk of gastric ulceration in elderly patients on NSAIDs (such as naproxen) as they are particularly at risk. Bronchospasm should not be a high-risk problem as the patient is not allergic to NSAIDs nor is she asthmatic. She may also be at risk of renal failure from NSAIDs due to her age and history of hypertension. One option would be to prescribe a proton pump inhibitor such as omeprazole alongside the NSAID (to protect the gastric mucosa) or opt for alternative pain relief such as paracetamol or codeine.

6. B. This patient is in an Addisonian crisis, likely due to sudden interruption of long-term high dose systemic steroid therapy. It may also be triggered by an underlying infection or a major trauma, when the long-term steroid dose is not increased to compensate for the additional stress. Management is to correct the hypotension (fluids) and restart steroid therapy (IV hydrocortisone initially, then oral steroids). This highlights the importance of patients carrying steroid cards.

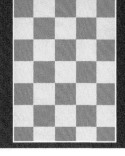
Chapter 1 Principles of haematology

Blood cells

1. H. This description refers only to memory B cells.
2. K. Only T lymphocytes are categorized in this particular manner, depending on whether they express principally CD8 or CD4 at their cell membranes. Both have specific and different immune functions.
3. F. Basophils represent the smallest component of bloodstream white cells. They are derived from CFU-Baso progenitor cells, which themselves are derived from CFU-GEMM (the myeloid progenitor cell).
4. A. The only blood cell that has the capacity to transport gases in bulk is the red blood cell, which contains haemoglobin molecules. These are capable of binding and releasing oxygen in appropriate pO_2 environments.
5. E. Eosinophils are the primary effector cell for attacking parasitic organism, in particular helminths. When in the bloodstream, they typically travel between bone marrow and sites of inflammation and infection.
6. J. Lymphocytes include plasma cells, memory B cells, CD8 and CD4 T cells and natural killer (NK) cells. The largest of these is the NK cell. Of these lymphocytes, the NK cell contributes the most to innate rather than adaptive immunity.
7. B. Enucleate blood cells consist of either platelets or red cells. However, platelets play a far more prominent role in haemostasis.

Chapter 2 Red Blood cells and haemoglobin

Abnormalities of the blood film

1. J Acanthocytes, where red cells display an irregular outline, are associated with liver disease.
2. I Rouleaux are seen in any scenario characterized by raised erythrocyte sedimentation rate due to increased globulins (erythrocyte sedimentation rate). This would be significantly raised in acute temporal arteritis.
3. C As the spleen normally removes these nuclear inclusions (Howell-Jolly bodies) from circulating red cells, functional or physical absence of the spleen permits their persistence.
4. K The film correlate of an increased RDW is anisocytosis. Target cells may be present due to iron deficiency, but this is not the most discriminatory finding in this example.
5. L This man has glucose-6-phosphate dehydrogenase deficiency. The Mediterranean variant confers susceptibility to acute haemolysis if broad (fava) beans are ingested. Diabetic ketoacidois, infection and sulphonamides (sulphamethoxazole component of septrin aka cotrimoxazole) are oxidative stress factors well-known to provoke intravascular haemolysis in these patients. This has caused the acute fall in his haemoglobin.

Chapter 3 Red blood cell disorders

Haemolytic anaemia

1. D Although the DIC will provoke MAHA (option I), the primary diagnosis is acute transfusion reaction. ABO compatibility is usually due to human error and is catastrophic but entirely preventable. ABO incompatibility is a type of alloimmune haemolysis.
2. B This patient is in a typical ethnic origin for sufferers of G6PD deficiency. He had no prior knowledge of his condition due to being well and asymptomatic until experiencing significant oxidative stress. Failure of the pentose phosphate pathway results in a reduced pool of available reduced $NADP^+$, which is required to regenerate glutathione (a key intracellular antioxidant molecule). Haemoglobin has become denatured and oxidized, precipitating in Heinz bodies intracellularly.
3. G The skin discolouration arises as a result of vascular sludging. The jaundice is caused by unconjugated hyperbilirubinaemia. The pain is due to Raynaud phenomenon. This lady has cold autoimmune haemolytic anaemia. As a victim of multiple autoimmune diseases, she is at high risk of developing further autoimmune phenomena. The monoclonal antibody rituximab (anti-CD20) is effective in idiopathic cold AIHA.
4. I There is a high risk of DIC in patients with severe burns. The haemolysis seen secondary to DIC is secondary to red cell destruction due to shearing and mechanical damage in capillaries and arterioles from collision with fibrin strands. This type of haemolysis is referred to as macroangiopathic haemolysis. It is a feature

of thrombotic thrombocytopenic purpura, haemolytic uraemic syndrome and DIC.

5. H Cephalosporins are one of the most common causes of drug-induced haemolytic anaemia. The three mechanisms represent different routes leading to a drug-induced haemolytic anaemia.

Complications of sickle cell anaemia

1. I Severe pain may be a feature of a painful infarctive crisis even before any external evidence of tissue hypoxia is present. Acute painful crises are characteristic of sickle cell anaemia. Often examination is normal. A high requirement for analgesia is also a feature of recurrent painful crises in these patients.

2. A General anaesthesia is a stressor that frequently provokes decompensation in individuals with poor physical fitness. Perioperative features such as dehydration, fasting and hypothermia under anaesthesia combine to make general anaesthesia a major risk factor for precipitating various types of sickle cell crisis. This gentleman is experiencing acute chest syndrome. Oxygen supplementation, IV antibiotics, rehydration, warming and analgesia are the priorities. Exchange transfusion may be required and his case must be urgently discussed with a haematologist. The intensive care team should also be made aware because he might need mechanical ventilation if his respiratory function deteriorates further.

3. D Significant increase in susceptibility to infection in sickle cell anaemia has resulted in a minor infection leading to catastrophic complications. This patient is peri-arrest due to septic shock arising from gastroenteritis. She requires resuscitation and circulatory support if she is to survive.

4. E Splenic sequestration crises typically present in patients younger than 2 years of age. The girl is from a high-risk geographic zone for sickle and is presenting with features that can be attributed to a sickle crisis. It is therefore appropriate to assume sickle status until proven otherwise in this example. Primary resuscitation, however, is the same as it would be for anyone with such extreme anaemia and hinges on restoration of the oxygen-carrying capacity of the blood with volume expansion, transfusion and circulatory support if necessary.

5. F This patient's sister has had Parvovirus B19 (also called erythema infectiosum, fifth disease or slapped cheek syndrome). This is benign and self-limiting, although it can provoke a transient pure red cell aplasia. In sickle cell anaemia patients, however, it can result in aplastic

anaemia, which has precipitated this patient's anaemic and thrombocytopenic symptoms. He will also have leucopoenia and, given the fever, will need admission and intravenous antibiotics, as the leucopoenia will compound his preexisting high susceptibility to serious infection.

Chapter 5 Haematological malignancies

Haematological malignancies

1. G. The age and manner of presentation are typical for chronic lymphocytic leukaemia. The film is characteristic and diagnostic.

2. B. The presenting symptoms are secondary to anaemia. The dramatic weight loss should signal the possibility of a malignancy. The massive splenomegaly is secondary to extramedullary haemopoiesis, since normal bone marrow is replaced by nonfunctional fibrosis. The film appearance itself is diagnostic, but the mention of the 'dry tap' also supports a diagnosis primary myelofibrosis.

3. C. Myelodysplasia (MDS) is a disease of the elderly, and often is discovered when unexplained cytopenias are incidentally discovered, as in the case described. The ringed sideroblasts in combination with unilineage dysplasia on bone marrow examination confirms the myelodysplasia diagnosis and further subclassifies it as MDS with ring sideroblasts.

4. K. Painless lymphadenopathy and mild splenomegaly are characteristic lymphoma findings on examination, but alone are not sufficient to differentiate lymphoma from other haematological malignancies. A cyclical fever, though rare, should make the practitioner think of Hodgkin lymphoma, where it is termed a 'Pel-Ebstein' fever. Alcohol-induced painful lymphadenopathy is also rare symptom, but when present is highly specific for Hodgkin lymphoma. The lymph node biopsy (investigation of choice in lymphomas) is diagnostic; Reed-Sternberg cells are only seen in Hodgkin lymphoma.

5. D. An infection that has failed to respond to community-prescribed antibiotics suggests impaired immune function, the acute critically unwell presentation and the cytopenias are features typical for an acute leukaemia. The presence of myeloid blasts differentiates myeloid from lymphocytic leukaemia, and the mention of the high proportion of myeloid blasts on marrow examination rules out an atypical presentation of myelodysplasia.

Chapter 6 Haemostasis

Integrating clinical assessment, full blood count, blood film and coagulation assay investigations

1. **L** This lady has two confirmed autoimmune conditions, once of which is SLE, both autoimmunity and SLE in particular are associated with antiphospholipid syndrome (option L). Recurrent DVT and recurrent miscarriages is also a history suggestive of this condition. This test should ideally be repeated in 12 weeks to confirm the diagnosis.

2. **H** This lady would be at high risk for thrombosis (obese, cancer, immobility) and was prescribed thromboprophylaxis - unfractionated heparin, as she had reported a LMWH allergy. This choice was erroneous as unfractionated heparin would most likely recreate any adverse effects of LWMH. Pain and necrotic skin change at the injection site, a new thrombosis (venous > arterial) and thrombocytopenia (option H), particularly a fall >50% of baseline following exposure to heparin suggests heparin-induced thrombocytopenia (HIT). The timing, 5–10 days postexposure, is characteristic. The rash experienced on the previous exposure may have been a less dramatic presentation of HIT that was not picked up.

3. **D** The paramedics' information suggests a substantial impact to the right temporal zone, common in a lateral impact with a window. The agitation and confusion are characteristic of a severe head injury. However, the unclear but worrying history of multiple transfusions and a bleeding disorder, as well as the joint contractures and difficult veins in a young patient are strongly suggestive of haemophilia. The old laboratory results support this; normal platelets and PT with prolonged APTT suggests either factor VIII or IX deficiency. In an acute intracranial bleeding scenario, he needs to have the deficient factor restored to 100%, particularly as he needs neurosurgical evacuation of the haematoma. However, in this case, without knowing which factor to replace, a combination of PCC and cryoprecipitate is the emergency treatment of choice. Known haemophilia A (factor VIII deficiency) would warrant cryoprecipitate, known haemophilia B (factor IX deficiency) would warrant PCC if recombinant factor were unavailable (rare in the UK – most laboratories have at least one emergency dose of factor VIII and factor IX). Since haemophilia B does not feature on the previous list, haemophilia A (option D) is the only correct option.

4. **E** Prolonged bleeding postdental extraction, easy bruising, nosebleeds, menorrhagia are all examples of mucocutaneous bleeding and hints at a deficit in platelet number or functionality. Impaired platelet functionality arises in von Willebrand disease (vWD) because of the role of von Willebrand factor (vWF) in the transient tethering phase of primary haemostasis. Death from bleeding in a first-degree relative in this case suggests an inherited rather than spontaneous mutation. Type 1 vWD, the most common type, exhibits reduced levels of vWF (the assay measures 'vWF antigen concentration') as in this example. Factor VIII is reduced, as its survival in the circulation is markedly shortened by the relative absence of vWF, its carrier protein.

5. **A** This lady has suffered her first thrombotic event, which could have been easily attributed to the OCP and her weight. Fortunately, she mentioned the maternal family history of a thrombophilia. The available options antithrombin deficiency and factor V Leiden would both correlate clinically, however the haematologist's explanation specifically refers to the mechanism of action of antithrombin deficiency; thus option A is the correct answer. Thrombin is also usually inhibited by antithrombin in addition to activated factors IX, X and XII. Obesity and hyperlipidaemia are risk factors for antithrombin deficiency.

Chapter 7 Transfusion products

Integrating interpretation of laboratory results with decision-making regarding transfusion of blood products, plasma derivatives and recombinant factors

1. **M** The group matched A Rh +ve initially looks to be the optimal transfusion product for this symptomatic anaemic lady postobstetric haemorrhage. However, a history of significant febrile or allergic reactions to red cell transfusion should prompt use of washed red cells in future transfusion. The only correct option is therefore M. As a group A individual, she can safely receive blood from group O or A donors, and as she is Rh +ve herself the Rh status of the donation is of no concern.

2. **L** The Hb is not dramatic in this context, nor are the platelets. Fibrinogen is low, but not worryingly so: this level would not preclude stable clot formation. There is however evidence of multiple clotting factor deficiencies as seen by the significantly prolonged PT and APTT

values. FFP, which contains clotting factors and fibrinogen in physiologic proportions, will significantly improve the PT, APTT and the fibrinogen. FFP from a group A donor is ideal, and the Rh status of the donor is unimportant. The FFP from the O −ve donor would likely contain anti-A antibodies and is therefore unsuitable. Type O patients can only receive plasma from another type O donor. Remember that FFP differs from red cells in that the universal FFP donor is AB.

3. D   A platelet count <20 × 10^9/L with risk factors for bleeding (in this case sepsis) warrants platelet transfusion. Patients with known HIV that are CMV −ve require CMV −ve blood products, therefore D is the correct option.

4. G   This man has a gastrointestinal bleed, oozing puncture sites and spontaneous subcutaneous haemorrhages. In the context of overwhelming sepsis, disseminated intravenous coagulopathy (DIC) is highly likely. Whilst he may ultimately require red cell and platelet transfusion if these values continue to trend downwards (very likely), and FFP as well, the most important priority is replacement of fibrinogen with cryoprecipitate since this is what is most exacerbating failure of haemostasis in this patient. This patient with DIC is actively bleeding with a low fibrinogen and therefore should be administered cryoprecipitate to restore his fibrinogen levels and facilitate clotting.

5. K   All Rh −ve women of childbearing age must receive Rh −ve red cell transfusions if required (see Chapter 7: The Rh antigen [previously termed 'Rhesus antigen'] system). However, in this scenario there is no indication for any transfusion of red cells. Rh −ve women are routinely administered anti-D immunoglobulin at specific points perinatally, including soon after delivery. Future pregnancies with a Rh positive fetus would potentially be at risk from maternal anti-Rh antibodies (developed by fetal blood from a Rh +ve fetus entering the maternal circulation) so the anti-D is administered to minimize the chance of antibody generation. Refer to the passages describing the Rh antigen in pregnancy.

Chapter 9 The innate immune system

Concerning innate immunity

1. I.   Neutrophils circulate in the blood and migrate to tissues—they are a key phagocyte of bacteria. Macrophages are also phagocytes, but they reside in tissues, developing from circulating monocytes.

2. A.   The mucociliary escalator helps to remove pathogens from the respiratory epithelium. It is paralysed by tobacco smoke, predisposing smokers to lower respiratory tract infections.

3. E.   Natural killer cells share a common progenitor with B and T cells, however they are a member of the innate immune system (they have no memory and are not specific in their action). They can kill antibody coated cells, independent of the major histocompatibility complex (antibody-dependent cell-mediated cytotoxicity).

4. B.   Mast cells are similar to basophils, but unlike basophils they reside in tissues. Mast cells that are situated near blood vessels can quickly cause the vasodilation that is typical of allergy.

5. J.   The low pH of the stomach is lethal to many pathogens. Normal gut flora does prevent pathogenic colonization but only in the colon; the stomach and small intestine are relatively free from microbes.

Concerning complement

1. G.   The membrane attack complex is a set of complement proteins which, on stimulation of the complement cascade, form a polymer that destroys pathogens by punching holes in the cell membrane.

2. I.   The classical pathway is a rapid complement activation pathway, initiated by the presence of antibody.

3. F.   C1 esterase inhibitor is deficient in patients with hereditary angioedema.

4. E.   Anaphylotoxin stimulates the release of histamine, which causes increased vascular permeability and attracts white blood cells to the site of infection.

5. J.   The processes involved in the complement cascade are regulated by complement inhibitors.

Chapter 10 The adaptive immune system

Concerning cell surface molecules

1. G.   Antigens are substances specifically recognized by receptors of the adaptive immune system.

2. J.   Collectins are a family of pattern recognition molecules that recognize and opsonize pathogens in solution.

3. C.   MHC class I molecules recognize antigens from intracellular pathogens.

4. E.   Intracellular or phagocytosed antigens expressed simultaneously with MHC are

recognized by the T cell receptor on the surface of T lymphocytes.

5. B. Toll-like receptors are a family of related molecules found on mammalian cell surfaces; they activate the innate immune system after exposure to a pathogen.

Concerning tolerance

1. Central tolerance. This is the induction of apoptosis in any developing lymphocyte that binds strongly to autoantigen.
2. IL-10. Secreted by Tregs in response to self-reactive T cells.
3. Peripheral tolerance. This may be through pollen injections or oral/sublingual therapy, but the overarching process is by inducing peripheral tolerance to the allergen.
4. Costimulation. APCs express costimulatory molecules, allowing them to present antigen and activate the T cell, but not all circulating cells express costimulatory molecules.
5. IFN-γ. This would also be involved in the response to intracellular pathogens.

Concerning B and T lymphocytes

1. F. To become fully active and begin releasing antibody, B cells must be stimulated by T helper cells.
2. J. B and T cells originate from lymphoid stem cells in the bone marrow.
3. C. Plasma cells are a mature type of B lymphocyte. They contain vast amounts of endoplasmic reticulum in order to produce a large quantity of immunoglobulin.
4. A. CD8 is a cell surface marker expressed on cytotoxic T cells.
5. G. Cytotoxic T cells recognize antigen in conjunction with MHC class I molecules.

Chapter 11 The functioning immune system

Concerning the immune system in action

1. G. This response is also the basis of type I hypersensitivity.
2. A. Phagocytes destroy most extracellular bacteria with the help of C3b and antibody.
3. H. INF-α and -β inhibit transcription and translation of viral proteins in neighbouring cells.
4. D. MHC class I molecule present intracellular antigens to CD8+ T cells.
5. C. Granulomas typically appear as an accumulation of lymphocytes and macrophages around a central area of caseous necrosis.
   E A patient with a single episode of *Strep. pneumoniae* pneumonia

Chapter 12 Immune dysfunction

Immune dysfunction

1. I. This test measures the levels of immunoglobulin.
2. B. A rise in C-reactive protein would imply an acute immune response (appendicitis) and may be elevated before any change in the white cell count.
3. G. This test measures previous exposure to *Myobacterium tuberculosis* or the bacille Calmette-Guérin (BCG) vaccine. Previous exposure to either results in a firm, red lesion at the site of injection 48–72 hours later. It is caused by infiltration of macrophages and T cells. The tuberculin skin test is being superseded by a blood test, including gamma interferon release assays (IGRA).
4. C. This test is used extensively in medicine. It is used to detect antibodies such as in detecting anti-HIV antibodies.
5. D. Nickel hypersensitivity is a delayed type (IV) hypersensitivity reaction. Patch testing is used to diagnose this type of hypersensitivity. As opposed to skin prick testing which is used in type I hypersensitivity.

Concerning hypersensitivity

1. F. This hypersensitivity is a result of soluble antigen and antibody interactions.
2. J. All patients with a suspected or proven case of anaphylaxis should be seen by a specialist in allergy clinic.
3. E. Allergic rhinitis, also known as 'hay fever': there is high morbidity in sufferers. Management includes antihistamines and local (intranasal) corticosteroids.
4. H. Other forms of type II hypersensitivity include haemolytic disease of the newborn and autoimmune haemolytic anaemia.
5. C. Occurs following a group A beta haemolytic streptococcal infection of the throat or the skin (impetigo).

Concerning autoimmunity

1. G. Most patients with SLE have antibodies against double-stranded DNA.
2. I. Type I diabetes is caused by destruction of β-cells in the islets of Langerhans. Different HLA alleles are implicated in its pathogenesis, as is low level pancreatic inflammation.
3. H. HLA-B27 is also associated with reactive arthritis and psoriatic arthritis (spondylarthropathies).
4. E. This negative selection occurs in the thymus for T cells and in the bone marrow for B cells.

5. B. The antibodies stimulated the thyroid stimulating hormone (TSH) receptor, resulting in hyperthyroidism.

Chapter 13 Medical intervention

Concerning immunological interventions

1. C. These are classic side-effects associated with long-term systemic steroid use. While beclomethasone is a steroid, when used in an inhaler it is unlikely to cause systemic side-effects, although local immunosuppression can cause throat infections with *Candida,* for example.

2. B. The patient appears to have a rheumatic condition, most likely rheumatoid arthritis. While NSAIDs, corticosteroids and infliximab are all important parts of the treatment of rheumatoid arthritis, it is crucial that patients are properly assessed early by rheumatologists, who can then start the appropriate therapy.

3. H. TPMT metabolizes azathioprine and variations in enzyme levels are present in the population, potentially causing severe immunosuppression.

4. E. Calcineurin is involved in the upregulation of IL-2 receptors in T cells and is required for their activation. Calcineurin inhibitors such as tacrolimus and ciclosporin cause immunosuppression by disrupting this pathway.

5. F. Infliximab is used in various rheumatological conditions, as well as inflammatory bowel disease. Adalimumab is another anti-TNF-α drug.

Concerning the immune system in action

1. G. This response is also the basis of type I hypersensitivity.

2. A. Phagocytes destroy most extracellular bacteria with the help of C3b and antibodies.

3. H. IFN-α and $-\beta$ inhibit transcription and translation of viral proteins in neighbouring cells.

4. D. MHC class I molecules present intracellular antigens to CD8+ T cells.

5. C. Granulomas typically appear as an accumulation of lymphocytes and macrophages around a central area of caseous necrosis.

Active immunity Resistance to an infection or disease that develops as a result of prior infection or vaccination.

Adaptive immunity An immune response that is slow to respond but produces lasting immunity and is adapted to produce the most effective eradication of the pathogen.

Adjuvant A substance that enhances the immune response to a vaccine.

Agglutination The process by which suspended bacteria, cells or particles clump together.

Allergen An antigenic substance that stimulates an immediate hypersensitivity reaction.

Antineutrophil cytoplasmic antibody (ANCA) A type of autoantibody directed against proteinase-3 (cANCA) or against myeloperoxidase (pANCA).

Antibody A protein produced by B lymphocytes in response to the presence of an antigen.

Antigen Molecules that are recognized specifically by receptors on cells of the adaptive immune system.

Antigen-presenting cells Cells capable of presenting antigenic material to cells of the adaptive immune system.

Autoimmunity Occurs when the body's own defences are targeted against normal body components.

Apoptosis Programmed cell death.

Atopy Possessing a genetic predisposition to allergy.

Chemotaxis The movement of cells in response to chemicals, often to a site of infection.

Collectins A family of pattern-recognition molecules, present in solution, that stimulate the innate immune system in response to a pathogen.

Complement A series of enzymatic reactions stimulated by the presence of a pathogen.

Cytokine Intercellular molecules used to transmit messages from one cell to another.

Degranulation The release of the preformed secretory granule contents by fusion with the plasma membrane.

Ecchymoses (bruises) Diffuse flat haemorrhages under the skin.

Erythropoietin A hormone, secreted by the kidney, that regulates erythropoiesis.

Haemorrhage Loss of circulating blood.

Haematocrit The relative volume of erythrocytes in the blood.

Haematoma Distinct local swelling caused by loss of blood into a muscle or subcutaneous tissue.

Haptens Small molecules that need to be bound to a large carrier molecule in order to become immunogenic.

Human leucocyte antigen (HLA) The human form of major histocompatibility complex (MHC): cell surface proteins that present antigen.

Hypersensitivity The inappropriate response of the immune system to an antigen.

Immunity A state of relative resistance to a disease.

Immunoglobulin (Ig) A protein substance secreted from plasma cells in response to infection.

Immunoglobulin domain An amino acid sequence, common to many proteins that are involved in pathogen recognition.

Inflammation Localized response to tissue damage characterized by redness, swelling, pain, oedema and increased white cell count.

Interferon A cytokine that is targeted against viruses and intracellular bacteria.

Innate immune system Produces a nonspecific response to an infection or disease.

Major histocompatibility complex (MHC) A cluster of genes encoding for cell surface receptors that present antigen on the surface of cells.

Monoclonal antibody Identical immunoglobulin that has been synthetically produced to target a specific antigen for therapeutic or diagnostic purposes.

Opsonin A substance that binds to a molecule to enhance its uptake by a phagocyte.

Passive immunity The passage of immunity from one individual to another.

Pathogen An organism that causes disease.

Pattern recognition molecules Are present either in solution or on the surface of cells and are capable of recognizing molecules characteristic of infection.

Packed cell volume (PCV) A measure of the proportion of blood occupied by red blood cells.

Petechiae Punctate haemorrhages <2 mm in diameter, usually clustered.

Polymorphism Slight differences in the genetic material of individuals within a population.

Purpura Any condition with bleeding into the skin or mucous membrane.

Sepsis Immune dysregulation caused by infection, potentially resulting in organ failure and death.

Thymus A mediastinal organ in which T cells develop.

Tolerance The ability of the immune system to ignore molecules that it has the capacity to attack.

Toll-like receptor A family of pattern recognition molecules on the cell surfaces that stimulate the innate immune system in response to a pathogen.

Urticaria Also called hives or nettle rash, characterized by an area of red inflammation and raised white bumps.

Vertical transmission Transmission of an infection from mother to fetus.

Vaccine A suspension of antigenic material injected to produce immunity against infection and disease.

Note: Page numbers followed by *f* indicate figures, *t* indicate tables and *b* indicate boxes.

TITLES AVAILABLE IN THE CRASH COURSE SERIES

- Psychiatry
- Metabolism and Nutrition
- Anatomy & Physiology
- Pharmacology
- Haematology & Immunology
- Neurology
- Cardiology
- General Medicine
- Pathology
- 1000 SBAs and EMQs for Medical Finals
- Rheumatology & Orthopaedics
- Obstetrics & Gynaecology
- Paediatrics

- Respiratory Medicine
- Medical Research, Audit and Teaching: the Essentials for Career Success
- Endocrinology
- Gastrointestinal System
- Renal and Urinary System
- Medical Ethics and Sociology
- Cell Biology and Genetics
- Quick Reference Guide to Medicine and Surgery
- Surgery
- Muscles, Bones and Skin
- Infectious Diseases

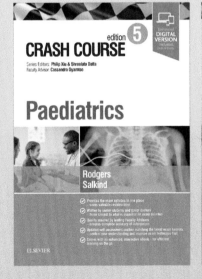

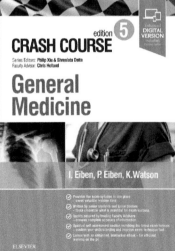

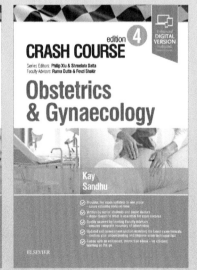

Printed and bound by CPI Group (UK) Ltd, Croydon, CR0 4YY

03/10/2024

01040305-0003